Advance Praise for *Sizzling Sex for Life*

"*Sizzling Sex for Life* is the most practical, authoritative, and comprehensive sexuality guide ever written."

—Eli Coleman, PhD, chair of the Human Sexuality Program, University of Minnesota, the nation's largest training program for sexuality professionals

"I have been a fan of Michael Castleman's sexuality writing for decades. His sex writing ranks among the best—engaging and great for the general public. *Sizzling Sex for Life* is accurate, beautifully written, and very accessible. It covers every issue clients bring to me, including many that are highly controversial. I can't wait to recommend the book to my sex therapy colleagues, clients, and friends."

—Elizabeth Rae Larson, MS, DHS, LMHC, director at Seattle Institute for Sex Therapy, Education, and Research

"*Sizzling Sex* is my new go-to book for all things sexual, and I will be recommending it to friends, clients, and students alike. This book is solidly grounded in the latest research (indeed, over, 2,500 studies!), yet is written with wit and humor and in a very fun and accessible writing style. *Sizzling Sex* is a truly ground-breaking, comprehensive guide to male sexuality from birth (e.g. circumcision) to the end stages of life (e.g. sex in nursing homes). It goes beyond similar books of this genre, focusing not only on the causes and resolution of sexual problems, but also on timely and important topics such as pornography, consensual nonmonogamy, and sex education—and again, with all conclusions reached and advice steeped in data but presented in a way that had me nodding along and laughing out loud. It is indeed so complete in its coverage of issues, I will be requiring it as reading in my university Human Sexuality class. Any man who reads this book is bound to become more sexually aware, satisfied, and comfortable—as well as a much better lover to women partners. Indeed, I'd venture that any man who reads this book (either in part or in whole) will also become a better person and partner in general, as it is full of sage advice for both sex and life. While written for men, women who love men will also gain an enormous amount of knowledge about both their own sexuality, and male sexuality, from reading this book. This book is truly brilliant."

—Laurie Mintz, professor of psychology at the University of Florida, Gainesville, and author of *Becoming Cliterate* and *A Tired Woman's Guide to Passionate Sex*

"*Sizzling Sex* is a meticulously researched, beautifully written, wonderful compendium that provides deep insights into how men think, feel, and behave sexually. This book is a must-read for men and their partners."

—James C. Wadley, PhD, chair of the Lincoln University counseling department

"I wish every man I've ever known had read this book! It's practical, positive, sexy, funny, kind, and humane. What a terrific, helpful, and reassuring resource."

—Katie Kleinsasser, communications consultant, Planned Parenthood of New York City

"A real stunner! I particularly like its wonderful comprehensiveness, and the brilliant, very accessible way Castleman discusses sex research. After forty years as a sex therapist and author of several sex books myself, I still found it fascinating and remarkably informative."

—Isadora Alman, MFT, sex therapist, author of *Doing It: Real People Having Really Good Sex* and *What People Keep Asking Me about Sex and Relationships*

"What an extraordinary book! I wasn't surprised. I've been a huge fan of Castleman's sexuality writing for years. But *Sizzling Sex for Life* goes way beyond his previous work. It's fantastic—so comprehensive and so sensitive to both men and women, and completely evidence-based. I'm confident that *Sizzling Sex for Life* will be the leading sex guide for years to come. I plan to recommend it to everyone I know."

—Diana Wiley, PhD, sex therapist

"*Sizzling Sex for Life* proves that Michael Castleman is a sexuality genius. Such breadth! Such depth and wisdom! The style is warm, friendly, witty, sensitive to women, and totally accessible to general readers—quite a feat since the book discusses so much sex research. I particularly liked Castleman's sage advice about sexual coaching. I love this book!"

—Joan Price, author of *Better Than I Ever Expected: Straight Talk about Sex after Sixty*

"*Sizzling Sex for Life* is a wise, wonderful, gentle encyclopedia of sex—everything you want to know all in one book, including a whole lot you won't find anywhere else."

—David Hersh, PhD, founder of Hersh Centre for Sexual Wellness

"The best, most comprehensive guide I've ever seen for creating great sex. Packed with great information and practical tools to solve problems and enhance erotic pleasure."

—Rachel Needle, PsyD, codirector of Modern Sex Therapy Institutes

"I loved every word of *Sizzling Sex for Life*. It's so comprehensive, so accessible, such an inviting, nonjudgmental read, so well researched and organized. It addresses men beautifully, but is also very sensitive to women. I especially loved the chapters on porn—so sensible and refreshing. I can't wait to recommend the book to my students, sex therapy clients, and radio listeners."

—Laurie Betito, PhD, president of Sexual Health Network of Quebec,
host of sexuality talk show *Passion*

"Lots of smiles and several laughs in *Sizzling Sex for Life*. And it's so authoritative, entirely evidence-based, backed up by 2,500 research papers, very commendable. I will definitely recommend it to clients, colleagues, and friends. It has so much great information about so many subjects. Castleman's book is an adventure in life-long pleasure that enlightens and thrills as a great sex guide should."

—Norelyn Parker, PhD, sex coach

"Very comprehensive. Very impressive. I plan to recommend *Sizzling Sex for Life* to my sex therapy clients, colleagues, and friends. I especially loved the chapters on anal play, BDSM, and consensual non-monogamy. Clients often raise these issues, and now I can refer them to the wonderful discussions in this book."

—Zita Nickeson, LCPC, CST, sex therapist

"*Sizzling Sex for Life* is wonderful—comprehensive, exhaustively researched, and beautifully written. I love the way Castleman thoroughly debunks the whole idea of sex addiction. Great book!"

—David Ley, PhD, clinical psychologist and author of *The Myth of Sex Addiction*

"*Sizzling Sex for Life* provides excellent, practical, down-to-earth advice—and Castleman backs it up by citing more than 2,500 studies. I especially applaud his insightful discussions of sexual controversies, notably school sex ed and pornography. And in addition to encouraging lovers to coach each other, he offers insightful suggestions—what to say, how, and when. Reading *Sizzling Sex for Life* is like talking with a wise older brother who has a ton of sexual experience, two tons of good sense, and a sweet sense of humor."

—Marty Klein, PhD, publisher of the *Sexual Intelligence* newsletter, author of *Ask Me Anything*, *America's War on Sex*, and more

"*Sizzling Sex for Life* deserves to be a huge success. It's amazingly comprehensive, deeply researched, superbly written, myth-busting, and fun to read. I love Castleman's emphasis on pleasure—and he provides solid, step-by-step, relationship-enhancing encouragement to fully enjoy it. The book is also very strong on the religious roots of so-called sex addiction. *Sizzling Sex for Life* is a major contribution to sex education and therapy."

—Stella Resnick, PhD, sex therapist and author of *Body-to-Body Intimacy*

"What a great book! I'm so glad Michael Castleman took on this mammoth project. I wish everyone would read the chapters on sexual assault prevention, pornography, and sex addiction—all very eye-opening, sex-positive, and so helpful!"

—Charla Hathaway, founder of BodyJoy sex and intimacy coaching center

"*Sizzling Sex* is phenomenal beyond words. So exhaustively researched, so well-written. I especially enjoyed Castleman's advice that men should always kiss both sets of lips, and the way he debunks so many sexual myths—that masturbation is harmful, that athletes shouldn't have sex before the big game. I am very excited to recommend *Sizzling Sex* to my clients. I know it will help them gain a really comprehensive sex education, understand lovemaking on a deeper level, and enjoy better sex—sizzling sex—throughout their lives."

—Lisa Thomas, LCSW, LMFT, sex therapist

"Castleman charms his readers with a historical approach to sexual issues and an obvious love of language. *Sizzling Sex* offers clever wit as well as essential education for those who want to become sensitive and joyful lovers. This book provides reassurance and wisdom from an established expert whose writing style reflects his message of bringing playfulness, acceptance, and compassion into the bedroom."

—Kate McNulty, LCSW, AASECT-certified sex therapist, author of *Love & Asperger's*

"Such a great book. As a parent of two teens, I really appreciated the chapters on school sex education, virginity loss, and hooking up. I applaud Castleman's emphasis on sex education based not on fear of pregnancy and infections, but on pleasure, and hope his insights encourage parents to discuss sex with their teens. I also loved his step-by-step recommendations for those who think they might be sex/porn addicts."

—Louanne Weston, PhD, sex therapist

"What a wonderful self-help book for men—and women. I totally agree with the main message: 'Make love the way most women prefer by doing the *opposite* of what you see in porn.' Another takeaway is the importance of a healthy lifestyle. I appreciate the book's sense of humor and the engaging, real-world way it speaks to men's sexual sensibilities. Great book!"

—Linda Weiner, LCSW, Washington University

"This is the book we've been waiting for! *Sizzling Sex* is a much needed, well-researched, beautifully written book on the sexuality of men and anyone who loves them. *Sizzling Sex* answers all important sex questions, debunks tons of myths, explains women's sexuality to men, and informs everyone how to have great sex. Castleman delivers a comprehensive resource packed with advice you just can't help but share. A must-have for all sex educators, therapists, and anyone who wants better sex!"

—Heather McPherson, LPC-S, LMFT-S, CST,
founder of Sexual Health Alliance and Respark Therapy & Associates

"Michael Castleman's magnum opus, *Sizzling Sex for Life,* is a fun, insightful, easy-to-read book that helps everyone understand sexual issues and create more pleasurable sex lives. It's an important book for anyone who wants to have sizzling sex. It's also very useful for sex educators, counselors, and therapists. I've already sent several clients its well-documented information for some of their issues. In one case, a client believed that using lubrication meant that his girlfriend wasn't into him. I was able to send him statistics from *Sizzling Sex* showing that vaginal dryness doesn't necessarily indicate lack of arousal. I also found the chapters on pornography very perceptive. I know I will refer to *Sizzling Sex* time and time again. Bravo!"

—Mimi Gelb, MS, LMFT, CST, sex therapist

"I really enjoyed *Sizzling Sex* and think it's wonderful for both general readers and therapists! It's a very easy, enjoyable read that provides comprehensive, yet digestible sex information relevant to both men and women. It can be read cover-to-cover, or most chapters can be read as stand-alone pieces. I really like Castleman's use of the word 'loveplay' instead of 'foreplay,' as well as his chapter on novelty as key to sizzling sex."

—Kim Glenn, MA, CST, sex therapist

"*Sizzling Sex for Life* is wonderful, provocative, fiercely intelligent, and witty—quite possibly the only self-help sexuality guide any man will ever need. Castleman provides elegant advice on sexual communication and practical solutions to common sex problems. I highly recommend this fascinating, thought-provoking book to readers who seek to deepen their understanding of sexuality and become better lovers. I will definitely recommend it to my patients."

—Nazanin Moali, PhD, sex therapist, host of *The Sexology Podcast*

"*Sizzling Sex* is a practical, comprehensive, much-needed encyclopedia of sexuality. Imagine, everything from talking to young children about sexuality to sexual self-therapy for adults—all in one well-written volume. If you ever anticipate needing any guidance about any sexual issue, keep a copy of *Sizzling Sex* on your shelf."

—Mark Schoen, PhD, founder of SexSmartFilms.com

"*Sizzling Sex for Life* is absolutely wonderful. I've very much enjoyed reading it and will certainly recommend it to my couples and sex therapy clients. I particularly enjoy the simple, easy-reading writing style. The self-help and coaching information is also great. I can imagine this being bedside reading for many individuals and couples who want to become better lovers. I appreciate how easy it is to skim through the pages to find topics of interest. It is such a thorough, comprehensive, and user-friendly book. Reading *Sizzling Sex* was an absolute pleasure!"

—Julaine Maxwald, psychoanalyst

"This book is my favorite reference for all things male. The many insights and the practicality of advice provide an incredible guide. Each chapter is a treasure of information substantiated by comprehensive research. This is an invaluable resource not just for sexuality clinicians and educators, but for everyone."

—Cheryl D. Walker, MA, APC, sex therapist

"I have already found *Sizzling Sex* immensely helpful, particularly with clients who love data and want to know the science behind their experiences. I'm so glad Castleman advocates scheduling sex! This is the first thing I recommend to couples. The chapter about men supporting women through menopause is excellent. So is the discussion of pornography. *Sizzling Sex* is a much-needed resource. It's thorough, evidence-based, and sex positive, which are the characteristics I look for when recommending books to clients."

—Madelyn Esposito-Smith, LPC, CST, sex therapist

"*Sizzling Sex for Life* is a joy to read! I especially appreciate Castleman's focus on women's sexuality. It's so obvious that the best way for women to enjoy sex is to *teach* or *coach* their partners how they like to be pleasured, and the erotic pace they enjoy. That never occurred to me as a twenty-year-old virgin many, many years ago! Castleman returns to that idea often, as it applies to virtually every sexual encounter. And *pace* is so critical, whether it involves kissing and caressing, oral play, or anything else. Women are the experts on their own pleasure, and it's so great that Castleman has made the idea a cornerstone of *Sizzling Sex*. It's what sets his book apart from all the other sex guides I've read over the years. Not to mention that his endearing sense of humor cracked me up every time—my favorite: 'Boner Basics.'"

—Linda Newhart Lotz, MSW, PhD, assistant professor, Valencia College

"Castleman's writing is superb. *Sizzling Sex for Life* is a great destination for anyone looking to explore sexual issues. Self-help books usually go into great detail about one narrow area. In contrast, *Sizzling Sex* is so comprehensive. I also love how Castleman presents a historical perspective on sex. It's engaging and sex-positive and normalizes the diversity of human sexuality. I very much look forward to recommending *Sizzling Sex for Life*."

—Alicia Beltran, LCPC, CST, sex therapist

"*Sizzling Sex* is a wonderful, straightforward compilation of important sex research findings imbued with humor and compassion. I so appreciate the discussion of women's orgasms and how they are best produced. I also appreciate the section on female sexual pain. I've never seen this topic included in any sexuality book directed at men—bravo! And the comprehensive discussion of pornography is greatly needed by both men and women. In summary, *Sizzling Sex* is absolutely phenomenal! I look forward to recommending it to clients, colleagues, and friends."

—Sandra Lindholm, PsyD, CST, sex therapist

"*Sizzling Sex for Life* is a passport to the best sex! It celebrates human sexual pleasure non-judgmentally, and welcomes readers to explore theirs and savor it, no matter what their age. Castleman demonstrates that the large majority of human sexual behavior is normal, and that we should slow down and enjoy the pleasure. Reading it is like having an extended conversation with an older brother with a good sense of humor who tells it like it is."

—Andrew Hancock, LCSW, CST, sex therapist

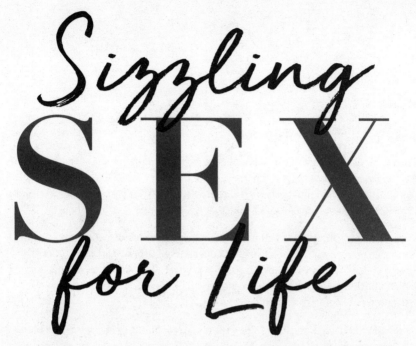

Sizzling SEX for Life

EVERYTHING YOU NEED TO KNOW TO
MAXIMIZE EROTIC PLEASURE
AT ANY AGE

MICHAEL CASTLEMAN
FOREWORD BY DR. PATTI BRITTON

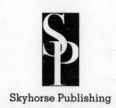

Skyhorse Publishing

Skyhorse Publishing books may be purchased in bulk at special discounts for sales promotion, corporate gifts, fund-raising, or educational purposes. Special editions can also be created to specifications. For details, contact the Special Sales Department, Skyhorse Publishing, 307 West 36th Street, 11th Floor, New York, NY 10018 or info@skyhorsepublishing.com.

Skyhorse® and Skyhorse Publishing® are registered trademarks of Skyhorse Publishing, Inc.®, a Delaware corporation.

Visit our website at www.skyhorsepublishing.com.

10 9 8 7 6 5 4 3 2 1

Library of Congress Cataloging-in-Publication Data

Names: Castleman, Michael, author.
Title: Sizzling sex for life: everything you need to know to maximize
    erotic pleasure at any age / Michael Castleman.
Description: New York, NY: Skyhorse Publishing, [2021] | Includes
    bibliographical references and index. | Identifiers: LCCN 2020044626 (print) | LCCN
2020044627 (ebook) | ISBN
  9781510762558 (hardcover) | ISBN 9781510762565 (ebook)
Subjects: LCSH: Sex instruction.
Classification: LCC HQ31 .C3158 2021 (print) | LCC HQ31 (ebook) | DDC
    613.9071—dc23
LC record available at https://lccn.loc.gov/2020044626
LC ebook record available at https://lccn.loc.gov/2020044627

Cover design by Daniel Brount
Cover images from Shutterstock

Print ISBN: 978-1-5107-6255-8
Ebook ISBN: 978-1-5107-6256-5

Printed in the United States of America

For my sex-positive parents, Mim and Lou Castleman.

For my wonderful, fifty-year partner in life, love, and lovemaking, Anne Simons.

And for David Fenton, who, in 1974, coaxed a reluctant health journalist to write his first article about sex.

"Sex is perfectly natural, just not naturally perfect."
—Sex therapist Thea Synder Lowry
(1932–2002)

Contents

Foreword   xiii

Introduction   xiv

Part I
The Ten Ingredients of Sizzling Sex

1. Why Be Sexual? *Pleasure!*   3
2. Getting in Shape for Sizzling Sex   8
3. The Lifelong Joy of Self-Sexing   16
4. Affirmative Consent: "Yes, I Want to Be Sexual with You"   25
5. Gentle, Extended, Mutual, Whole-Body Massage: The "Language" of Sizzling Sex   30
6. Sexual Coaching Made Easy: How to Ask for What You Want   42
7. The Magic of Lubricants: Better Sex Quickly—Guaranteed   47
8. Secrets of Sizzling Oral Sex   51
9. Novelty: Sizzling Sex Feels New and Different   59
10. Sexual Fantasies: Revel in Your Erotic Imagination   64

Part II
From Infancy to Old Age:
Sexual Issues Throughout the Lifespan

11. Does Circumcision Reduce Men's Sexual Sensitivity?   73
12. A Parents' Guide to Toddlers' and Preschoolers' Natural Sexual Curiosity   77
13. Childhood Sex Abuse: Recovery and Sizzling Sex Are Possible   86
14. Age of Consent: How Old Is Old Enough?   94
15. Teen Pregnancies Have Plummeted, But School Sex Education Doesn't
    Work—Huh?   99
16. Men Who Want Sizzling Sex *Must* Participate Fully in Birth Control   107
17. Men Who Want Sizzling Sex *Must* Prevent Sexually Transmitted Infections   125
18. The Virgin's Guide to Happily Losing It   134
19. Today's Young Adult Hookups Used to Be Called Dating   145
20. How to Prevent Sexual Assault and Harassment   153
21. If the Woman You Love Gets Raped   161
22. "You're Insatiable!" "You Never Want To!" How Sex Therapists Recommend
    Overcoming Desire Differences   164
23. Sizzling Sex During Pregnancy, Nursing, and Parenting   173
24. Over Time, Does Sexual Quality Decline?   178
25. My One and Only? Infidelity and Sex Work   182
26. Chronic Illness and Disabilities: Sizzling Sex Is Always Possible   189
27. Sex and Drugs: Many Spoil Lovemaking, Some Enhance It   201
28. How Men Can Support Women through Menopause   210
29. No One Is Ever Too Old for Sizzling Sex   215
30. How to Approach Sex Problems: From Self-Help to Sex Coaching to Sex Therapy   225

Part III
A Guide to Resolving Men's Sex Problems

31. Penis Size: Look Your Largest—Safely and Inexpensively   231
32. The Cure for Premature Ejaculation: How to Last Longer   238
33. Trouble Climaxing? How to Resolve Orgasm/Ejaculation Problems   247
34. The Man's Guide to Firm Erections, and How to Treat Erectile Dysfunction 252

Part IV
The Man's Guide to Women's Sexuality

35. Men and Women: More Similar Than Different   273
36. A Man's Guide to Women's Bodies   275
37. Women's Desire: Possibly Similar to Men's but Often Different   288
38. Why So Many Women Have Trouble with Orgasm   297
39. A Man's Guide to Women's Sexual Pain   304

Part V
Other Ways to Play

40. A Consumer's Guide to Vibrators   311
41. Other Sex Enhancements   317
42. Anal Sex—without Pain   322
43. Hall Passes, Threesomes, Swinging, Sex Clubs, and Polyamory:
        The Curious Couple's Guide to Consensual Nonmonogamy   330
44. BDSM: A Loving Introduction to Bondage, Discipline, and Sadomasochism   338
45. Minority Sexual Orientations, Minority Gender Identities: Lesbian, Gay,
        Bisexual, Transgender, Queer, Nonbinary, Intersex, and Asexual   347

Part VI
What Everyone Should Know about Pornography

46. The Main Problem with Porn: It Misleads Men about Themselves, Women,
        and Lovemaking   357
47. The Deep Evolutionary Roots of Porn—and Another Art Form Many Women Love 363
48. How Much of Porn Is Violent? Does Porn Contribute to Sexual Assault?   371
49. Porn's Impact on Adolescents   377
50. The Three Differences between Women Porn Actors and Other Women   381
51. Men, Porn, and the Controversy Surrounding "Sex Addiction"   385
52. The Anguish Some Women Feel about Porn   407

Acknowledgments   412
About the Author   414
Bibliography and References   415
Index   416

Foreword

A S A SEXOLOGIST, I have always had a soft spot in my heart for men—heterosexual, gay, queer, trans, or however one identifies as a man. Being a man poses enormous challenges. Men are not socialized to cope well with their emotions. Studies have repeatedly shown that most men suffer sexual performance anxiety. Men also need help shedding the cloak of performers and finding their paths to sexual self-realization—how to be fully sexually human, to express their full pleasure potential, and to connect with other human beings in loving, sexual ways.

Many of my clients have been single men trying to navigate the choppy waters of dating or enhancing their sexual patterns, or coupled men seeking to please, be pleased, and succeed as lovers. My clinical and educational approach is sex positive and based on empowerment. I encourage men and those who love them to find the truth of who they are, discover how to overcome years of self-doubt and poor sexual skills, and resist the barrage of messages (especially from porn) about what it means to be skilled, loving, sexual men. Yet even with all the help my profession provides, many men feel lost when it comes to having satisfying sex or feeling good about their sexuality.

Which brings me to the book you hold in your hands. *Sizzling Sex for Life* is an entire library of sexual self-empowerment. It's filled with upbeat, supportive, sexually illuminating information carefully nuanced for today's complex sexual world. Michael Castleman has become our go-to source for practical advice and insights into evidence-based research about all things sexual. His book is far reaching, depathologizing, permission giving, sex positive, nonjudgmental, and friendly to all sexual identities, styles, and preferences. Written with wit and flair, it's filled with straight talk and compassionate self-help advice that encourages intimacy and erotic exploration. It is a must-have resource for every sex therapist, counselor, educator, and researcher—and for anyone who wants sizzling sex.

Decades ago, sex therapist Bernie Zilbergeld released *The New Male Sexuality*, which was the bible on the topic for years. Now, *Sizzling Sex for Life* offers the single most comprehensive roadmap for men and their lovers to great sex over the entire life span.

I'm confident you'll agree that this book explains everything men—and women—need to know about sexual issues and fulfillment. It is sure to bring hope, great pleasure, and deeper intimacy to men and their partners.

—Patti Britton, PhD, MPH, past president of the American Association of Sex Educators, Counselors, and Therapists, cofounder of Sex Coach U, which trains and certifies sex coaches worldwide, and author of several books, including *The Art of Sex Coaching* and *The Complete Idiot's Guide to Sensual Massage*

Introduction

THIS IS MY third—and last—sex book. It culminates a fifty-year career as a sexuality journalist and counselor.

After college, this English major spent seven years working as a counselor at clinics specializing in family planning and sexual infections—in Ann Arbor, Michigan (1973–75) and San Francisco (1976–79).

Family planning was, and still is, a largely female profession. Back in the 1970s, condoms were still hidden behind druggists' counters, and few men used them. Most women in the field doubted that men would set foot in a clinic that gave away "rubbers" and counseled men to support women's use of other contraceptives. But in 1976 several visionary women in the San Francisco Health Department persuaded the Carter administration to fund the Men's Clinic, the nation's first birth control facility for men, I was among its founding staff. Our challenge—could we bring men in?

In the 1970s, the big news in sexuality was the invention of sex therapy by William Masters, MD, and Virginia Johnson. Their book, *Human Sexual Inadequacy* (1970), documented their success treating men's premature ejaculation (PE) and women's difficulties working up to orgasm. Before Masters and Johnson, psychologists considered such dysfunctions symptoms of deep emotional turmoil. But psychotherapy rarely helped. Masters and Johnson showed that PE and orgasm difficulties could usually be cured quickly, consistently, and permanently with a combination of accurate sex information and less genitally fixated lovemaking based on leisurely, playful, mutual whole-body massage.

The University of California's San Francisco Medical Center offered the new sex therapy. A faculty member served on the advisory board of the Men's Clinic. We pitched him on training us to teach men how to last longer, thinking the service might attract our target audience and allow us to promote condoms. He was game and off we went.

The Men's Clinic offered PE counseling for free and, when necessary, referrals to sex therapists (10 percent of cases). Men from all walks of life arrived in surprisingly large numbers—even a member of the Hell's Angels motorcycle club—all eager to learn dependable ejaculatory control. Once our clients gained the sexual confidence they craved, they often asked, "Is there *anything else* you want to tell me?" That's when we pulled out the condoms. We distributed thousands. The clinic attracted media attention. Geraldo Rivera visited for a segment on *Good Morning America*.

After the Reagan administration defunded the Men's Clinic, I earned a master's in journalism from UC Berkeley (1979). My thesis, "Uncovering the Condom Industry," documented condoms' quietly increasing popularity, debunked the myth that they reduce sensitivity, and urged pharmacists to display them openly. *Consumer Reports* incorporated my research into its first-ever report on condoms in 1980 (condoms remained hidden behind pharmacists' counters until the mid-1980s when the AIDS epidemic made safe sex a national priority).

The 1970s also marked the blossoming of the women's movement. It resonated deeply with my wife, then girlfriend, Anne. Three of that era's pioneering women's sexuality books made big impressions on me: *Our Bodies, Ourselves* by the Boston Women's Health Collective (1971), *For Yourself: The Fulfillment of Female Sexuality* by sex therapist Lonnie Barbach, PhD (1975), and *The Hite Report: A Nationwide Study of Female Sexuality* by sex educator Shere Hite (1976).

These books—and conversations with Anne and many women in and out of family planning—revealed that, like most men, I knew little about how most women prefer to make love. But I was eager to learn.

I wrote my first sex book, *Sexual Solutions* (1980), in my late twenties. It focused on teen and young adult men. Its message was that the sexual style most women say they prefer is identical to what sex therapists recommended to prevent and cure most of men's sex problems. I was a young man advising my peers: if you make love the way most women enjoy, you'll suffer fewer sex problems. Your partners will also enjoy sex more. They'll have orgasms consistently. And you'll get kudos—an erotic win-win.

Sexual Solutions led me into several important organizations: the American Association of Sex Educators, Counselors, and Therapists; the Society for the Scientific Study of Sexuality; and the Society for Sex Therapy and Research. Their members' collective wisdom has influenced me profoundly.

One fan of *Sexual Solutions* was the writer of *Playboy* magazine's advice column, the "Advisor." He recruited me into the informal network he consulted when faced with questions he found challenging. Ten years later, he asked me to answer the sex queries. I spent five years answering more than one thousand questions from 1991 to 1995.

The *Playboy* Advisor:
"Authoritative" Answers That "Discourage Misogyny, Bravado, and Violence against Women"

Today, *Playboy* is a relic of pre-internet times. But from its launch in 1953 through the 1990s, it was hugely popular with young men.

Playboy was also controversial. Supporters, mostly men, loved its photos of nude women—oh, and its cartoons, articles, and interviews. Critics, overwhelmingly women, called it pornography that destroyed women's self-esteem and duped men into thinking that women were hotter to trot than the vast majority actually were.

In 1998, these two perspectives collided at a cocktail party for the sociology department at the University of Louisville, Kentucky. A woman professor accused *Playboy* of promoting sexually misinformed misogyny. A male professor countered that, while the magazine could be criticized, its "Advisor" column was accurate and respected women. *Impossible*, she replied. He retorted, *Wanna bet?*

Their friendly wager evolved into an analysis of every "Advisor" answer from the column's inception in 1960 through 1997—including my five years. Their conclusion: Advisor answers were consistently "authoritative" and "discouraged misogyny, bravado, and violence against women." Thank you.

I wrote my second sex book, *Great Sex* (2004), after turning fifty, thirty years into my relationship and a father of two. I'd left family planning for journalism specializing in health and sexuality.

Great Sex reflected a sexual landscape transformed by four events:

- The increasing popularity of vibrators (starting in the late 1970s)
- The devastating impact of AIDS (starting in 1980)
- The introduction of Viagra (1998)
- The arrival of the internet, which, by 2000, made tons of pornography available for free. By comparison, *Playboy* looked quaint.

Great Sex updated *Sexual Solutions*, incorporating twenty more years of sex research. It reaffirmed my original message: *when men make love the way most women prefer, everyone benefits.* It also addressed the new world of ubiquitous free porn, telling men: porn is like the chase scenes in action movies—exciting and fun to watch, but *not* the way to drive. I urged men not to imitate it, but to do the *opposite* of what they saw in porn—instead of porn's all-genital sex, *Great Sex* advocated lovemaking based on leisurely, playful, mutual whole-body massage that eventually focuses between the legs.

Contrary to what many women believe, porn-viewing men don't hate women. They watch largely as a masturbation aid. Most men engage in solo sex considerably more than most women. Self-sexing is more enjoyable with erotic fantasies. Men's own get stale, so they turn to porn. The problem is that porn presents erotic fantasies, cartoon versions of sex. Unfortunately, many men consider it a how-to manual. I discuss how porn misleads men in chapter 46.

Great Sex intrigued the editors at *Psychology Today*, who, in 2009, invited me to blog on their website. I've posted twice a month ever since (PsychologyToday.com/blog/all-about-sex).

In 2010, I launched GreatSexGuidance.com, where I answer sex questions from people of all ages and sexual inclinations worldwide. Over the past four decades, I've answered more than twelve thousand questions—and have felt gratified by the thank-you notes.

Sexual Self-Help Usually Works

This is a sexual self-help book, a genre some deride as simplistic and ineffective.

I have tremendous respect for sex therapy and often recommend it, but at one national sexology conference, I heard a prominent sex therapist insist that self-help books were useless, that his practice overflowed with couples who'd gained nothing from them. Duh! When self-help works, people don't need sex therapists.

In addition to being myopic, this gentleman had also failed to keep up with sexology research. Many studies show that self-help improves lovemaking:

- Dutch researchers divided men with premature ejaculation or erectile dysfunction (ED) into two groups, wait list or self-help. The latter explored a website that presented standard sex therapy recommendations. After six months, the wait-list group reported scant improvement, but among the self-helpers, the majority reported substantial benefit.
- This same team offered other men with PE or ED twelve weeks of web-based sex information and brief email Q&A. Months later, two-thirds reported significant improvement.
- Then these same investigators recruited 117 women suffering vaginal muscle spasms that make intercourse painful or impossible (vaginismus). They were randomized to a wait list, a self-help book, or professional therapy (ten two-hour group sessions). After a year, no one in the wait-list group improved. But the inexpensive self-help book worked almost as well as the much more costly professional therapy.

- German researchers assigned seventy women with vaginismus to a wait list or to a website that provided information and other recommendations. After six months, the self-help group reported significantly less discomfort and more enjoyable sex.
- One of women's leading sexual complaints is little or no libido. University of Florida researchers placed twenty-two such women on a wait list and gave twenty-three others a self-help book, *A Tired Woman's Guide to Passionate Sex* by sexologist Laurie Mintz, PhD. It presents a self-help version of sex therapy for low libido. In the wait-list group, 5 percent reported increased desire; the book users, 54 percent. Among low-desire women, sex therapy usually helps some 50–60 percent while, depending on the study, drug treatment (flibanserin) helps 15–50 percent. The self-help book was approximately as effective as the drug or professional therapy—but cost less and caused no side effects.
- Finally, researchers at Concordia University in Illinois analyzed seventy studies of self-help. It showed little benefit for weight loss and drug addiction, but remarkable effectiveness for sex problems.

It's no surprise that sexual self-help usually works. A great deal of sexual misery stems from mistaken beliefs. With authoritative information, many people benefit quickly.

It's also no surprise that professional therapy works somewhat better. It can be tailored to individual needs, and many studies show that, independent of the therapy itself, a supportive, face-to-face relationship with a trusted professional is beneficial. But in a nation of 325 million, sex therapists and coaches number only a few thousand, and their services cost more than many can afford. Self-help books work almost as well for the price of a pizza.

Self-help books provide substantial benefit to around two-thirds of readers. For the other third, sex coaching or therapy help about two-thirds. This leaves around 10 percent of sexual issues resistant to therapy—usually because of medical conditions or psychological problems.

If you have a sex problem:

- Think twice before giving much credence to internet sex information. Some is accurate, but much is not, and it can be difficult to distinguish the good from the bad. Look for research citations—and not just one study, but several—the more the better.
- Try a self-help book or two. Many provide practical, reasoned, research-based information. But some are wanting, especially books about curing alleged sex/porn addiction. Again, look for citations. *Sizzling Sex* is entirely evidence based. I cite more than 2,500 research papers—see GreatSexGuidance.com/references.
- If difficulties persist, consult a sex educator, coach, or therapist, or a sexually informed medical provider. To find practitioners near you, see chapter 30.

Sex-Negative, Sex-Positive
Americans hold two views of the carnal dance:

- Sex-negative folks call hip-locking fine—occasionally—for married couples who want to conceive children and cement holy wedlock. But they disapprove of recreational sex, both solo and partnered, insisting that it causes crushing guilt, shame, abuse, and sex addiction.
- Sex-positive thinkers counter that while testing the mattress might cause personal and relationship difficulties, overall for the large majority of people, sex is usually

pleasurable. Whether for procreation, relationship affirmation, or just for fun, it's normal, healthy, nurturing, often therapeutic, and usually emotionally satisfying.

Unfortunately, our culture leans toward sex negativity. In contrast, *Sizzling Sex for Life* is sex positive. Sure, sex can cause problems. So can winning the lotto. Sex ranks among life's top pleasures. Sex-negative crusaders have vastly exaggerated its downsides. For example, they claim:

- **Legions of internet pedophiles have plunged us into an epidemic of child sexual exploitation.** To combat this alleged scourge, in 2009, forty-nine state attorneys general created a task force to study the threat and recommend responses. The task force concluded that internet-fueled child sex abuse was "not a significant problem."
- **Child sex abuse leaves victims sexually incapacitated for life.** Child sexual mistreatment is despicable and its perpetrators should be imprisoned. However, with therapy and supportive lovers, many if not most childhood sex abuse survivors can recover psychologically and enjoy satisfying lovemaking, even sizzling sex.
- **Teens are more promiscuous than ever. Teen pregnancy is a national crisis.** Actually, compared with their parents and grandparents, today's teens are less sexually active and more likely to use contraception. Research by the Centers for Disease Control and Prevention show that since 1990, the teen pregnancy rate has fallen substantially.
- **Internet pornography is filled with violence against women that contributes to sexual assault.** Actually, porn is less violent than most cop shows, action movies, and video games. The research consistently shows that as porn has become more easily available, the rate of sexual assault has decreased (chapter 48).
- **Almost all women in porn are survivors of childhood sex abuse.** Actually, the one study that looked into this shows that women porn actors are no more likely than other women to have suffered sexual abuse. They work in porn largely because it pays well and they enjoy sex more than most women (chapter 50).

The Woman Who Invented Sex Therapy Had No Professional Credentials

Officially, the pioneers of sex therapy were William Masters, MD, and his research assistant, Virginia Johnson. But as Thomas Maier relates in their joint biography, *Masters of Sex*, Masters was consumed with research and had little interest in applying their findings therapeutically. Johnson developed their model for sex therapy and deserves most of the credit for inventing the field.

Today, sex therapy certification requires:

- State licensure as a mental health professional
- Additional training in sexual issues
- Hundreds of hours of mentor-supervised practice

Johnson would not have qualified. The first sex therapist was a former nightclub singer who never graduated from college. She was also a highly sexual woman who loved physical intimacy and had an intuitive feel for communicating the elements of satisfying lovemaking.

- **Sex trafficking is a huge problem.** Human trafficking is reprehensible, but it's nowhere near as rife as antitrafficking activists claim. They cite figures from the International Labor Organization that 21 million people worldwide are currently subject to forced labor, of whom 22 percent, overwhelmingly women, are forced into sex work—4.6 million women. However, the best source of information on this crime, the United Nations Office on Drugs and Crime, estimates 55,000 trafficked persons worldwide annually, 59 percent of whom are women, with 58 percent of them sexually exploited—19,000. Of course, even one person trafficked for sex is one too many, but comparing these figures—4,600,000 versus 19,000—it's clear that those who see sex trafficking everywhere have exaggerated the problem.

Some, Many, Most

Only one sexual generalization is universally valid: Everyone is sexually unique. If you've had more than one lover, were any two erotically identical? Sexuality is as individual as our DNA.

Beyond individual uniqueness, it's impossible to make sweeping assertions. Consider the conventional wisdom that men are obsessed with doing the deed, while women can take or leave it. Actually, when couples consult sex therapists for desire differences, in one-third to half of cases, the spouse who wants more sex is the woman.

Even when research quantifies some aspect of sexuality, questions remain. For example, an estimated 1 percent of Americans identify as transgender. That's a tiny proportion of the population, but it's more than 3 million people. Are "some" Americans transgender? Or "many?"

Throughout this book, I endeavor to provide a sense of proportion. My estimates come directly from the research literature.

In any sex guide, generalizations are unavoidable. But only one is truly valid. Everyone is sexually unique.

Sex? Or Gender?

Passport applications ask one's sex—male or female. But actually, that's gender. Historically, sex and gender have been conflated, but they are not synonymous. Gender describes one's individual identity. Sex, in the sense of erotic orientation, describes who you'd like to undress.

Sexual preference might be heterosexual, gay/lesbian, bisexual, or asexual. The common abbreviation for folks who are sexual but not exclusively hetero is LGBTQ—lesbian, gay, bi, transgender, and queer. But transgender and queer describe gender, not sexuality. Transgender and queer individuals may embrace any sexual orientation.

Gender is a spectrum—there have always been more than two genders, but until this century, people who identified as transgender, queer, or nonbinary (neither male nor female) were largely ignored, or if noticed, often stigmatized, persecuted, and sometimes murdered. In recent years, as the transgender/queer/nonbinary population has become more visible and vocal, historical assumptions about gender have been upended.

The best research shows that 90 percent of Americans are exclusively heterosexual and cisgendered—"cis" meaning they embrace the gender assigned at their birth. Ten percent are lesbian/gay or bisexual. Around 1 percent is transgender. And approximately 1 percent is asexual.

This book largely addresses the sexual issues facing cisgendered heterosexuals—nine out of ten people. But a great deal of sex information has little if anything to do with gender and sexual preference. Part I's ten ingredients of sizzling sex apply to pretty much everyone who is sexual, independent of gender or sexual orientation. The same goes for much of the rest of this book.

I abhor all discrimination based on gender and sexual preference, and hope that everyone of all genders and erotic inclinations can obtain the sex information they need, here or elsewhere, and enjoy sizzling sex.

Comprehensive

In 1974, I was writing health articles for a community newspaper in Michigan. For Valentine's Day, the editor asked me to write an article he wanted to title "How to Make Love." I was all of twenty-four and no expert. At first, I refused. But the editor coaxed, and Anne encouraged me.

I read Masters and Johnson and interviewed several sexologists. I enjoyed that assignment more than I expected, in part because sex is endlessly fascinating, and in part because writing that piece led to the quick, happy resolution of a problem that had bedeviled the young me, premature ejaculation. With the Masters and Johnson program and Anne's help, in a month, I was cured. I thought, *I can't be the only one. Men should know about this.* I've covered sex research and therapy ever since.

In *Sizzling Sex for Life*, I have endeavored to discuss sexuality comprehensively. Of course, no single work can cover everything, but I've strived for comprehensiveness from cradle to grave.

Most sex books flow from the pens of therapists who cite studies, but usually frame their narratives around case studies. Many are valuable. Several clinician friends have written such books, which I've enjoyed and value. But as a journalist with training in epidemiology, I've chosen a different path—a thorough investigation of what's known about sex based on (1) research published over the past seventy years and (2) decades of conversations with some of the nation's leading sex educators, researchers, counselors, coaches, and therapists.

Of course, we'll never know everything about sex, but recent decades have seen an explosion of sex research, very little of which has reached the public. I've done my best to remedy that.

For Life

Until 1998, the year the Food and Drug Administration approved Viagra, most people assumed that after a certain age—sixty, seventy, whatever—people became "too old" for sex. Actually, there's no expiration date for lovemaking, solo or partnered.

I recall a headline from around 1990 (before Viagra): "After 70, Sex Stops." The researchers asked elders if they still had intercourse. The large majority said no. The researchers equated intercourse with sex, and assumed their respondents were no longer sexually active. In fact, for many if not most older adults, erection difficulties, vaginal dryness, medical conditions, and aches and pains make intercourse difficult or impossible, even with lubricant and erection drugs. Seniors who remain sexual usually jettison intercourse in favor of "outercourse": kissing, cuddling, mutual whole-body massage, hand jobs, fingering, oral sex, toys, and possibly some kink. Sexy elders still get it on, but usually *without* intercourse, and enjoy their lovemaking just as much, sometimes more.

Sizzling Sex for Life addresses not only older lovers, but everyone. Most children engage in sex play, but sex doesn't become a social issue until kids go to school. School sex education teaches nothing about pleasure. It's not sex-positive lovemaking instruction, but sex-negative dangers-of-sex jeremiads. I discuss sex and young people in chapters 11–18. Those chapters also guide parents in how to discuss sex with their children. That's not easy. I speak from experience, having two now-adult children. If you feel tongue-tied talking about sex, *hide this book* where your kids will find it—and, let's hope, read it.

A focus on pleasure also contributes to public health. Despite decades of anticigarette campaigns, 15 percent of Americans still smoke. Warnings about future risk of heart disease and lung cancer haven't moved them to quit. We might do better if billboards blared this little-known truth: *Men who smoke have trouble getting it up. Women smokers have trouble with sexual responsiveness.*

For Men
In mixed gender company, most men speak one way, while in all-male settings, they speak differently, especially about "plowing the furrow." This book usually employs clinical terms, but I also use men's earthier language. For instance, in part VII's discussion of pornography, I use the four-letter words intrinsic to men's experience of porn. If you feel offended, feel free to stop reading. But to get through to men, I use the terms most likely to resonate for them.

And the Women Who Love Them
While I write for men, I've also striven to be sensitive to women, to inform men of the many research breakthroughs of the past few decades—most by women sex researchers—that have shined new light on how women experience erotic pleasure. Sadly, many men are in the dark about this, so I've tried to explain what many women wish they could pound through thick male skulls.

Equally sadly, many women are in the dark about how men experience sexual issues and pleasure, particularly porn. I've also endeavored to inform women about men's experience of sexuality.

My Wish for Men: Kiss Her Lips—Both Sets
The core messages of my two previous sex books remain germane: make love the way most women prefer by doing the opposite of what you see in most porn. In addition, *Sizzling Sex for Life* adds one more erotic precept for men. Spend a good deal of time every time kissing her lips—both sets, upper and lower, your tongue dancing with hers and all around her vulva and external clitoris. Some women don't relish cunnilingus—ask. But assuming the woman in your bed enjoys receptive oral, always provide what men call "eating pussy."

Gentlemen, eat more pussy. Feast on it every time. It's delicious, fun, and key to most women's orgasms and satisfaction.

Since the late 1940s dawn of sex research, one finding has been reconfirmed hundreds of times. Men climax during 95 percent of partner intercourse experiences, but depending on the study, women's rate of coital orgasms is only 50–70 percent. Over time, as many women languish unsatisfied, they may turn off to sex and resent their partners, possibly threatening their relationships.

Why do so many women have trouble with orgasm? The conventional wisdom says women are the more emotionally complicated gender so more can go wrong. However, with all due respect to women's psychological intricacies, the research shows that women have difficulty working up to orgasm largely because so many men—and women—mistakenly believe that intercourse is what produces it.

Gentlemen, you may feel obsessed with penis size, getting it up, and how long you last, but what's between your legs is actually *less* important to most women's sexual satisfaction than how you use your lips and tongue. The key to most women's orgasms is gentle, extended clitoral caresses with fingers, tongue, and toys. Provide that generously every time. Eat more pussy—and also use your tongue to discuss the moves you both enjoy.

I want to be clear: I don't speak for women. For way too long, from popes to Freud to TV psychologists, men claiming to be experts have told women how they're "supposed to" experience sex—and have gotten it horribly wrong. Fortunately, the recent sexuality literature is replete with studies by women sexologists about women's experience of sex—and what they wish men knew. Few of their findings have reached the public—until now.

Women often complain that men don't listen to them. Occasionally, my wife has uttered those very words. But for the past four decades, I've done my best to hear what women say about erotic pleasure. My mission is to present that information in terms that work for everyone.

AARP Publishes a New Word

For decades, AARP has published a great deal of sex information for older adults. For five years (2010–14), I wrote a monthly sex column for the organization's website. In 2013, almost fifty years after Masters and Johnson described the physiology of whoopee, an editor called to say that as far as anyone there could tell, my upcoming column contained a word AARP had never previously published: *clitoris*. I didn't know whether to laugh or cry.

My Wish for Women: Please Lighten Up about Men Stroking to Porn

The best current evidence—from a woman-led research team—suggests that one-quarter of women (25 percent) believe porn is poison, spawn of Satan that degrades women, promotes rape, debauches adolescents, destroys relationships, spurs divorce, and causes sex addiction. Believe it or not, none of this is true. None of it.

Many women believe that only degenerate men watch porn. Actually, virtually all men with internet access have—and do. Canadian researchers wanted to compare the sexual attitudes of men who either had or had never watched porn. They couldn't find a single man who hadn't seen it. Porn is one of men's top internet destinations for just one reason. From sinners to saints, virtually all men go there—and watch with one hand busy.

The best research shows that porn does not cause the many social woes often blamed on it. Only a small fraction of porn contains actual violence. Since the late 1990s when free porn exploded on the internet:

- The nation's sexual assault rate has plummeted 58 percent.
- Teen pregnancies have dropped 70 percent.
- Teens' use of condoms has reached an all-time high.
- The divorce rate has declined 40 percent.
- The sex addiction industry claims porn addiction is an epidemic. Actually, the best estimate is that around two men per thousand (0.2 percent) view porn compulsively, a minuscule fraction of men.

Sexually compulsive men and women need professional help—and effective assistance is available (chapter 51). But virtually all men have seen porn. Legions watch frequently, many daily. The sky hasn't fallen.

Unfortunately, in a culture as reflexively sex negative as ours, the minority of women who detest porn get substantially more media attention than the large majority who don't believe it heralds the collapse of civilization. I doubt that my words can change the minds of women convinced porn is poison. But I hope part VII reassures most women that for the vast majority of men, as long as it doesn't interfere with life responsibilities and partner lovemaking, porn is largely benign, and self-sexing to it is no reflection on men's sanity or their devotion to the women they love.

* * *

Sex is one of life's greatest pleasures. It can also drive people crazy. I hope *Sizzling Sex for Life* reduces confusion and misery and enhances erotic pleasure and satisfaction for lovers of all ages and erotic inclinations.

I wish you sizzling sex.

PART I:
The Ten Ingredients of Sizzling Sex

CHAPTER 1:
Why Be Sexual? *Pleasure!*

WHY DO THE horizontal tango? Reasons differ, of course, but I believe I speak for the great majority of my brethren when I say that most men crave it. While the male libido may not always boil over on the front burner, it's usually simmering in back—*only one thing on their minds*.

Men's lust confounds many women. Some call it perverse. Actually, libido is hormonal. In men, it's a function of testosterone. Similar hormones, androgens, fuel desire in women.

Most women understand how it feels to be influenced by hormones. Many suffer hormone-related premenstrual syndrome, menstrual cramps, and discomforts of pregnancy, the postpartum period, nursing, and menopause. During these ups and downs, many women ask men's forbearance. "It's not me. It's my hormones." But when it comes to emotions induced by testosterone—lust, competition, aggression, porn viewing—many women withhold reciprocal indulgence. They believe men should rise above biology and maintain equanimity in the face of what some women call "testosterone poisoning."

The male sex hormone isn't necessarily toxic, but it's more intoxicating than many believe. In the nonsexual realm, it fuels rage, bullying, violence, and war. Sexually it makes many men appear insatiable. It sends them to porn and sex workers. And it drives some to commit abominations—child sex abuse and sexual assault and harassment.

What Transgender Men and Women Teach

The most eloquent testament to the power of testosterone comes from the small set of humanity who have rejected the gender they were assigned at birth (cisgender) and transitioned to the other. A former colleague of mine had gender affirming surgery and expressed astonishment at its sexual impact. "As a man," she explained, "I thought about sex constantly. My libido often felt irresistible. If I didn't get sex, I masturbated, daily, for years. Now that I'm a woman, I still enjoy sex, but don't think about it much and hardly masturbate at all. If given a choice between sex with a man or talking with my girlfriends, I'd usually choose the girls."

One of the most public transgender men is Chaz (née Chastity) Bono, child of singer/actor Cher and the late singer/politician Sonny Bono. Chaz Bono took testosterone and felt flabbergasted. As a woman, he'd ruminated about sex only occasionally. But as a man, he says he thinks about it almost constantly. When his girlfriend declines his frequent invitations, he self-sexes much more than he ever did as a woman.

Why does testosterone make men so libidinous? We evolved that way to perpetuate the species. The Bible recognizes the evolutionary imperative. In Genesis, God's first commandment to humanity is *Be fruitful and multiply*.

As a result, in the West, from ancient times until the twentieth century, there was only one moral reason for sex—procreation in the context of marriage. Sexual conservatives insist this is still the case.

But if procreation were the sole acceptable reason for lovemaking, throughout history most women would have done the deed only a few dozen times, from their midteens through twenties (births to women over thirty were rare until the late twentieth century). Men would have had sex for more years, but still not very often.

Meanwhile, there's no reason to believe that down through the ages children abstained from sex play, or that men waited until girls could become pregnant, or that adults obeyed the procreation-only edict for fear of God. In Genesis (38:11–26), Judah, one of Jacob's twelve sons, beds a harlot, not for procreation, but because of lust.

From Three Reasons to 237

Beyond children, two other motives for lovemaking eventually emerged: marital harmony and erotic pleasure. Self-proclaimed guardians of decency endorsed the former and condemned the latter.

Then in 2007, University of Texas researchers asked hundreds of volunteers to list all the reasons they or those they knew had ever engaged in sex. The 442 respondents, age seventeen to fifty-two, came up with way more than three reasons—234 more.

The myth is that emotionally and sexually, men and women are polar opposites. The adage goes: women have sex to become intimate while men become intimate to have sex. There's some truth to this. But what's more remarkable about men's and women's replies is their similarity.

Women's Top Fifteen Reasons for Partner Sex
(From most to least cited)

1. I felt attracted to the person.
2. I wanted to experience physical pleasure.
3. It feels good.
4. I wanted to show affection.
5. I wanted to express my love.
6. I felt sexually aroused and wanted release.
7. I felt horny.
8. It's fun.
9. I was in love.
10. I felt swept up in the heat of the moment.
11. I wanted to provide pleasure.
12. I wanted closeness/intimacy.
13. I wanted the pure pleasure.
14. I wanted an orgasm.
15. It's exciting, adventurous.

Men's Top Fifteen Reasons
(From most to least cited)

1. I felt attracted to the person.
2. It feels good.
3. I wanted to experience pleasure.
4. It's fun.
5. I wanted to show my affection.
6. I felt sexually aroused and wanted release.
7. I felt horny.
8. I wanted to express my love.
9. I wanted an orgasm.
10. I wanted to provide pleasure.
11. The person turned me on.
12. I wanted the pure pleasure.
13. I was swept up in the heat of the moment.
14. I desired closeness/intimacy.
15. It's exciting, adventurous.

Meston, C. M., and D. M. Buss. "Why Humans Have Sex." *Archives of Sexual Behavior* 36 (2007): 477.

Note that neither men nor women mention procreation. Having children was one of the fifty *least* cited reasons for partner lovemaking. Once the only legitimate reason, procreation has become almost parenthetical to lovemaking.

In addition, the three most frequent reasons have nothing to do with either lust, which supposedly rules men, or commitment, which purportedly animates women. All genders' top three reasons focus on attraction and pleasure.

Finally, these respondents prioritized lust identically (number 7) and felt very similar about using sex to express love (number 5 for women, number 8 for men) and feeling close/intimate (number 12 for women, number 14 for men). Far from inhabiting different planets, Mars and Venus, both men and women live on the planet between them, Earth.

Compared with women, men were more likely to respond to women's physical appearance: desirable body, attractive face, she turned me on. This confirms research showing that most men become aroused visually.

Women were more likely to go all the way based on its contribution to intimacy. This supports a great deal of research showing that most women—but by no means all—prefer sex in the context of committed relationships.

So why do men and women lock genitals? For many more reasons than most people think, but rarely for the biblical reason, and primarily for pleasure, which contributes to happiness:

- Dartmouth scientists asked 16,000 Americans what makes them happy. Sex ranked at or near the top of the list. Moving from sans sex to weekly whoopee made people feel as good as having an extra $50,000 in the bank.
- University of Toronto investigators surveyed 30,645 adults about sex and happiness. Compared with abstinence, increasing sexual frequency up to once a week made them increasingly happier. With more sex, respondents stayed happy, but didn't become happier.

Play with Me

If sex makes people happy and lovers do it primarily for pleasure, what is sex? Adult play.

Almost all adults engage in nonerotic recreation: hobbies, sports, travel, and so forth. But mention "play," and what comes to mind is childhood frolicking.

Youngsters' play offers grown-ups important insights into sex. Picture a playground with swings, slides, sandbox, carousel, and climbing structure. What does it mean if one child loves the swings while another prefers the sand box? Nothing at all. Different kids play differently. That's just who they are. And it's fine. No single playground activity is better than any other. None is "normal" while others are "deviant." They're all perfectly acceptable, enjoyable ways to play.

No Significant Regional Differences

Some places have reputations as sexually "wide open," anything goes. Actually, what happens in Las Vegas or elsewhere also happens everywhere else. Sexual minorities gravitate to cities, so homosexuality, swinging, and BDSM are more visible in urban areas. But unconventional sex thrives everywhere. Search "swing clubs" or "BDSM" and any locale. You might be surprised.

But when adults play naked and horizontally, stern judgments arise. Suddenly, sex-negative doyens of decency call a few activities "good/normal" and everything else "bad/deviant." They insist that "normal" sex is heterosexual, married, infrequent, monogamous, procreative or marriage affirming, noncommercial, same generation, in private, without porn or sex toys, and vanilla (no BDSM). Sex that's "deviant" is homosexual, unmarried, recreational, promiscuous, commercial, solo or in groups, cross generational, in public, and with porn, toys, and BDSM.

These judgments reflect a serious misunderstanding of play. Down through the ages, accusations of deviance and perversity have caused enormous misery, including imprisonment, torture, and execution. For what? For frolicking in parts of the playground where many normal, healthy, loving people enjoy playing.

The Two Definitions of "Normal"

Many sex questions boil down to "Am I normal?" That depends on one's definition. "Normal" may mean socially acceptable. Or it may mean conventional, what most people do. Or healthy, unlikely to cause harm. It's quite possible to be "normal" using one definition but not the others.

Ninety percent of people are exclusively heterosexual. Lesbians, gays, bisexuals, and asexuals are different—in that sense, "abnormal." But in terms of mental health, they're perfectly "normal." They're also increasingly socially accepted. And any problems associated with their sexual orientation, for example, a higher rate of suicidal thoughts, has nothing to do with how they play in bed, per se. Rather, it's all about their membership in stigmatized sexual minorities.

Most Americans Have Sampled Unconventional Sex

There is no normal, conventional sexuality. Everyone is unique, playing in distinctly individual ways. If conventional lovemaking involves adult heterosexual kissing, cuddling, and vaginal intercourse, with maybe some oral sex, most Americans have played in unconventional ways.

- More than half of children play sex games with other kids. *Show me yours, I'll show you mine.* The best evidence shows this is harmless.
- More than half of boys admit masturbating by age fifteen, more than half of girls by seventeen (the true prevalence of solo sex is undoubtedly higher—many people don't admit it).
- At some point in life, 15–20 percent of American men patronize sex workers.
- Many Americans with chronic conditions or disabilities can't play conventionally but with a little creativity can still enjoy sizzling sex.
- Many elderly lovers can't accomplish intercourse but love playing in other ways.
- By age fifty, 40 percent of Americans have experimented with anal play (usually fingering, not penis-anus intercourse).
- Approximately 20 percent of Americans have engaged in consensual nonmonogamy.
- University of Minnesota investigators surveyed 775 college students (243 men, 532 women). Those admitting unconventional sex were 46 percent.
- Indiana University researchers surveyed 2,021 American adults and discovered that many enjoyed elements of BDSM: spanking (30 percent), dominant/submissive role-playing (22 percent), restraint (20 percent), and whipping/flogging (13 percent). The investigators also found that 43 percent had played in public.
- In fantasy, unconventional sex is even more popular. The number one erotic fantasy is sex with someone other than one's regular partner. More than half of Americans admit fantasies involving BDSM. And more than half of women fantasize being forced into sex.

We Must Think Twice before Labeling Anything "Deviant"

Here's an irresistible headline: "New Survey Shows How Americans Have Sex." Who wouldn't read that article?

We're all fascinated by everyone else's sexuality. We want to know what's "average," "typical," and "normal," that is, conventional, so we can compare ourselves to the supposed norm. But the deeper researchers delve into sexuality, the greater the variation they've documented. Everyone is erotically unique.

And if there's no normal, it's difficult to call much "deviant." Deviance implies a significant departure from "normal," which doesn't exist. Now, the legal system defines some sexual variations as crimes, notably sexual assault and adult sex with children. Aside from these horrific acts, there is no "normal" or "abnormal," so we should think carefully before calling anything "deviant."

Sexual Inclinations: Not Predictable

Anyone can be into anything. Most social conservatives oppose abortion, porn, premarital sex, school sex education, homosexuality, and consensual nonmonogamy. But plenty of conservatives enjoy anal play, sex toys, BDSM, threesomes, swinging, and porn. There's even an evangelical swing group, Liberated Christians, in Phoenix, Arizona.

If sociologists know your zip code, education, occupation, religion, and income, they can predict with reasonable accuracy your politics and the media you view. But they would know next to nothing about your sexuality. Anybody can enjoy anything. Erotic pleasure is individual.

CHAPTER 2
Getting in Shape for Sizzling Sex

MENTION THE BEDROOM rock 'n' roll, and you probably don't think of meditating, yoga, a salad, a walk, or extra sleep. But standard health advice boosts libido and enhances sexual ability and pleasure:

- Get regular exercise—the equivalent of a brisk thirty- to sixty-minute walk each day.
- Eat mostly plant foods—at least five daily servings of fruits and vegetables, preferably more. Cut down on meats. Consume fewer whole-milk dairy products. Minimize fast foods and eliminate junk foods.
- Maintain healthy weight.
- Incorporate stress management into your life.
- Don't use tobacco.
- Don't consume more than two alcoholic drinks a day.
- Sleep at least seven hours a night.

Here's why. Physiologically, enjoyable sex requires:

- A healthy nervous system, so you can respond to erotic touch and enjoy it
- A healthy heart and blood vessels (cardiovascular system), so extra blood can raise erections in men and enable clitoral sensitivity and vaginal lubrication in women
- Deep relaxation, which boosts sexual enjoyment and helps the nervous and cardiovascular systems function at their erotic best

Before around forty, most people can smoke, drink, loll on the sofa, wash down bacon cheeseburgers with ice cream, and gain weight—and still enjoy decent sexual function. But that lifestyle slowly ravages the body, and after forty or so, the damage catches up with you. If you'd like to enjoy great sex from youth to triple digits, embrace a healthy lifestyle when you're young and maintain it throughout life. Or start today, no matter how old you are. You'll add years to your life and life to your years.

Of course, even exemplary health habits don't preclude sex-sabotaging illness or injury. But a healthy lifestyle boosts your chances for lifelong sizzling sex.

Regular Moderate Exercise
Exercise supports healthy arterial function, which increases blood flow to the genitals. It boosts libido-fueling testosterone in men and androgens in women. Exercise is also critical to weight control. It promotes deep relaxation, improves sleep, elevates mood, and contributes to self-esteem and well-being, all of which enhance libido and sexual enjoyment:

- Massachusetts researchers asked 1,709 men over forty about their lifestyle and sexual satisfaction. Those who exercised the most reported the best sex and the fewest sex problems.
- University of California, San Diego, investigators surveyed the sex lives of seventy-eight sedentary men with an average age of forty-eight. Then the men took hour-long walks four days a week. After nine months, their fitness improved and so did their sex lives—more libido, greater arousal, increased sexual frequency, and better orgasms.
- Singapore scientists enrolled ninety obese men, with an average age of forty-four, in exercise programs of either low or moderate intensity. Six months later, both groups reported better sex, but the moderate-intensity group showed greater improvement.

Regular moderate exercise produces similar sexual benefits in women.

It doesn't matter what type(s) of exercise you choose. Do anything you enjoy: walking, swimming, yoga, tennis, gardening, cycling—whatever gets you moving for at least thirty minutes a day, at least several days a week, ideally daily.

It's never too late to start exercising. Even very old folks who have led largely sedentary lives show improved health and fitness with modest walking, stretching, and lifting weights no heavier than cans of beans.

Many Americans believe that exercise is useless unless it's aerobic—sweat-inducing workouts that boost heart rate considerably. Optimal aerobic fitness does, indeed, provide a winning edge for serious athletes and soldiers in combat. But for those who simply want the health, longevity, and sexual benefits of exercise, aerobic workouts are not necessary.

Kegel Exercises: Better Orgasms

In 1948, urologist Arnold Kegel, MD, was treating women with stress incontinence, embarrassing urine leakage triggered by coughing, sneezing, or laughing. He thought the cause might be weak urinary sphincter muscles that could not stay closed under the abdominal pressure caused by these actions. Those muscles are part of the pelvic floor muscle group between the legs. Kegel theorized that strengthening them might cure stress incontinence. He was right.

The women who practiced Kegel's exercises also reported an unexpected benefit—better orgasms. The pelvic floor muscles, notably the pubococcygeus (pew-boh-coxee-GEE-us, a.k.a. PC), are the ones that contract during orgasm. As they become stronger, so do orgasms—in all genders.

To do Kegels, first identify your PC—it's the muscle you contract to interrupt urinating or to squeeze out the final drops. PC contractions also cause anal tightening.

Sex therapists recommend doing both slow and quick Kegels. For slow ones, flex your PC and hold it contracted for a slow count of three, then relax. For quick Kegels, contract and relax your PC as rapidly as possible. Begin with five slow contractions and five quick ones three times a day. Slowly work up to twenty-five slow and fast three times a day.

Kegels can be practiced anywhere. Only you know you're doing them. It usually takes a month or two of daily Kegels to notice enhanced orgasms.

Or women can do Kegels using ben-wa balls (chapter 41).

Few yoga classes are aerobic, but even mellow, meditative yoga improves sex. Korean researchers recruited forty-one women, aged thirty to sixty, who had high cholesterol, blood pressure, blood sugar, and triglycerides (blood fats). Twenty participated in gentle, hour-long yoga classes twice a week. The rest did not. Twelve weeks later, the yoga group showed lower cholesterol, triglycerides, blood sugar, and blood pressure—and reported greater sexual desire and arousal, more vaginal lubrication, and improved sexual satisfaction. University of British Columbia investigators reviewed a dozen studies of yoga's impact and declared the ancient discipline "enhances sexuality."

No matter how you exercise, regularity is more important than intensity. It's better for health and sex to take daily forty-five-minute walks than to hike for several hours twice a month.

As you plan your exercise regimen, don't forget horizontal workouts. Sex takes only about as much energy as walking up a few flights of stairs, but an hour of lovemaking burns 100–150 calories, equivalent to sixty minutes of strolling or stretching.

Does Sex Trigger Heart Attacks?

In 1979, former New York governor Nelson Rockefeller had a heart attack at age seventy-one in the arms of a woman who was not his wife. His twenty-six-year-old lover faced a mistress's nightmare. Should she slip away, allowing him to be discovered later with his reputation intact? Or call 911, hoping to save him—and reveal his infidelity? She dialed 911, but Rockefeller died.

Despite Rockefeller's experience, sex-related heart attacks are rare:

- Belgian researchers reviewed thirty-six studies of activities shortly before heart attacks. More than half the people (56 percent) were doing nothing special. The rest were:

  - Getting angry while driving (7.4 percent)
  - Exercising (6.2)
  - Drinking alcohol or coffee (5.0)
  - Breathing polluted air (4.8)
  - Suffering emotional distress (3.9)   Nawrot, T. S., et al. "Public Health
  - Getting angry, not driving (3.0)   Importance of Triggers of
  - Eating a big meal (2.7)   Myocardial Infarction: A
  - Making love (2.2)   Comparative Risk Assessment."
                                               Lancet 377, no. 9767 (2011): 732.

- Swedish scientists interviewed survivors of 699 heart attacks. Only 1.3 percent were sex related, and they clustered among the least physically fit.

- German investigators analyzed 38,000 autopsies. Deaths attributable to sex— 0.0026 percent, less than three per thousand.

- Tufts researchers reviewed fourteen studies and concluded that for every hour spent in the throes, heart attack risk rises "three per 10,000 person-years." If 10,000 people make love at their usual frequency for a year, we could expect three heart attacks, a tiny risk. And among those who played sexually more than once a month, risk was even lower, just one per 10,000 person-years—really tiny.

More Fruits and Vegetables

It's not necessary to become vegetarian, but those who eat the most fruits and vegetables report the greatest libido and sexual satisfaction:

- Italian researchers surveyed 215 adults' sex lives, then told half to eat as usual. The other half adopted a near-vegetarian Mediterranean diet. After eight years, the Mediterranean group reported significantly fewer sex problems.
- Another Italian team surveyed the sexual function of fifty-nine women. Half made no diet changes. The rest adopted a Mediterranean diet. After two years, the Mediterranean group reported significantly better sex.
- Greek researchers surveyed 350 men under forty about diet and sex problems. As their consumption of fruits and vegetables increased, their sex problems decreased.
- A third Italian team reviewed dozens of studies of a near-vegetarian diet and found that it helped prevent erectile dysfunction.
- Finally, Australian investigators analyzed eighty-nine studies of lifestyle and sexual function involving 348,865 participants. As participants' diets became healthier— more fruits and vegetables and less meat, dairy items, fast foods, and junk foods—ED risk declined significantly.

Plant foods contain antioxidant nutrients that help keep the cardiovascular and nervous systems healthy.

Forget the myth is that eating red meat is manly. The cholesterol and saturated fat in meats and whole-milk dairy foods accelerate the growth of deposits (atherosclerotic plaques) that narrow the arteries, limiting blood flow into the genitals. Cholesterol and saturated fat are also found in egg yolks, fast foods, junk food, deep-fried foods, and rich desserts.

It's easier to transform your diet than you might think. Have some fruit with breakfast. Eat at least one salad a day. And one night a week, instead of a meat-centered meal, try a hearty vegetable-bean soup. Make a big pot and you'll also get a few lunches out of it.

Maintain Healthy Weight

Plenty of overweight people enjoy active, fulfilling sex lives. In personals ads, they're known as BBW/BBM—big beautiful women and men. But most studies show that losing 5–10 percent of body weight improves sex—for a person weighing 200 pounds, that's ten to twenty pounds:

- At Duke University's weight loss program, a forty-four-year-old man shed forty-seven pounds. "To my amazement—and my girlfriend's delight—I suddenly had the sexual energy of a twenty-year-old lifeguard." Comments like his prompted Duke staff to survey the sexual effects of weight loss on seventy men with an average age of forty-two. Moderate weight loss—5–10 percent—significantly improved their libidos and sexual satisfaction.
- Brown University researchers tracked 229 obese women in a weight-loss program. After a year, they lost an average of fifteen pounds and reported better sex and fewer sex problems. Those who lost the most weight experienced the greatest sexual improvement.
- English researchers analyzed thirty-two studies of sex after weight loss. Most reported a major postloss increase in sexual desire and function.

- A North Carolina weight control researcher reviewed forty-seven studies of sexuality after significant weight loss. The large majority showed substantially increased libido, arousal, and sexual function and satisfaction.

Losing weight enhances sex in many ways:

- **Improved self-esteem.** People feel more attractive and radiate increased desirability, so they also look sexier to potential lovers.
- **Less fatigue.** It takes work to carry extra pounds. As weight increases, so does fatigue, which increases as the day wears on. Most people make love at night, so extra weight robs you of energy just when you want to get it on.
- **Less pain.** Carrying extra weight is hell on the leg joints. Many studies show that extra pounds mean more arthritis. Pain kills libido. Weight loss reduces joint pain, which boosts libido and enhances sexual pleasure.
- **Lower cholesterol.** University of South Carolina researchers checked the cholesterol levels of 3,250 men, then surveyed their sex lives. The higher their cholesterol, the more likely they were to report ED. In women, high cholesterol reduces clitoral responsiveness and vaginal lubrication.
- **Less diabetes.** Diabetes increases risk of ED and impairs clitoral sensitivity. Weight loss can reverse type 2 diabetes, which accounts for 95 percent of the disease.

Of course, losing weight isn't easy. You've probably heard that nine out of ten dieters regain what they lose. But this means that 10 percent lose weight for good. How? They learn from their mistakes.

"Permanent weight control is a learning process," says James Hill, PhD, of the University of Colorado Health Sciences Center in Denver. "People try a diet, lose a little, regain it, and feel they've 'failed.' But they haven't failed. They're learning by trial and error. Over time, they figure out what works for them."

Hill cofounded the National Weight Control Registry (NWCR), a database of people who have lost at least thirty pounds and kept it off for at least a year. Since 1993, the NWCR has collected more than seven thousand success stories. The average registrant has lost sixty-six pounds and kept if off for five years.

Ultra-Strenuous Workouts Suppress Libido

For sizzling sex, stick to moderate exercise. University of North Carolina researchers surveyed exercise habits and libido among 1,077 adult male athletes. Regular moderate exercise produced peak sexual desire. With increasing intensity and duration, fatigue depresses libido.

How? "They stop dieting," Hill explains. "Dieting involves major short-term changes that are usually impossible to maintain long-term. Our mantra is 'small changes for life.' Figure out what diet modifications you can live with—then stick with them."

Most people who keep weight off also walk. A lot. Exercise burns calories. "It's almost impossible to keep weight off without regular exercise," Hill says. "Walking is registrants' top physical activity. Most walk daily and take the stairs instead of the elevator."

Losing weight and maintaining the loss are two different challenges. "People lose weight in many ways: low-carb, low-fat, low-calorie, Weight Watchers," Hill explains. "But most maintain lower weight on a low-fat, low-calorie diet with lots of walking."

Daily Stress Management

The American Psychological Association surveyed more than two thousand US adults and concluded that the nation is seriously stressed out. Stress is also a major cause of sex problems. Stress management helps resolve them:

- Brown University researchers taught meditation to forty-four college students complaining of sex problems. Twelve weeks later, they reported less anxiety and improved lovemaking.
- Swedish investigators surveyed the quality of life of 152 adults, then taught half to meditate. Six months later, the meditators reported more enjoyable lovemaking.
- University of British Columbia researchers surveyed cancer survivors who complained of libido loss and poor sexual function. Half learned to meditate. After six months, the meditators reported better sex.

Stress triggers release of two hormones, cortisol and adrenaline, that direct blood away from the central body, including the genitals, to the arms and legs for escape or self-defense. Stress management opens the arteries of the body's core, including the genitals, providing the extra blood that produces erections and clitoral sensitivity.

Proven stress relievers include exercise (aerobic or nonaerobic, e.g., yoga), meditation, music (playing or listening), massage, laughter, hot baths, gardening, having a pet, visualizing relaxing scenes, and spending quality time with friends, family, or a lover. Incorporate one—or more—into your daily life. Ideally, combine them: walk your dog. Garden with your partner. Take the family to a comedy show.

No More Than Two Alcoholic Drinks per Day

From Shakespeare's *Macbeth*: Alcohol "provokes the desire, but it takes away the performance." How true. Alcohol is the world's leading cause of drug-related sex impairment.

The first drink is disinhibiting. It increases receptivity to carnal invitations. But when those of average weight drink more than two beers, cocktails, or glasses of wine in an hour, alcohol depresses the nervous system and interferes with sexual responsiveness. A "drink" is one 12-ounce beer, one shot of 80-proof spirits, or five ounces of wine, a standard wine glass about half full.

If you regularly consume more than two drinks a day, or if you ever binge on alcohol—consuming several drinks in one sitting—ask your doctor for help cutting back.

Quit Tobacco

Smoking damages the cardiovascular system. It raises blood pressure and accelerates the growth of the arterial deposits that reduce blood flow to the genitals. Smoking is also associated with sex-impairing nerve damage, especially among diabetics. And it's linked to sedentary lifestyle, obesity, and sleep problems, all contributors to sex problems.

- Boston University researchers compared the sexual function of 119 male smokers and nonsmokers, ages eighteen to fifty-eight. The smokers reported significantly more sex problems—even those in their twenties.
- Korean scientists surveyed 900 women about smoking and sex. The smokers reported substantially more sex problems.

- Rutgers researchers analyzed eighty-three studies of smoking's sexual impact. Male smokers suffered high risk of erection impairment.

The bad news is that after quitting, risk of lung cancer remains high for many years. The good news is that smoking-related sexual impairment largely disappears within a few years of quitting.

If you smoke, ask your doctor about quitting.

A Good Night's Sleep

An estimated 30 percent of Americans have trouble sleeping. Insomnia reduces libido and raises risk of anxiety and depression, both sex killers. In addition, the medications used to treat sleep problems may impair lovemaking.

Blame it on Thomas Edison. Before electric lighting, a 1910 survey showed that Americans slept an average of nine hours a night. Then in 1913, Edison introduced his light bulb. Americans started staying up later—and sleeping less.

There is no "normal" amount of sleep. Individual needs vary. But experts agree that to function optimally, the vast majority of adults need at least seven hours a night. Many require eight or more.

With age, time spent in deepest sleep declines, which impairs sleep quality. British researchers asked 2,568 men and 1,376 women over age fifty about their sleep quality and sexual function. As sleep quality declined, so did the likelihood of men's erections, as well as arousal and orgasms for both men and women.

Should Athletes Abstain before the Big Game?

Athletic folklore abounds with coaches forbidding sex the night before big games. However, many world-class athletes have done the deed the night—or a few hours—before contests and have emerged victorious. Olympic long jumper Bob Beamon typically abstained the night before but broke his rule before the 1968 Olympics. He set a world record. Basketball great Wilt Chamberlain said he had his 100-point game a few hours after sex. And the Minnesota Vikings coaches separated players from their partners the night before the team's four Super Bowls. Their record: 0–4.

Researchers at Cal State San Marcos tested a dozen male athletes' leg strength before and shortly after sex and found no significant differences. Sex is no more strenuous than walking up two flights of stairs. Coaches don't forbid stair climbing, so how did the prohibition originate? It began in the ancient world, when the goal of sports was not just victory, but also spiritual purity, which required abstinence.

New York Yankees manager Casey Stengel once said, "It's not the sex that hurts. It's staying up all night chasing women." Before contests, athletes need rest—and sex can help. Former champion triathlete Bob Arnot, MD, always had sex the night before triathlons. It helped him sleep.

However, some people, especially many women, find that sex keeps them awake. Canadian ski racer Kerrin Lee-Gartner abstained from sex with her husband the night before the 1992 Olympics because it interfered with her sleep—but they made love the morning of her race, and she won gold.

If sex helps you sleep, go ahead, play the night before. But if it keeps you up, postpone.

But regular exercise improves sleep, as does quitting smoking and limiting alcohol. Nicotine is a stimulant and alcohol disrupts sleep.

In addition, one sleep problem, obstructive sleep apnea, is a strong risk factor for ED. Apnea is caused by excess tissue in the throat, often the result of obesity. The hallmark symptom is loud snoring punctuated by choking silences when excess throat tissue blocks that passage, momentarily interrupting breathing. This sets off biological alarms that rouse the person, restoring breathing. But frequent rousings destroy sleep and substantially increase risk of ED. Chinese researchers analyzed nine studies involving 1,275 participants. Apnea doubled risk of erection problems in men and sexual difficulties in women.

If your bedmate says you snore with periodic silences, ask your doctor for a sleep study. If you sleep alone and feel drowsy during the day, a sleep study might also be indicated.

Sleep apnea can be effectively treated with a device that gently pushes air down the throat, a continuous positive-airway pressure machine (CPAP). Swedish researchers prescribed CPAPs for 401 men with apnea and ED. Their sexual function improved significantly. A Chinese study of 207 men with apnea and ED showed similar results.

Even those who don't have apnea benefit sexually from more sleep. Many Americans are chronically sleep deprived. University of Michigan investigators surveyed how long 171 women slept each night. As their time spent asleep increased, so did their libidos the day after and their odds of partner lovemaking.

*   *   *

Finally, Australian investigators analyzed 92 studies of 346,865 adults' lifestyle and sexual function. As smoking and alcohol consumption decreased, and as exercise, stress management, and plant-based diet increased, the results showed substantially more sexual energy and pleasure.

CHAPTER 3
The Lifelong Joy of Self-Sexing

OVER THE PAST seventy years, sex research has consistently shown that gentle massage from head to toe is the foundation of sizzling sex. How do we become familiar with it? By being cuddled as children, and by touching ourselves during masturbation, also known as solo sex, self-sexing, onanism, and the world's oldest pastime—not to mention hundreds of imaginative colloquialisms (page 17).

Masturbation is the foundation of satisfying sex and the world's most widely practiced type of lovemaking. Unfortunately, since biblical times, it has also been heavily stigmatized. *You'll go blind, insane, grow hair on your palms, and wind up in Hell!*

However, since Alfred Kinsey's studies in the late 1940s, playing solo has become somewhat more accepted. That's progress, but the pace has been glacial. Jacking off—and jilling—remain largely unmentionable. When was the last time you discussed your solo sex frequency and techniques? Mention taking matters into your own hands and people laugh nervously, then shut up. We still have a long way to go before do-it-yourself sex becomes as celebrated as it should be.

Solo sex is our original sexuality. It introduces children to erotic pleasure. It provides convenient comfort, joy, and stress relief throughout life—for free at your fingertips. Assuming it doesn't interfere with one's responsibilities and relationships, self-sexing causes no harm, except possibly chafing—use saliva or a commercial lubricant to avoid this.

Masturbation is also therapeutic. It's fundamental to resolving premature ejaculation in men and orgasm difficulties in all genders. It's critical to recovery from childhood sexual abuse. It even helps prevent prostate cancer. Chinese researchers analyzed twenty-one studies of sexual frequency and prostate cancer risk involving 55,490 men. Two to four ejaculations per week, solo or partnered, significantly decreased risk.

If you feel ambivalent about making love with yourself, it's difficult to have great sex with anyone else.

The Sin of Onan

Ancient Mediterranean cultures regarded masturbation as inevitable, therefore acceptable. The Hebrews were an exception. Consider this story from Genesis. Judah, son of patriarch Jacob, had two sons, Er and Onan. Er married Tamar but died before they had children. The ancient custom of levirate marriage required Onan to marry his widowed sister-in-law and give her sons who would become his dead brother's surrogate heirs. But Onan objected. Er was the firstborn. In ancient Hebrew culture, he would have received a double portion of his father's inheritance, two-thirds of the estate. Onan would have received one-third. With Er gone, Onan inherited everything. If he fathered a son by Tamar, that boy would become the honorary firstborn and *he* would inherit the double portion, leaving Onan with only one-third of what he would have received had

Slang Terms for Solo Sex

The more popular an activity, the more ways to describe it. The number of synonyms for masturbation confirm its tremendous popularity.

Compared with most women, most men yank considerably more. Consequently, men have more terms. A modest sampling:

Men: Beat off, beat the meat, bop the baloney, buff the banana, choke the chicken (or Cyclops), clean your rifle, crank the shank, date Ms. Palm, do your homework, fist your mister, flick your Bic, flog the log (or your dog), hide the sausage (or salami) jackin' the beanstalk, jerkin' the gherkin, jerk off, get your rocks off, give it a tug, go blind, grease pipe, honk your horn, mash the mango, moanin' with Onan, peel the banana, play a flute solo (or pocket pool, or pinball, or five-on-one), polish the banister (or rifle, or sword), pull the pole, procrasturbate, shake the sausage, slam the ham, slap the sausage (or salami), spank the monkey, stroke off, stroke the bloke, take matters into your own hands, tease the weasel, tenderize the tube steak, tickle the pickle, varnish the flagpole, wank, whack it, whip your willy, yank the crank (or shank).

Women: beat the bush (or around the bush), butter the biscuit (or muffin), cuddle the kitten, dial the pink phone, diddle Miss Daisy, feed the beaver, feel the love, finger paint, get to know yourself, gild the lily, girls' night in, give yourself a hand, jill off, ménage a moi, muffin buffin', paddle the pink canoe, pet the kitty (or poodle), polish the pearl, push your button, roll the dough, rub one out, rub the nub, scratch the snatch, tame the shrew, tiptoe through the two lips, unbutton the fur coat.

Tamar produced no sons. When Onan and Tamar shagged, instead of ejaculating inside her, he "spilled his seed on the ground." Onan's action infuriated God, who struck him dead.

Theologians of several faiths largely agree that Onan committed two sins, one small, the other large. His minor infraction was rejection of levirate marriage. His major sin was nonreproductive sex.

Why forbid recreational sex? That's a matter of theological and historical opinion, and who you believe wrote the Bible—the Almighty or humans. I'm persuaded the authors were human, and that they banned nonprocreative sex to distinguish the ancient Hebrews from their neighbors, and to boost their chances of survival. The biblical Israelites were a small, struggling ethnic group surrounded by imperialistic powers constantly threatening conquest. To have any hope of independence, they had to field as large an army as possible, which required sons. Consequently, the authors of the Five Books of Moses had God decree that the only legitimate sex was procreative. Onan did not pull pipe, but by "wasting" his seed, he threatened national survival and outraged the Lord.

Onan's execution proved it was anathema for a man to ejaculate anywhere but inside a vagina. Christianity also reviled the sin of Onan—and generalized it from decrying just masturbation to condemning all recreational sex. We're still contending with the fallout. Consider the derivation of "masturbation." It comes from two Latin words: *manus*, hand, and *stuprare*, to sully—using the hand to defile oneself.

As if religious dictums weren't sufficiently stifling, in 1760, Swiss physician Samuel Tissot published *Onanism: A Treatise on the Diseases Produced by Masturbation*. Without a shred of evidence, he claimed that stroking not only offended God, but also depleted men's bodies of precious semen, which caused debility, insanity, illness, and death. Translated into many languages, the book became a bestseller and demonized masturbation throughout much of the world.

Have you ever eaten a graham cracker? It was invented by Rev. Sylvester Graham (1794–1851), an early American health activist whose popular pamphlet "On Self-Pollution" (1834) promoted vegetarianism because eating meat triggered masturbation. Graham also urged his followers to reject white flour and use only whole wheat. In the 1860s, one of his disciples created a whole-grain cracker and named it after the sinister minister.

Have you ever poured milk on a bowl of corn flakes? They were invented by John Harvey Kellogg (1852–1943), the physician-proprietor of a prominent health spa in Battle Creek, Michigan. Like Graham, Kellogg insisted masturbation was the root of all evil. He urged parents to punish children for solo sex and deter it by feeding them the breakfast cereal he concocted.

Another staunch opponent of buffing the banister was Sigmund Freud (1856–1939). He called it "the primary addiction," postulating that it contributed to a host of psychological woes.

The contemporary bible of mental illness is the *Diagnostic and Statistical Manual of Mental Disorders* (DSM), published by the American Psychiatric Association since 1952. It condemned self-pleasuring as "deviant" until 1968.

Finally, in 1994 when AIDS was a global health calamity, a reporter asked US Surgeon General Jocelyn Elders, MD, if, given the AIDS risk of partner sex, it might be appropriate to promote masturbation to young people. She replied, "Masturbation is part of human sexuality. Perhaps it should be taught." Despite her tepid endorsement, congressional conservatives went ballistic and Elders was forced to resign.

How Often Do Americans Masturbate?

No one knows. An old joke declares that 98 percent of people admit they masturbate—and the other 2 percent are lying.

Underestimation of self-sexing appears to be rampant. Solo sex has been stigmatized for centuries. Social and religious conservatives continue to condemn it. Few sexual liberals celebrate it. And most people feel embarrassed admitting or discussing it. As a result, we can assume that many, if not most, people underestimate their frequency.

Two widely cited studies corroborate this. For a 1994 survey, University of Chicago researchers asked 3,432 Americans age eighteen to fifty-nine how often they masturbated, and then in 2007, they asked another 3,005 Americans age fifty-seven to eighty-five. Replies varied wildly.

In 2009, Indiana University researchers surveyed self-sexing among 5,865 Americans age fourteen to ninety-four. Again, replies were all over the place. But compared with the Chicago group's findings, the Indiana team found masturbation much more common.

Consider one age group, those thirty to thirty-nine:

Survey	Men 30–39 saying they ever masturbated	Women 30–39 saying they ever masturbated
Chicago	67%	49%
Indiana	93%	80%
Difference	26%	31%

Laumann, E. O., et al. *The Social Organization of Sexuality: Sexual Practices in the United States.* Chicago: University of Chicago Press, 1994.

Lindau, S. T., et al. "A Study of Sexuality and Health among Older Adults in the United States." *New England Journal of Medicine* 357 (2007): 762.

Herbenick, D., et al. "Sexual Behavior in the United States: Results from a National Probability Sample of Men and Women Ages 14–94." *Journal of Sexual Medicine* 7, suppl. 5 (2010): 255.

Why such large differences? Both surveys used representative samples and asked similar questions. The Chicago study preceded the Indiana effort by almost twenty years, but American sexual mores usually change slowly, especially when the subject is as unmentionable as self-sexing.

The most plausible explanation turns on how the researchers polled their subjects. The Chicago group interviewed them face-to-face. The Indiana team used telephone interviews supplemented by an anonymous questionnaire. When facing interviewers, many deny or underestimate stigmatized activities. But as social distance increases, interviewees are more likely to admit it. The Indiana team avoided face-to-face interviews in favor of more distant phone interviews and questionnaires. Not surprisingly, the Indiana survey showed substantially more solo sex.

Meanwhile, it's unlikely that the Indiana results capture the whole truth. Despite greater social distance, given enduring embarrassment about stroking, it's virtually certain that many respondents understated their frequency. I bet the true prevalence of self-sexing is greater than the Indiana findings.

So how common is masturbation in the US? Hard to know, but it's a safe to say it's quite common, the world's most popular type of sex.

The Demographics of Diddling

In addition to gender and age, other factors also affect the likelihood of masturbation. Sex researchers generally agree that:

- Testosterone-driven men tickle the pickle considerably more than estrogen-infused women polish the pearl. However, more than half of American women now own vibrators. While some use them in partner lovemaking, most deploy them exclusively solo.
- Healthy individuals usually masturbate more than those with illnesses or chronic medical conditions.
- With increasing education, people usually feel more comfortable about rubbing the nub.
- Religious liberals usually masturbate more than religious conservatives.
- Compared with those who refrained from sex play as children and adolescents, those who played doctor and spin the bottle usually masturbate more as adults.
- As sexual fantasies increase, so does frequency of masturbation.
- As mental health deteriorates, women usually push the button less, but most men report no less choking of the Cyclops.
- As age increases, self-sexing usually declines, but many late-life adults continue to masturbate, some elderly men daily.
- White people report more masturbation than African Americans, Asians, and Hispanics. However, this probably reflect whites' somewhat greater comfort admitting it.

While diddling continues to be stigmatized, some evidence suggests that over the past sixty years, it has either become more accepted or people feel more comfortable admitting it. German researchers surveyed university students in 1966 and thirty years later in 1996.

"At age 15, did you masturbate?"

1966: Women, 20 percent. Men, 50 percent.

1996: Women, 60 percent. Men, 80 percent.

"At age 19, did you masturbate?"
   1966: Women, 30 percent. Men, 85 percent.
   1996: Women, 85 percent. Men, 95 percent.

Myths and the Truth about Self-Sexing

MYTH: **Masturbation is a refuge for those without partners.**
TRUTH: Actually, compared with singles, coupled individuals usually masturbate *more*. With extended singlehood, sex, including self-sexing, moves to the back burner. But a relationship usually keeps sex up front and hands become more likely to wander.

MYTH: **Masturbation uses you up sexually.**
TRUTH: This myth holds that at birth, we're each granted some predetermined number of orgasms, and once we run through them, that's it. Nonsense. You may want sex only a little or a great deal, but biologically, there's no limit on erotic pleasure or number of orgasms. Masturbation can't use you up. Nor does it deplete sperm or semen. The testicles of normal, healthy, postpubertal men make sperm continually, and unless men have prostate surgery, the gland always secretes seminal fluid.

MYTH: **Masturbation causes erectile dysfunction.**
TRUTH: Self-sexing, per se, does *not* cause ED. However, it's linked with some erection difficulties for two reasons. First, the stigma. Doing what's taboo causes anxiety, which boosts blood levels of the stress hormone, cortisol. This hormone directs the discretionary blood supply out to the limbs for fight or flight, and away from the central body, including the genitals. When anxiety reduces blood flow through the penis, this may contribute to erection impairment. But the cause of this type of ED is not sanding wood. It's the stress engendered by internalizing social disapproval.

The other reason self-sexing may be linked to ED involves what happens *after* men come. Erections subside, and men enter the recovery ("refractory") period. They find it difficult or impossible to raise subsequent erections for a while—only minutes in some teens, but in many elderly men, twelve hours or longer. Men uninformed about the refractory period may blame masturbation for any difficulty raising their next stiffie. But the same thing happens after orgasm with partners. Even daily masturbation does not increase risk of ED.

MYTH: **Masturbation increases prostate cancer risk.**
TRUTH: This myth dates from a British study showing that frequent young adult ejaculations—both solo and partnered—are associated decades later with increased risk of prostate cancer: "Frequent masturbation during men's twenties and thirties was a marker for later increased prostate cancer risk."

If Stroking Produces Only Weak Erections

Beyond men's refractory periods, weak erections while self-sexing might result from fatigue, drug use, emotional stress—or possibly cardiovascular disease, especially if you smoke, are overweight, or have high cholesterol or blood pressure. Erection problems can be the first sign of cardiovascular disease. If you raise only weak erections solo, see your doctor.

However, other studies show that as ejaculations increase, risk of prostate cancer *decreases*. A Harvard-National Cancer Institute (NCI) study compared risk in two groups—men who reported four to seven ejaculations a month versus those who reported twenty-one or more. The latter were 67 percent *less* likely to develop the disease. The researchers concluded: "Frequency of ejaculation is not related to risk of prostate cancer."

Which study should we believe?

- Larger subject pools produce more reliable results. The Harvard-NCI study had 222,426 participants, the British study just 840. The Harvard-NCI study is more believable.
- Prospective studies are more reliable than retrospective research. Prospective trials move forward in time. Researchers examine participants at the outset and then periodically after. Retrospective studies look backward in time. Researchers ask subjects to recall past events. But memory can play tricks, especially when asking men in their fifties to estimate how often they polished the pistol during their twenties. Prospective trials are the gold standard of medical research. The Harvard-NCI study was prospective, the British study retrospective. The Harvard-NCI study is more believable.
- Biological plausibility increases believability. As men's number of sexually transmitted infections increases, so does prostate cancer risk. Ejaculation flushes the prostate, expelling pathogens that may contribute to cancer. So we would expect frequent ejaculations to reduce risk across the lifespan. That's what the Harvard-NCI study showed. It's more believable.
- Corroboration. Several other studies corroborate the Harvard-NCI conclusion. No other studies support the British report.

The only reasonable conclusion: Masturbation reduces prostate cancer risk.

MYTH: Masturbation causes mental health problems.
TRUTH: One oft-cited report analyzed several studies that explored how people felt after intercourse and solo sex: "Intercourse was a significant predictor of both men's and women's satisfaction with their mental health. Masturbation was associated with less happiness and more depression."

If you spent your youth hearing that self-sexing is unnatural, perverted, and a one-way ticket to Hell, its association with unhappiness and depression makes perfect sense. Yes, solo sex is linked to mental health problems, but it doesn't *cause* them. The cause is society's vilification of this normal, natural, healthy diversion.

If your religion demonizes masturbation, that's between you and your deity. But sexuality authorities agree that stroking—or using vibrators—doesn't cause mental health problems.

Advanced Stroking for Men: Slow Down and Savor
Some young men participate in "circle jerks," group masturbation sessions. Men love to compete, so circle jerks sometimes become contests—who can come first. If you enjoy this, have fun. But such competitions train young men to come quickly.

Other elements of jerkin' the gherkin also reinforce rapid ejaculation: some men feel anxious about getting caught self-sexing and stroke hurriedly. And once stroking yields to partner lovemaking, many young men worry that partners might change their minds, so they shoot first and worry about ejaculatory control later.

Through the lifespan, rapid, involuntary, premature ejaculation (PE) is men's number-one sex problem. In every age group, it spoils lovemaking for one-quarter to one-third of men.

Fortunately, men who have trained themselves to come quickly can usually *retrain* themselves to last as long as they'd like, in part by slowing the pace when they masturbate.

In addition, some men and many women have trouble working up to orgasm. Extended self-pleasuring is the foundation of the sex therapy programs that resolve these problems.

Advanced Stroking for Women: Consider Increasing Your Frequency

The best evidence suggests that 5 percent of women are highly sexual, as horny as many men. They stroke like men, too—often.

But 95 percent of women self-sex less. In the Indiana study (page 18), when asked if they'd masturbated during the previous year, only 54 percent said yes, considerably less than men's 72 percent.

Ladies, your solo sex frequency is totally up to you. But if you want sizzling sex during partner lovemaking, you might consider self-sexing more.

Researchers with the US Army surveyed the sexual satisfaction of eighty-two military wives. As their masturbation frequency increased, so did their self-esteem, libido, ease of arousal, likelihood of orgasm with their husbands, and overall sexual satisfaction. Sex takes practice. Solo sex teaches us how to respond to erotic touch—not just between the legs, but everywhere. That knowledge is indispensable to satisfying sex.

It's virtually certain that your guy regularly takes matters into his own hand. What's good for the gander is also good for the goose. Whether you're single, cohabiting, married, separated, divorced, or widowed, masturbation to orgasm is fun and satisfying and enhances partner lovemaking at any age.

Masturbation While Coupled? Sorry, Ladies, You Can't Satisfy All His Sexual Needs

It's possible that some men object to their lovers buttering the biscuit. But during my almost fifty years of answering sex questions, no man has ever raised this issue. Most men love to see women losing themselves in Eros, and if it's solo, men are more likely to applaud—and want to watch—than feel threatened.

Meanwhile, I've received hundreds of inquiries from women—some curious, others distraught—wondering why, now that they're coupled, their men have continued to wank. *Shouldn't I satisfy all his sexual needs?* Sorry. He has needs that transcend your relationship, notably the lifelong very male need for solo sex, which, by definition, is a do-it-yourself enterprise.

Men and women often attach different meanings to masturbation. For most men, it's little more than self-soothing, a quick, convenient, economical, enjoyable way to relax. But some women consider their men's masturbation a form of infidelity, especially when they stroke to porn (part VII).

Whatever it means to you, scratching that itch is our original sexuality. It's one of the first ways children learn to experience pleasure. Left to themselves, most kids are enthusiastic wankers. Why not? It's such fun. Your man masturbated for years, possibly decades, before he met you. Partner sex doesn't replace masturbation. The two are complementary. Why give up apple pie once you've tasted blueberry?

For self-soothing, men often masturbate while women are more likely to talk with friends. People have every right to self-soothe. Unfortunately, some women feel threatened by men's diddling. These women have succumbed to the romantic fallacy that lovers should meet each other's every need. Actually, whether single or coupled, at every age, everyone has the right to masturbate.

Stroking and partner sex both involve genital play, but the two are different. When self-sexing, you have just one person to please and self-touch provides immediate feedback that allows quick adjustments to maintain pleasure. But in partner sex, you have to be sensitive to your lover, provide pleasure, communicate what turns you on and off, learn how your partner enjoys being caressed, and make sexual compromises to keep your lover happy. As heavenly as partner lovemaking can feel, it's more complicated than self-sexing, and is not the same as self-pleasuring, a need many men feel deeply and frequently.

The vast majority of men masturbate from their teens through elderhood. There's little, if anything, women can do to change that. Compared with singles, coupled men usually masturbate *more*. If you object to his stroking, it's highly unlikely he'll stop. He'll just retreat into deeper secrecy that compromises emotional intimacy. I wish more women would accept male masturbation graciously, even if they don't understand it.

The Future of Remote Sex

Masturbating for each other is especially handy when lovers are apart. Remote sex is nothing new. Ever since literacy, separated lovers have touched each other from afar through erotic mail, which recipients often held in one hand while doing something else with the other. A good deal of correspondence between husbands and wives survives from the Civil War, some of it quite steamy. In 1863, Union chaplain Rev. James Cook Richmond wrote home: "I am rising stiff at the thought of your twin hillocks with their rosy blossoms, and the sweet hairy valley between your perfect legs. It makes my mouth water to think my mouth will soon plant infinite kisses on both sets of your lips."

During the twentieth century, remote sex migrated to the telephone. Dear Abby has recommended phone sex for long-distance lovers.

Of course, remote sex is not the real deal, but the body's sexiest organ is the mind, and remote sex excites it. Now, web-enabled sex toys extend the possibilities as never before.

Welcome to teledildonics, a.k.a. cyberdildonics. The woman wields a dildo embedded with touch sensors. The man slips into a penis sleeve capable of pulsating and squeezing. They link their toys using an app and connect through FaceTime. When she strokes or sucks or inserts the dildo, he sees it on his screen and his sleeve pulses and contracts, delivering sensations remarkably close to actual erotic play. Or the man has an artificial vulva-vagina-clitoris embedded with touch sensors and the woman has an app-enabled vibrator. As he strokes or licks, her vibrator reacts and she can "feel" his caresses.

Teledildonics is still in its infancy, and app-enabled sex toys aren't cheap—around $600 per pair (kiiroo.com or lovense.com). But as teledildonics matures, prices are likely to drop, and "I'll call you tonight" may acquire a whole new meaning.

"He'd Rather Masturbate Than Have Sex with Me"

Almost everyone enjoys an occasional scoop of ice cream. But if ice cream is all you eat, that's a problem.

The same goes for solo sex. Frequent masturbation, even daily or more, is usually fine, as long as it doesn't turn you into a recluse or interfere with school, work, life responsibilities, or partner sex in a relationship. But over the decades, many distraught women have messaged me expressing hurt, sorrow, and anger that their men would rather stroke than make love with them.

My heart also goes out to women rejected for Ms. Palm and her five daughters. In long-term relationships, couples have a responsibility to negotiate a mutually comfortable sexual frequency. If anyone routinely strokes to the exclusion of partner lovemaking, that's a problem.

My suggestion: Schedule partner sex dates in advance. That way you both prioritize horizontal time together and men (and some women) can still slam the ham at other times. If scheduling becomes contentious or doesn't work, consider sex coaching or therapy.

For Deeper Intimacy, Masturbate for Each Other

"Intimacy" means self-revelation—disclosing who you really are, warts and all, and discovering the same about your partner. What's more self-revealing than showing your lover how you make love to yourself? Few sex resources discuss this, but the Indiana researchers delved and showed that masturbating for and/or with a lover is surprisingly popular. In most age groups, more than 40 percent of Americans have played that way:

Age	Men saying they've ever masturbated for/with a partner	Women saying they've ever masturbated for/with partner
14–15	6%	9%
16–17	20%	20%
18–19	49%	39%
20–24	55%	47%
25–29	69%	64%
30–39	68%	63%
40–49	62%	56%
50–59	52%	47%
60–69	37%	36%
70+	32%	18%

Herbenick, D., et al. "Sexual Behavior in the United States: Results from a National Probability Sample of Men and Women Ages 14–94." *Journal of Sexual Medicine* 7, suppl. 5 (2010): 255.

Now, watching each other polish the jewels may not be your cup of tea. But if the two of you feel so inclined, this underappreciated path to self-revelation is likely to deepen your intimacy.

All Partner Sex Contains Elements of Solo Play

As our original sexuality, masturbation contains the seeds that eventually blossom into partner lovemaking. Self-sexing teaches us to respond to erotic touch, explore the full range of our sexuality, and work up to orgasm. Stroking with partners can enhance intimacy. And solo play is central to sex therapy for several common sex problems. If you feel bad about making love with yourself, it's difficult to feel good about it with anyone else.

CHAPTER 4
Affirmative Consent: "Yes, I Want to Be Sexual with You"

ONCE MASTURBATION HAS familiarized you with your erotic self, the bedrock foundation of sizzling partner sex is genuine consent offered freely—no pressure, coercion, or incapacitation from alcohol or other drugs and no fear of shaming or retaliation for refusing. Satisfying sex requires deep relaxation. It's difficult, often impossible, to relax without authentic consent. If you want to excel as a lover, as things heat up, you need to hear some variation of *Yes, I want to be sexual with you.*

But between the ideal of true consent and the horror of sexual assault lies a vast realm of ambiguity on the part of one or both potential lovers. If the hesitant partner clearly says no, then continued insistence becomes either harassment or rape. But if a potential lover says, *I don't know . . . maybe . . .*, then the pursuer becomes a persuader on a mission and coaxing may cross the line. Pursuers, usually men, wine and dine their ambivalent targets, usually women, often with emphasis on the wine. Alcohol increases the likelihood of an eventual *yes*—though it also substantially increases risk of sexual assault, erection problems, orgasm impairment, and later regret.

In contemporary America, plenty of women of all ages pursue men. But usually, it's the other way around—men pursuing women, seeking their consent . . . and sometimes deplorably forcing sex without it.

Going back to ancient times, many relationships have involved mutual love and respect: for example, in Genesis, the marriages of Sarah, Rebecca, Leah, and Rachel to Abraham, Isaac, and Jacob. Nonetheless, in Western cultures and legal systems, until around a century ago, consent—that is, women's consent—was never considered an issue. Women had no right to refuse. Men *owned* their wives and daughters as property and exerted complete control over their lives, bodies, and sexuality. In some cultures, that's still the case.

The Long and Winding Road to Consent

Until recently in history, few women except sex workers enjoyed real control over their sexuality. In Genesis, Abraham's nephew, Lot, lives in Sodom. He's sitting at the town gate when two angels dressed as travelers arrive. In the ancient world, hospitality was a major virtue, so Lot invites them into his home.

But the wicked men of Sodom mass at Lot's door, demanding to "know" the two strangers, that is, gang rape them. Lot begs them to depart. They refuse and threaten to break down his door. Lot tries to save the strangers by offering up his virgin daughters in their place. Then angels save the day by striking everyone in the mob blind. Soon after, God destroys Sodom and neighboring Gomorrah. But before the thunderbolts fly, the two strangers/angels lead Lot and his family to safety. Why? Lot protected them, making him a "righteous man." Of course, viewed through a contemporary lens, Lot is a monster. He offered his daughters to rapists. However, in his world, women had little value and Lot was "good."

Ancient fathers had life-and-death power over their daughters. If fathers decided that any of their female offspring had shamed the family—by eloping, refusing arranged marriage, seeking divorce, or getting raped by anyone but them—patriarchs could punish their daughters however they saw fit, including execution, with legal impunity and cultural support. In some countries, this is still the case—so-called honor killings of wayward girls. Advocacy organizations estimate that honor killings currently claim the lives of twenty thousand young women worldwide annually.

Until the twentieth century, when women married, control of their sexuality passed to their husbands, who were legally free to "take" them whenever they wanted regardless of their wives' wishes. There was no such thing as marital rape. By marrying, women implicitly consented to satisfying their husbands' lust on their husbands' terms. It was also legally impossible for men to rape servants or slaves. When their masters wanted sex, they could not refuse. Providing sex on demand was their lot in life.

In ancient Rome, rape became a crime—but not against its many women victims. In the Eternal City, the victims were the fathers and husbands, who owned raped women. Forcing sex on them damaged the owners' property.

The Christian Bible sounds somewhat more progressive. Paul tells the Corinthians, "The husband should give his wife her conjugal rights, and likewise the wife to her husband. For the wife does not have authority over her body, but the husband does. Likewise the husband does not have authority over his body, but the wife does." Nice words, but there is no evidence that early Christian women had any real right to refuse incest or marital sex. Their immortal souls may have belonged to God, but their bodies belonged to their fathers or husbands, who could do as they pleased.

In Europe, from the Middle Ages through the Renaissance, rape was rarely considered a crime—as long as the couple hailed from the same social class. Men forcing sex on women was usually viewed as a mating ritual, with men often abducting women and "taking" them in lieu of formal marriage proposals. In the small villages of medieval Europe, victims could almost always identify their attackers, and their families confronted the rapists. If perpetrators wed their victims, all was well, case closed.

But if assailants refused to marry, they could insist on trials and claim the women had consented. Consent defenses usually prevailed, even if women could point to injuries suffered trying to fend off attackers. Women's testimony carried scant legal weight. Only in cases of severe injury or several witnesses testifying that women had been steadfast in their resistance could men be convicted of rape. In such cases, they were fined—again, not for violence against women, but for damaging their owners' property. Rapists were punished severely only when plebeian men assaulted upper-class women. Those men were tortured and executed.

As the centuries passed, sexual assault evolved from a property crime against women's masters into a violent crime against women as human beings. But women who dared bring charges were typically vilified and shunned. Their attackers usually got off with consent defenses. And marital rape remained impossible. Well into the twentieth century, Western women could not legally refuse sex with their husbands.

After World War I, as women slowly gained legal rights, marital rape became an increasingly noticeable crime. Many husbands didn't get the memo—sexual assault remained common in marriage. Not until the 1970s did US law criminalize marital rape. The last states to do this, Oklahoma and North Carolina, did so in 1993.

For millennia, patriarchal societies viewed women as little more than baby incubators and sex toys. Only recently has that really changed.

In addition, sexual consent can be tricky. The human heart is fickle. People change their minds. Memories may differ. Alcohol muddies the waters. And contemporary men's leading sex educator, pornography, depicts women almost universally eager for anything and everything.

Until the 1970s, few lovers expected explicit consent. Most relied on nonverbal cues, with passionate response to unfolding erotic escalation implying permission to go further. But this caused problems. Lingering Victorian sensibilities held that "good girls" shun sex and have to be coaxed into it. Some men who thought they were coaxing were, from women's perspective, assaulting them.

This led late twentieth-century feminists to popularize a new norm, *no means no. Feel free to coax—but if we say "no," you must stop.* Unfortunately, *no means no* didn't make much impression on many horny, drunk, testosterone-crazed young men coming on strong to drunk young women with blossoming libidos and a deep need to feel desired. The former took to plying the latter with liquor until they were too plastered to say *no.* And without an explicit no, these men assumed *yes.*

Meanwhile, the demographics of higher education and the military began to change. During World War II, only a tiny fraction of armed forces personnel were women. Today, it's 15 percent. As recently as the 1990s, colleges were mostly male. Now women comprise 57 percent of undergraduates and 59 percent of grad students. In 1975, women accounted for only 23 percent of college faculty, today 42 percent. In 1975, few college presidents were women, today 23 percent. Women's increasing numbers have led to greater clout and increasing demands for sexual rights.

In the military, in higher education, and in American culture as a whole, women have become fed up with the problems inherent in *no means no* and have promoted a new standard, *yes means yes*—clear, unambiguous consent for every sexual escalation—"affirmative consent."

The push for affirmative consent has triggered backlash. Critics complain that repeatedly asking permission is awkward and kills romance. Others dismiss the idea as political correctness run amok. Some detractors urge young men to insist that young women sign "sex contracts" so they can't be charged with rape.

Meanwhile, supporters contend that affirmative consent is a trifling inconvenience given that many women, especially teens and young adults, must contend with unwanted sexual attention and the threat of sexual assault.

Does Affirmative Consent Prevent Sexual Assault?

In 2014, California became the first state to require both high school sex education classes and college orientation programs to promote affirmative consent that requires initiators to ask, *Is this okay?* at every step up the erotic ladder. Many other states are considering similar legislation. And increasingly, colleges and the military incorporate affirmative consent into disciplinary actions around alleged assaults: *Did she clearly consent to fellatio?*

I'm 100 percent in favor of affirmative consent. It's key to sizzling sex. But affirmative consent plays little if any role in sexual assault prevention. In recent years, many colleges and the military have implemented remarkably effective rape-prevention programs. Within a year or two, these efforts have consistently reduced assaults by half or more. But they hardly mention affirmative consent (chapter 20).

Most Men Lust, Most Women Want to Feel Desired

In today's America, the vast majority of men of all ages understand that sexual assault is a serious crime. But boys continue to become young men in a culture that socializes them to act on their desires, to be sex seekers and initiators. Meanwhile, the vast majority of women of all ages understand that they have legal rights, including inviolable control over their bodies. But girls continue to become young women in a culture that insists they charm men by appearing attractive and desirable.

Unfortunately, once young men and women become interested in each other, few are adept at the subtle art of sexual negotiation. They lack the life experience to feel comfortable proceeding from friendship through courtship to sex, let alone sizzling sex, and their learning curve often involves heartache and possibly trauma. For teens and young adults, genuine consent often becomes a casualty of naivete.

By the time people reach their midthirties, they've usually matured sufficiently to navigate the choppy waters of Eros. Men become less driven by testosterone. Most learn to respect women. And the large majority of men age out of violent crimes. In addition, women understand more about their assault risk and become better skilled at avoidance. As a result, women's rape risk declines:

Women's age	Proportion of reported sexual assaults
12–17	15%
18–34	54%
35–64	28%
65+	3%

National Sexual Assault Hotline

Affirmative Consent Means Better Sex

While the occasional quickie can be fun, sexuality authorities agree that the most satisfying lovemaking unfolds slowly and playfully. A slow pace is critical to most women's responsiveness. Studies of women's lovemaking preferences consistently show that most want at least twenty minutes of kissing, cuddling, and nongenital caresses before proceeding to genital play.

Unfortunately, a slow pace comes less naturally to men, especially young men, who can rocket from neutral to intercourse in a flash. Young men need to know that rushed sex turns off most women and spurs them to tell friends Mr. Horndog is a lousy lay. Rushed sex also substantially increases men's risk of premature ejaculation, weak erections, and inability to ejaculate. The best, most mutually satisfying sex is leisurely and playful.

As things heat up, a slow pace allows plenty of time for initiators to whisper, *Is this okay?* It also creates opportunities for lovers to coach each other about the kinds of touch they enjoy. And it allows time to negotiate contraception and prevention of sexual infections.

Sexual assault is an abomination. Advocates of *yes means yes* might have more success incorporating the idea into young adult sexual culture if they emphasized another point: sizzling sex requires affirmative consent.

How to Deal with Mixed Messages

Affirmative consent presumes women are sure of their erotic intentions and capable of communicating them clearly. But some women of all ages, especially teens and young adults, are unsure and communicate ambivalence, especially if they've consumed alcohol.

As kissing deepens and hands begin to roam, escalating involvement offers ambivalent women both benefits and drawbacks. The benefits: pleasure, orgasm, confirmation of desirability, pleasing the man, and not being labeled a tease. The drawbacks: possible pregnancy, infections, and being shamed as a slut or prude. Women's uncertainty may preclude clear communication—and frustrate the hell out of libidinous men.

Gentlemen, if you want to be sure to avoid ambivalence, limit alcohol or don't drink, and always ask before escalating erotic touch. When in doubt, ask again. If you don't, you're at least a jerk, and possibly a felon.

Ladies, to minimize ambiguity, limit alcohol or don't drink, and speak your intentions clearly and out loud. Do not rely on body language. State your feelings explicitly—yes or no. Please do your best to avoid *maybe*. *Maybe* places you at significant risk of assault. Clearly state your limits. The same goes when women are the pursuers. Ladies, ask. Gentlemen, yes or no, but not maybe.

CHAPTER 5
Gentle, Extended, Mutual, Whole-Body Massage: The "Language" of Sizzling Sex

MENTION *SEX* AND most people imagine penis-vagina intercourse. Yes, doing the deed can be sizzling fun, and if you want children, it's usually necessary. But the vast majority of sex is not about procreation, but pleasure. Many couples enjoy fabulous lovemaking without the old in-out. The best partner sex is based on gentle, playful, mutual massage from head to toe.

Gentlemen, unless lovers explicitly request rough play and clearly specify their limits, forget everything you've ever heard about banging, nailing, hammering, or pounding women. Don't imitate the frenzied fucking you see in porn. For sizzling sex, your default position should always be slow, tender, mutual massage that eventually—after twenty minutes or so—extends to gentle, playful genital caresses.

In this book, "loving touch" means cuddling, kissing, caressing, fondling, hugging, nuzzling, petting, and snuggling. I'm not for a moment denigrating intercourse. But for satisfying intercourse, loving massage all over is a prerequisite.

When you get laid, get *laid back*. As you caress each other from head to toe, cultivate a slow pace—no faster than half speed. There's no rush. A leisurely pace enhances arousal, reduces risk of sex problems, creates space for negotiations, boosts erotic satisfaction, and gains you better reviews as a lover.

Touch: The Only Sense We Can't Live Without

During the nineteenth century, before safe, effective contraception and legal abortion, many hapless young women got knocked up—and abandoned their newborns at churches, hospitals, and police stations. The infants were warehoused in foundling homes, where most quickly died, presumably from disease.

Then New York physician Henry Dwight Chapin, MD (1857–1942), systematically observed hundreds of foundlings. At first, most appeared healthy, then for no apparent reason, they became listless, lost weight, wasted away, and died from what Chapin called "failure to thrive."

Chapin and his wife, Alice Delafield, a pioneering social worker, surveyed foundling homes in ten US cities and documented death rates of 95 percent for infants under one and 35–75 percent for those ages one to two. They suspected the culprit was malnutrition. They importuned foundling homes to serve better food. But when they did, their infant death rates hardly budged.

So the couple compared care at facilities with different death rates. At the most lethal, infants were left in cribs except during feedings. But at the facilities with lower death rates, nurses cuddled their wards. As cuddling increased, deaths decreased. Chapin and Delafield discovered that gentle, loving touch is crucial to infant survival.

Failure-to-thrive deaths rarely occur after infancy, but death from lack of touch at any age demonstrates the profound power of gentle flesh-to-flesh contact. Touch is an essential nutrient delivered through the skin. Infants can flourish without other senses, but without loving touch, they die.

The Source of Erotic Pleasure: C-Tactile Nerves

Enjoyment of gentle caresses is hardwired into the nervous system. Noxious sensations—bee stings, fractures—travel to the brain through pain nerves that trigger release of the stress hormone cortisol. But the skin also contains other nerves, C-tactile fibers, activated by pleasing touch. When cuddling and massage stimulate them, the body releases the hormone oxytocin, which increases feelings of relaxation, well-being, and attachment—emotions central to sizzling sex.

German researchers massaged forty-two women in various ways, then surveyed their libidos. Gentle touch that stimulated C-tactile nerves increased their desire.

Gentle touch also helps lovers get out of their heads and into their bodies. Our heads can be judgmental: *You're weird. You should be ashamed of yourself.* Negative self-talk interferes with the deep relaxation necessary for sizzling sex. Gentle touch enhances relaxation. It quiets the judgmental voice inside our heads and promotes whole-body pleasure from the scalp to the feet.

Many Men Lose Touch with Loving Touch

Most women intuitively understand that whole-body massage is fundamental to sizzling sex. But many men believe that sex equals hot beef injection and feel skeptical of whole-body caressing. Their doubts stem, in part, from the fact that as men leave childhood, many lose touch with gentle touch. Men slap each other's backs but are less inclined to touch affectionately as women do. Think back to your teens, to how arousing holding hands, kissing, or a hand on a thigh could feel. The entire skin surface is a sensual playground. Every square inch of skin can be sensually aroused. Why limit things to just a few spots?

Many men disdain massage-based lovemaking because it involves "foreplay," something you do before the main event. They wonder: *Why bother with preliminaries?* For the same reason athletes warm up before competitions. To function at their best, muscles and joints need warm-up time. Similarly, it takes time for lovers' bodies to become fully aroused, sexually functional, and capable of enjoying the erotic dance.

Many men, especially young guys, dismiss "all that touchy-feely crap." They engage in only perfunctory foreplay, most of it focused on women's breasts and genitals. In their headlong rush into intercourse, they ignore the rest of women's skin.

Rushing into intercourse turns off most women. Some enjoy occasional quickies (page 40), but the large majority say they prefer gentle, playful, extended, whole-body massage that eventually includes their breasts and genitals—but is not obsessed with them. In fact, to experience peak sexual arousal and orgasm, most women *require* whole-body caressing. "There's no way I'm going to get aroused with a minute or two of rubbing here and there," says New York sexologist Betty Dodson, PhD. "I need at least twenty minutes of gentle caresses all over—preferably more."

Rushed foreplay is also a one-way ticket to men's sex problems: premature ejaculation, erectile dysfunction, and trouble with ejaculation and orgasm—not to mention unresponsive lovers prone to late-night headaches who tell friends you suck in the sack. Popular songs extol doing it "all night long," but with genital-fixated, porn-style sex, many men can't even last a minute.

The penis is a sensitive fellow. The little guy loves getting excited, but if he gets too hot too quickly, he either ejaculates rapidly, or goes limp, or has trouble coming. Gentle loving touch distributes arousal around the entire body, which takes pressure off the penis. Men still become highly aroused—in fact, *more* aroused—but because they're turned on all over, their penises aren't the focus of all the excitement. This helps our sensitive buddies behave as we'd like.

Gentlemen, give slow, gentle massage a chance. Try this experiment: make two sex dates with your lover. First, do it your usual way, and take note of how you feel. Then, shortly before your second date, get professional massages or take turns massaging each other's heads, necks, shoulders, backs, and limbs for at least thirty minutes. Then make love. Chances are you'll enjoy postmassage lovemaking more.

Massage also slows the erotic pace. Take your time, then slow down even more. Your lover will thank you. So will your penis.

Consider combining mutual massage with pre-sex hot baths or showers, separately or together. Warm water is relaxing, and soaping and drying each other can be marvelous turn-ons.

Replacing rushed foreplay with leisurely, play-ful, whole-body caresses ranks among the most woman-pleasing lovemaking adjustments men can embrace. And once you adjust, I bet you discover that whole-body massage also enhances *your* erotic enjoyment.

Swedish? Or Deep Tissue?

In the US, two massage styles pre-dominate—Swedish and deep tis-sue. Both feel great, but Swedish is more sex enhancing. It involves light-to-moderate pressure and long, gliding strokes using the whole hand or the heel of the palm, and some kneading with the fingers.

Whole-Body Massage Boosts Men's Arousal

Extended foreplay offers men big benefits. Whole-body massage is key to firm erections, bomb-proof ejaculatory control, and earthquake orgasms—especially for men over fifty. University of Chicago researchers surveyed a representative sample of 1,352 older adults. Compared with men who routinely engaged in extended whole-body caressing, those who did not were:

- Twice as likely to report problems with arousal, erection, and orgasm/ejaculation
- Five times more likely to report unsatisfying sex

Extended mutual massage also:

- Boosted both men's and women's sexual and relationship satisfaction
- Reduced women's risk of sex problems

Other studies agree:

- Another Chicago team surveyed 27,500 adults age forty to eighty. As time spent engag-ing in nongenital touching increased, so did their arousal and sexual satisfaction.
- Scientists at the University of Utah showed 164 college students (91 men, 73 women) explicit videos that depicted either all-genital play or genital sex combined with kissing, cuddling, and nongenital massage. All genders rated the latter more arousing.

- Canadian researchers asked 2,000 heterosexuals which elements of lovemaking they considered most important to sexual satisfaction. They rated kissing, cuddling, and nongenital caressing almost as important as intercourse and orgasm.

When men spend more time providing whole-body massage, most women report feeling more desired, aroused, and satisfied. In addition, nongenital caresses release endorphins, the body's own mood elevators.

Gentlemen, for peak arousal and sizzling sex, spend the first twenty minutes or so touching everything *except* her breasts, butt, and vulva. If you make love with music playing, that's half a dozen typical songs. Then for another song or two, gently caress her breasts, tenderly toy with her nipples, and lovingly suck on them. Then ask if she feels ready for you to reach between her legs. I bet you both enjoy sex more.

Deep Breathing: The Crucial Complement of Loving Touch

As gentle, half-speed caresses relax the body, breathing naturally deepens. This enhances erotic relaxation and enjoyment—and helps lovers get out of their heads and into their bodies.

Deep breathing is central to meditation. It focuses the mind on the present moment. Lovemaking is similar. It also involves a break from everyday concerns and a focus on the sensual present.

Many men value being the "strong, silent type." They hesitate to breathe deeply during sex because it's audible. Sometimes silence is golden, but not when having a go. As arousal unfolds, deep exhalations naturally become soft love moans that enhance sex by communicating arousal. Erotic excitement is contagious. When you hear your partner breathing deeply and moaning softly, you become more aroused yourself. This creates a virtuous cycle—each partner's moaning excites the other and both become more turned on.

Massage Lotion? Or Sexual Lubricant?

As a rule, don't use massage lotions as sexual lubricants and vice versa. Massage lotions feel marvelous when rubbed into the skin, but they're rarely slippery enough to work well as genital lubricants. Sex lubes enhance intercourse, but often dry too quickly to enrich massage.

The combination of deep breathing and whole-body massage is more arousing than either alone. Celebrate your body's natural tendency to breathe deeply. Don't stifle love moans. Let your partner hear you. And feel free to vocalize—even scream—during orgasm.

Finally, deep breathing is a key element in treating several sex problems, notably premature ejaculation in men and orgasm difficulties in all genders.

The Other Senses Also Enhance the Dance

Sizzling sex is sensual. It involves all five senses. Touch may be the language of lovemaking, but mutual massage from head to toe feels even better when it includes sight, sound, smell, and taste:

- **Sight.** Compared with women, men tend to become more aroused visually, hence their fascinations with lingerie and porn. But other visual effects are also arousing; for example, candlelight creates a shimmering, romantic glow.

- **Sound.** In Greek mythology, Apollo is the god of both medicine and music. This makes sense. Music is a potent healer. Many studies show that music reduces anxiety, elevates mood, reduces pain, and improves quality of life. It's easy to bring music into your bedroom or anywhere you enjoy making love. Listen to anything you both enjoy.
- **Taste.** If you doubt the erotic power of food, check out the refrigerator scene in the movie *9½ Weeks*. Mickey Rourke and Kim Bassinger work themselves into a sexual frenzy feeding each other chocolate, strawberries, and Jell-O. Fine food and the conversation that accompanies it can make what happens after dessert even more delicious. Or take tasty treats to bed with you. Chocolate syrup and canned whipped cream tend to be favorites. Apply them anywhere (except inside the vagina), then lick them off.
- **Smell.** Fragrances have subtle but profound emotional power—hence the world's $29-billion-a-year perfume industry. A German study shows that as olfactory sensitivity increases, so do sexual pleasure and orgasm. Studies by neurologist Alan Hirsch, MD, director of the Smell and Taste Treatment and Research Foundation in Chicago, show that that certain fragrances—vanilla, lavender, and pumpkin pie (pumpkin, cinnamon, and nutmeg)—strengthen men's erections and contribute to erotic pleasure in all genders. Some people can't tolerate fragrances, but if you and your lover enjoy perfumes, try scented soaps, candles, and massage lotions.

The Mystery of Kissing

Many sex guides overlook a crucial element of loving touch: kissing. One reason is that kissing often occurs in nonsexual contexts with nonerotic meanings:

- Kissing a cheek (or air kissing) to say hello or goodbye
- Kissing children's boo-boos to heal them
- Kissing the Pope's ring or kings' hands or garments to signal reverence
- Kissing dice for good luck

In addition, kissing may signal betrayal, condemnation, or contempt:

- Judas's kiss that betrayed Christ
- The "kiss of death" that marked people for execution
- The phrase *Kiss my ass*

Nonetheless, locking lips often opens the door to locking hips. In chapter 1, among the 237 reasons why people have sex, liking the way the other person kissed ranked fairly high—number twenty-nine for women, thirty-nine for men.

The poet Percy Bysshe Shelley defined kissing as "soul meeting soul on lovers' lips." It's certainly possible for lips-only kissing to express love, but for soul to truly meet soul, most lovers engage in deep, open-mouth kissing with tongue play (a.k.a. French kissing). Some people consider deep kissing as intimate as intercourse (many sex workers refuse to kiss customers because, they say, it's "too intimate").

The earliest evidence of kissing appears in ancient Sanskrit texts (ca. 1000 BC). Early Europeans kissed, but the paucity of references in ancient Greco-Roman literature suggests that in those cultures, it was not routine. Later Europeans introduced smooching to the indigenous peoples of Australia, Tahiti, and several locales in Africa. In some Asian cultures, lovers kiss only in private, as public puckering is considered indecent.

Kissing makes many people feel self-conscious about their breath—hence the hundreds of millions of dollars spent annually on Life Savers, breath mints, and oral hygiene.

Zoologically, kissing is a mystery. Only two other species kiss like humans, chimpanzees and bonobos. But only humans and bonobos kiss deeply during sex.

It's not clear how kissing evolved. Some scientists say it originated with mammalian infant suckling. Human lips contain touch-sensitive nerves, and lip stimulation activates a surprisingly large area of the brain. However, all mammals suckle young, but only three species kiss.

Other scientists theorize that kissing evolved to bring noses close enough to sense others' pheromones, compounds that play a subtle but well-documented role in attraction and attachment. However, many species respond to pheromones, while only two kiss during sex.

Kissing boosts levels of three compounds in the body: endorphins, serotonin, and dopamine. Endorphins and serotonin elevate mood, while dopamine mediates libido. Kissing also increases blood levels of the calming hormone oxytocin, and decreases levels of the stress hormone cortisol. Consequently, kissing reduces anxiety, lowers blood pressure, and spurs emotional closeness.

Many people use kissing as a test of compatibility. In one survey, 59 percent of men and 66 percent of women said they'd ended budding relationships in part because the other person kissed badly or was stingy with kisses.

Massage: Beyond Sizzling Sex, Major Health Benefits

There's much more to massage than just sizzling sex. Massage releases oxytocin, which is calming, and endorphins, the body's own pain relievers. As a result, tender touch helps relieve pain, stress, and anxiety. It also boosts immune function, which helps prevent all illnesses.

Hippocrates, father of Western medicine, reportedly said, "The physician must be experienced in many things, but most assuredly, in rubbing." Modern massage research dates from the 1980s, when a study by University of Miami psychologist Tiffany Field, PhD, examined the effects of daily massages on premature infants in neonatal intensive care. Compared with untouched controls, massaged preemies grew faster and left the hospital sooner.

Field assessed the moods of eighty-four expectant mothers who complained of anxiety and depression. After twelve weeks of twice-weekly massages, they reported significant relief and improved relationships.

Some other findings:

- Carnegie Mellon researchers asked 404 healthy adults how often they hugged, then squirted live cold virus up subjects' noses. Those who hugged the most were least likely to catch the cold.
- Chinese researchers reviewed eighteen studies of massage for anxiety and depression. In every one, massage provided significant benefit.
- Korean scientists analyzed twelve studies of massage for cancer pain. Compared with cancer sufferers who remained untouched, those who received massage reported significantly less pain.

Among English speakers, open-mouth kissing wasn't called "French" until World War I, when large numbers of English and American soldiers fought in France and discovered how popular tongue play was there. The French call it the kiss of love (*baiser amoureux*) or kissing with the tongue (*baiser avec la langue*).

The vast majority of lovers enjoy kissing, but the research shows that women particularly value it. Many women say they can't feel satisfied without kissing before, during, and after genital play.

One study asked 1,041 adults how best to kiss. The vast majority said that fresh breath, clean teeth, and good grooming were essential. A large majority also valued soft, moist lips, deep breathing, mutual caressing, and assertiveness—not just passively accepting kisses but kissing back enthusiastically. Finally, most said the best kissing begins with mouths closed, and moves to deep kissing only as things heat up.

Forget *Foreplay*, Think *Loveplay*

Foreplay implies linear lovemaking: first some kissing, then hands on her breasts, next reaching between each other's legs, then intercourse and hopefully mutual orgasms. But linear lovemaking is formulaic and gets boring.

Loveplay is different. It's unpredictable, nonlinear, and never boring. It mixes things up in ways that feel new and different—and novelty is key to sizzling sex (chapter 9). In loveplay, nothing routinely leads to anything else. You might light some scented candles and share a glass of wine or listen to music while holding, kissing, and stroking each other's faces and necks. Next you might feed each other little snacks as you undress, while continuing to kiss and caress each other. Then you might shower together, dry each other, and share neck-and-shoulder massages. After that, you might retreat to bed, keep playing music, and lightly caress each other. Next, you might suckle each other's nipples, or trade foot massages, and after that, fondle each other's genitals briefly and then trade oral sex. After a while, you might have intercourse, then uncouple and feed each other more snacks, while continuing to kiss and caress each other. Next, you might return to oral or vaginal intercourse while your hands roam all over each other. And on and on. . . . None of this is "foreplay." It's all loveplay.

Compared with predictable foreplay, the novelty and creativity of loveplay feel more arousing. With loveplay, sex is always new and different—and more exciting and satisfying.

When couples jettison foreplay and embrace loveplay, both men and women become more deeply relaxed and erotically aroused and receptive. Men are less likely to have problems with erection, ejaculatory control, and orgasm/ejaculation. Women are less likely to have trouble with arousal, lubrication, and orgasm. And orgasms are more likely to feel ecstatic. Finally, leisurely, extended loveplay allows plenty of time to coach each other and discuss contraception and sexual infection prevention.

"I wish men would learn that sex feels best when it involves the whole body," Dodson says. "Sure, the genitals are important, but so is everything else. Guys who just want to fuck are clueless. Give me a lover who knows how to use his fingers, hands, lips, sex toys—and especially his tongue—all over me, creatively, with smiles and laughter for a nice long time."

So *That's* How It Feels

Can men ever know how women feel when their vulvas or clitorises get caressed? Can women ever know how fondling the head of the penis or the scrotum makes men feel? The short answer is no. If you don't have a clitoris, you can't know how touching it feels.

But there's more to it. All genders' genitals develop from the same embryonic cells—they're wired into the nervous system the same way. The genders don't differentiate until late in fetal development. While one gender can't know precisely how erotic touch makes the other feel, men and women can appreciate how the other gender experiences erotic caresses.

The Visible Clitoris = The Head (Glans) of the Penis. The embryonic cells that become the head of the penis in men become the head—the most visible part—of the clitoris in women. Each glans contains thousands of sensory nerve endings, a greater concentration of touch-sensitive nerves than any other part of the body. Clitoral caresses feel like touching the glans of the penis—except for one thing. The head of the clitoris is only about one-tenth the size of its penile counterpart, which makes every little bit of the clitoris *more sensitive* to touch.

This supersensitivity explains why, unless women specifically request otherwise, men should *always* caress the clitoris *very gently*. In porn, the men sometimes treat it roughly. Big mistake. Even when men caress and lick the clit lightly, many women can't take direct pressure on their buttons. There is nothing wrong with them. They're perfectly normal. If your lover has a supersensitive clitoris, don't fondle it directly. Instead, touch and lick *around* it, focusing on the bump only as they approach orgasm.

The Inner Vaginal Lips, Clitoral Shaft, Clitoral Crura, and G-spot = The Penile Shaft. The embryonic cells that become the shaft of the penis become several structures in women: the inner vaginal lips (labia minora), the clitoral shaft (the tissue that connects the head of the clitoris to the vulva), the clitoral crura (the "legs" of the clitoris that extend along the inner vaginal lips), and the G-spot, the erotically sensitive area an inch or two inside the vagina on its front wall (the top if she's on her back). Touching these areas feels to women like stroking the penile shaft feels to men.

Like the shaft, the inner lips, clitoral shaft, crura, and G-spot contain many nerves sensitive to erotic touch. They also contain erectile tissue. As women become sexually aroused, erection of these tissues parts the inner lips, exposing the clit, and makes the vagina more receptive to intercourse and the G-spot more sensitive to loving touch.

The Outer Vaginal Lips = The Scrotum. The outer lips develop from the same embryonic cells that form the scrotum. Touching them feels similar to how scrotum fondling feels to men.

The Vagina? Biologically, the vagina is the birth canal, babies' gateway into the world. Most people consider the vagina a key female sex organ. Some men believe it's the main one. But the embryonic tissue that becomes the vagina has no connection to the sexual tissues just discussed. It develops from the Müllerian ducts, tissue that degenerates and disappears as male fetuses develop.

The vagina contains touch-sensitive nerves, and many women enjoy great pleasure and intimacy from insertion of tongues and well-lubricated fingers, erections, and toys. But only around 25 percent of women are reliably orgasmic from vaginal touch alone (chapter 38). Most *need* direct clitoral caresses.

Pornography is obsessed with the vagina. The men in porn furiously pump fingers, erections, toys, and other things in and out. Actually, most women feel more sexually satisfied when men dial back the intensity of vaginal play and combine it with gently caressing the clitoris, vaginal lips, and G-spot.

Nipples. In porn, men often treat these sensitive little treasures roughly, pulling, pinching, and twisting them. If women explicitly request rough nipple play—for example, nipple clamps in consensual BDSM—then within their specified limits, provide the sensation they desire. But as a rule, treat women's nipples *gently*. Caress them with feathery touch and suck on them with lots of lips and tongue—no teeth unless specifically requested. Try this experiment: pull, pinch, and twist your own nipples. Chances are it doesn't take much to reach your comfort limit. Men who abuse women's nipples don't know squat about sex.

> ## Enjoying Receptive Anal Doesn't Mean You're Gay
>
> Some men avoid receptive anal touch for fear that it's "gay." It isn't. Gay men kiss. Is kissing gay? Plenty of totally heterosexual men enjoy receptive anilingus, sphincter massage, fingering, and toy insertion. Sexual orientation has nothing to do with the erotic moves you enjoy, just who you play with.

The Anus. The sphincter is rich in touch-sensitive nerves.

All Orgasms Are the Same . . . and Different

With sufficient relaxation, erotic focus, and loving caresses, most people eventually work up to orgasm (climax, coming, cumming). Men have one type, but Sigmund Freud postulated that women have two—clitoral and vaginal. During the 1980s, some sex researchers added a third for women, G-spot orgasms. Actually, male or female, there's only one type of orgasm, but depending on the circumstances and what triggers them, orgasms may *feel* very different.

In both men and women, orgasm involves rhythmic, involuntary, rapid, serial, wave-like contractions of the pelvic floor muscles that run between the legs and form a figure eight around the genitals and anus. Most orgasms involve four to ten contractions, though some women experience more. Contractions are typically separated by less than a second. One full set of contractions equals one orgasm. In addition, most orgasms include gasps, grunts, and convulsive spasms.

In women, the muscle contractions of orgasm are usually, but not always, visible as squeezing of the vaginal opening and anal sphincter. In some women, orgasm also releases fluid (female ejaculation). Most women who ejaculate produce a teaspoon or less, but some release more. Most women can have only one orgasm per romp, but a small minority can have two or more in rapid succession (multiple orgasm).

In men, orgasm typically includes ejaculation of semen. However, different nerves control orgasm and ejaculation. It's possible to have orgasms without ejaculating (dry orgasm), usually the result of spinal cord injury or prostate surgery. It's also possible to ejaculate without orgasm (numb come), usually because of fatigue, drugs, or feeling turned off by the partner or the sex.

Controversy surrounds some men's claims of multiple orgasms. If men can accomplish this, their numbers are tiny. Men in their teens and twenties can often raise new erections fairly quickly after orgasm and come again quickly. But as men age, the time between orgasm and the next erection (refractory period) grows longer. In elderly men or those with chronic medical conditions, it may take twelve hours or more.

If all orgasms result from serial contractions of the pelvic floor muscles, why has there been so much discussion of the supposed clitoral, vaginal, and G-spot varieties?

Freud made up his division of women's orgasms into clitoral and vaginal. There was—and still is—no evidence to support his assertion. In his view, clitoral orgasms were a sign of emotional immaturity. Mature women had vaginal orgasms. Nonsense. Physiologically, all orgasms involve pelvic floor muscle contractions. Some women can come from G-spot pressing, but those orgasms are physiologically the same as all others.

If all orgasms are the same, why do some feel weak and others earth-shattering? Why are some localized in the genitals, while others trigger whole-body convulsions?

Consider laughter. Physiologically, all laughter is the same, a reflex. But laughs may vary from quiet giggles to roaring guffaws. Or consider sneezes. Physiologically, they're all the same, but they vary from little snorts to explosions that rattle windows.

Orgasms may feel different for several reasons:

- **Stimulation.** Orgasm intensity may differ based on the trigger: clitoral caresses, intercourse, G-spot stimulation, vibrators, or other sex toys.
- **Context.** Orgasms in new, hot-and-heavy relationships may feel more intense than those years later. But not always. New love may also provoke anxiety. *Who is this person?* If long-term couples work to keep their lovemaking fresh, mutual trust and comfort may intensify their climaxes.
- **Duration.** Longer romps with more varied loveplay usually enhance orgasms.
- **Novelty.** New and different erotic moves add pleasure to lovemaking—and orgasm.
- **Fantasy.** Exciting fantasies during sex usually intensify orgasms.
- **Drugs.** For those with aches and pains, analgesics may reduce discomfort and add pleasure to orgasms. Some people say marijuana is O enhancing. But twisting the sheets while drunk often ruins orgasm.

Is Orgasm the Goal of Lovemaking?

Many people think so. Some believe without an O, why bother?

However, most sex coaches and therapists contend that the goal of sex is not orgasm but mutual pleasure, with or without orgasm. If lovemaking is whole-body massage plus orgasm, and for whatever reason orgasm doesn't happen, couples can still enjoy the pleasure of mutual erotic massage.

Orgasm may not be possible due to fatigue, disabilities, chronic medical conditions, or drugs: antidepressants, alcohol, sleep and antianxiety medications, and opioids, among others.

If you want orgasms but have difficulty getting there, start with self-help (chapter 33). If that doesn't work, consult a sexuality professional or sexually informed medical practitioner.

Try not to get hung up on the "kind" of orgasms you or your lover experience. Except for those deep into BDSM, the key to convulsive climaxes is to give and receive extended, gentle, playful, whole-body caresses that allow both partners to relax deeply and become sufficiently aroused to work up to happy endings—however they happen.

For a Happier Relationship, Savor Afterglow

Many sex guides ignore afterglow, the relaxed, dreamy, postorgasm period when many lovers feel particularly close. That's a shame. Cuddling during afterglow enhances sexual and relationship satisfaction.

University of Toronto researchers asked 335 adults (138 men, 197 women, age eighteen to sixty-four) how they felt about afterglow. They said small increases in postsexual cuddling produced substantial increases in sexual and relationship satisfaction.

The same team asked 101 couples to keep daily sex-and-relationship diaries for three months. When participants devoted extra time to postsex cuddling, they reported significantly greater satisfaction.

Afterglow was particularly important to women and parents of young children. Compared with most men, most women place more value on cuddling. Meanwhile, most parents of young children report a drop in both sexual frequency and nonsexual affection—and value them more, including afterglow.

Compared with women, men are more likely to fall asleep shortly after the mattress mambo. Many women complain about this, saying they feel robbed of postsexual cuddling they value.

Gentlemen, do your best to stay awake long enough to savor postplay cuddling. You'll probably feel better about your relationship—and chances are your sweetie will consider you a better partner and lover.

Secrets of Satisfying Quickies

Seven-course banquets can taste heavenly, but every now and then, fast food hits the spot. Sexuality authorities generally promote slow sex (this book included), but sometimes the clock is ticking, and some lovers enjoy rip-your-clothes-off quickies.

The upside of quickies—fast, furious, fun—is also their downside. Quickies don't allow much time to warm up to genital play.

Sexual function is rarely a problem for the vast majority of young men, who can raise erections at the drop of a zipper. But it's a different story for older men, whose erections rise more slowly, if at all. Hence, the adage: *What young men want to do all night takes older men all night to do.*

Sexual arousal is also problematic for many women of all ages. It takes a good deal of loveplay for many women to feel receptive to genital caresses. In addition, as women approach menopause, vaginal dryness may make quickies uncomfortable.

For most lovers of all ages, the intensity of orgasm often depends on the amount of time spent rolling in the hay. Don't expect your best orgasms from quickies.

On the other hand, if you like quickies, here's how to make the most of them:

- **Be as playful as time allows.** As you tear each other's clothes off, as much as possible, savor kissing, hugging, mutual massage, and whispered endearments. The more whole-body caressing, even in a short amount of time, the more satisfying your quickie is likely to be.
- **Heat up the anticipation.** Start warming up to romance before you rendezvous. If you travel to trysts, message beforehand about your eagerness to play. Or start with some phone sex.
- **Value the setting.** Lack of time is no reason to ditch an erotic ambiance. Arrange your quickies to include music, massage lotion, fragrance (perfume, flowers), and tasty treats.
- **Use lubricant.** Quickies don't allow many women sufficient time to produce natural vaginal lubrication. Saliva or commercial lubes help. Lubricants also increase the pleasure of genital touch and help many men's erections.

- **Keep a vibrator handy.** For many women and some men, a fast pace makes orgasm challenging. Vibrators and vibrating penis sleeves may enhance quickies.
- **Orchestrate surprises.** Novelty ignites erotic heat, especially during quickies.
- **Savor afterglow.** After your quickie, spend some time cuddling. If you must part quickly, savor afterglow by messaging.

CHAPTER 6:
Sexual Coaching Made Easy:
How to Ask for What You Want

I F I HAD a nickel for every time I've heard sex educators insist that the key to happy sexual relationships is "communication," I'd be rich. Yes, of course, communication is crucial. But as tongues start dancing, many people become tongue-tied. Compared with negotiating which movie to see, it's considerably more challenging to make sexual requests.

Part of the problem is the word *communication*. It implies proclamations. But speeches are rarely necessary. Effective erotic requests can usually be made using surprisingly few words.

Why speak up? Substantially better sex. University of Texas researchers analyzed forty-eight studies of 12,145 couples' sexual communication. As mutual coaching increased, both men and women reported enhanced desire and arousal. Women noticed more self-lubrication. Men enjoyed better erections. Women reported less pain during intercourse. And everyone was more likely to have orgasms and report sexual satisfaction.

No One Can Read Your Erotic Mind

Many people, especially teens and young adults, embrace the romantic notion that the moment lips lock, lovers become clairvoyant and intuitively understand what makes one another tick— and come. *If he really loved me, he'd know.*

That's naive. Mutual attraction never bestows the power to know your lover's mind. Unless you clearly state your likes and dislikes, your partner *can't* know what you find exciting—or repulsive.

Unfortunately, erotic mind-reading is a staple of popular media. On screens large and small, lovers rarely, if ever, discuss how they want to get it on. They jump into bed and every-thing proceeds perfectly. This is particularly true in porn, where no one ever negotiates any-thing. After perfunctory "hellos," the men unzip and the women fall to their knees. The same goes for romance fiction. The heroines bewitch their lotharios, who magically know precisely what drives their new ladies wild. With few exceptions, TV, movies, porn, and romance fiction all reinforce the absurd idea that love makes lovers psychic.

Of course, it's often difficult to say anything in the throes, let alone ask for adjustments. If you're critical, the other person might feel offended, or think you're carping or weird. As a result, many people who want erotic changes can't find the words. But clamming up robs you of pleasure while your partner remains in the dark about the caresses you actually enjoy—or don't care for.

Everyone is sexually unique. If you've had more than one lover, have any two made love identically? No one can read anyone's erotic mind. No one can possibly know what you like and dislike unless you reveal it. For sizzling sex, you *must* speak up. You're responsible for your own sexual pleasure and orgasms. No one else. You.

No One "Gives" Anyone Orgasms

Many people consider it their responsibility to "give" lovers fabulous orgasms. This wish is laudable, especially for men who hope to provide them to women. That's a big change from the nineteenth-century Victorian era when Western medical authorities proclaimed that women were incapable of sexual pleasure, so men had no responsibility to provide it. Men "took" sex from women, often considering their partners little more than passive receptacles for lust. Consequently, until well into the twentieth century, sex was usually something men enjoyed and many, if not most, women endured.

Today, we know that men and women are equally sexual and that satisfying lovemaking involves taking turns giving and receiving pleasure. Compared with Victorian ignorance, today's wish to "give" women thunderous climaxes represents progress. But no one gives anyone else orgasms. Each of us is responsible for our own erotic pleasure and satisfaction. When conditions are right, orgasms emerge from deep within us.

Orgasms are similar to laughter. Comedians can tickle our funny bones, but they don't "make" us laugh. They *help* us. They create the conditions that allow laughter. Like laughing, orgasms occur when our uniquely individual erotic needs have been met. For most people, those include trust, comfort, deep relaxation, possibly love, and extended loveplay.

During sizzling sex, lovers create the context that facilitates each other's orgasms. Each allows the other to dive into their pleasure and enjoy a happy ending. But we produce orgasms ourselves. That's why it's crucial to tell your lover what turns you on—and off.

Male Egos: Less Fragile Than Many Women Believe

Researchers at Western University in Pomona, California, convened ten focus groups—five male, five female—and asked how participants felt when women did not have orgasms. Everyone's top concern was the fear that the news would injure the men's delicate egos.

Gentleman, have you ever lost a foot race? Missed a basketball shot? Struck out in baseball? Of course you have. Did those disappointments obliterate your self-esteem? No, you kept trying, ideally with the help of coaches who identified your weaknesses and helped you improve.

The same is true in lovemaking. Ask for coaching. It's the *only* way to learn what pleases women and brings them to orgasm. If you want to help women to orgasms, you *must* appreciate the kinds of caresses that get each and every individual woman there. If they're afraid to tell you for fear of bruising your eggshell ego, you never learn what they need. Erotic ignorance is not bliss. You don't know it all. No matter if you're eighteen or eighty-eight, you have plenty to learn about every new partner—and quite possibly your longtime lover as well. Invite coaching. It's the only way to learn how to please.

And ladies, please don't just complain to girlfriends that your guy has a lot to learn. *Tell him.* If you don't, he *can't* know what you need. No matter what your age or the duration of your relationship, coaching your partner is the only way to receive the caresses you desire.

Men's egos are not as fragile as many women, especially young women, believe. Most men of all ages have a wealth of experience dealing with disappointment—everything from losing in sports to career setbacks to rejections from previous women. The overwhelming majority regroup and try again. Compared with the myriad ways men get shot down in life, sexual coaching is pretty benign. You're not rejecting him, just asking for a few adjustments. His ego will survive just fine. Eventually, he may even thank you for helping him become a better lover.

Start with Compliments

As we've seen, sizzling sex usually unfolds slowly. Slow sex facilitates erotic coaching. When lovemaking proceeds slowly, there's plenty of time to check in about what lights your fire—or extinguishes it. A leisurely pace also allows time to discuss contraception and sexual infection prevention. And it invites the erotic novelty that keeps whoopee fresh and exciting.

Of course, it's no fun feeling criticized, even gently. That goes double for doing the deed. Assuming you generally enjoy sex with your partner, before asking for changes, offer reassurance: *I love being with you.* Or *You're so desirable.* Or *I can't get enough of you.* Then say no more. That way your lover doesn't reflexively brace for a "but . . ." By offering unequivocal compliments, you gain valuable experience in sex talk. And kudos often lead to hotter humping.

Not that everyone should feel obligated to voice endearments in bed. Some people enjoy hearing them, others don't. But if the two of you typically say little or nothing, you might experiment with opening your mouths for more than kissing and oral sex. Everyone loves compliments, especially about how they make love.

"About Our Kissing . . ."

Of course, after compliments, there often lurks a "but . . ." That's fine. That's life. No one knows what you want unless you say so.

If you feel dissatisfied with any aspect of organ grinding, jot a list of everything you wish were different. Be specific. Not: *I wish she were sexier.* That's vague. Instead: *I wish I didn't have to place her hand on my penis. I wish she would take the initiative to fondle me.*

When your list is complete, rank your wishes in order from the easiest to discuss to the most challenging. Start with your easiest request, which often involves nongenital caresses, for example, kissing. Compared with genital touch, it's not as challenging to broach kissing. In addition, many people are particular about how they like to be kissed. A little discussion can quickly improve things. You might begin by asking, *About the way I kiss—do you like it? Would you prefer something a little different?* If your partner demurs, maybe you're the perfect kisser. Or you might probe a bit more. *How do you feel about how I use my tongue? I could lick your lips or not. Or stay shallow or slip it in deeper. What's your preference?* Negotiating nongenital moves provides great practice for discussing genital play.

Many people like to start kissing with mouths closed, reserving tongue play until things heat up. If a lover immediately slips you tongue and you don't feel ready, you might pull away momentarily and say, *I love our kissing, but can we keep our mouths closed a little longer, please?* Such discussions demonstrate that erotic coaching is no big deal, just a routine element of making love.

Distinguished Los Angeles sex educator Patti Britton, PhD, MPH, suggests two compliments for every critique in a "sandwich" format: start with praise. Proceed to your request. Then conclude with another compliment.

Recipients: Get What You Want—Using Just One Word

The word is *yes.*

If you feel reluctant or unable to coach using whole sentences, here's an effective one-word remedy. When you enjoy what's happening, say *yes.* When you don't, remain silent. That's it. Over a few months, that one word is quite likely to get you more of what you want and less of what you don't.

Many lovers try to communicate nonverbally with sighs and moans, but these signals may easily be misunderstood. If you moan in discomfort, your lover may misinterpret it as enjoyment. *Yes* is clearer, especially if you say it with feeling: *Oh, yes!* Lovers naturally provide more of whatever elicits a *yes* and less of what's greeted by silence.

Saying *yes* largely eliminates the need to utter words that cause difficulties: *No, don't*, or *Stop, you're hurting me!* It's easier—and better for relationships—to keep things positive. And once you start saying *yes*, your silence eloquently communicates that you're less than thrilled.

Yes can also help if you hope to receive caresses your lover is nowhere near providing. Say it when your partner does *anything close* to what you ultimately want. By reinforcing successive approximations of your goal caresses, your lover is likely to move toward what you want.

Of course, talking during sex might also cause conflict. One of you might prefer silence while the other enjoys a running commentary. One might prefer clinical terms—penis, vagina—while the other might prefer four-letter words. Discuss this. A good time is shortly after your orgasms as you both cuddle together during afterglow (see page 39).

If *yes* doesn't work for you, try *oooh* or *ahh*.

Initiators: Better Sex—Using Just Eight Words

The eight words are, *Is this okay? Would you prefer something else?* At every erotic escalation, initiators should ask these questions. They invite coaching. If the pace of loveplay is leisurely, they don't interrupt anything. And they recognize your partner's erotic uniqueness. Initiators might also follow up with, *Less intense? More?*

Don't wait for recipients to declare that some move is a turnoff. They might not feel sufficiently assertive or comfortable to tell you. At every step up the ladder, ask, *Is this okay? Would you prefer something else?*

Creative Afterglow

After mutual orgasms when you both feel satisfied and close, review what you enjoyed and ask for more. *When you were teasing my clit with your tongue, that was great. I'd love that every time.* Or *I love it when you go down on me, but my clit is so sensitive. Please lick around it, not right on it, until I'm close to coming, okay?*

Try to be positive about negatives. If a lover does anything you really can't stand, feel free to say so, but give it a loving spin. List a few moves you enjoy, then mention whatever you don't. *I really love the way you suck my cock, but when you suck on my balls, it's uncomfortable. Can we lose that?*

If Someone Takes "Forever" to Come

Some men and women take quite a while to work up to orgasm. Sometimes, it's situational. If you're drunk, in pain, under the weather, or suffering emotional stress, it may take longer than usual. But some people always take a long time. That's just who they are, and it's fine—unless it causes conflict. Coaching to the rescue.

If you're the one who takes "forever," here are some issues to discuss and adjustments to try:

- **Don't apologize. Analyze.** What do you think is going on? Apologizing acknowledges the issue but does nothing to resolve it. Examine your life and lovemaking. Look for reasons that might impede climaxing.
- **Ladies, did he gently caress your clit?** If not, chances are you won't come. A substantial research literature shows that at most only 25 percent of women are reliably orgasmic solely from intercourse. This is true no matter how deeply the people love each other and no matter the size of the man's penis or how long he lasts. To have orgasms, three-quarters of women *require* direct clitoral caresses by hand, mouth, or sex toy.
- **Limit depressants.** Alcohol is the big one. The amount required to suppress orgasm varies individually, but as drinking increases, likelihood of orgasm declines (pleasure,

too). Narcotics, antianxiety medication, and other drugs may also sabotage orgasm. Ask your physician or pharmacist if any drug(s) you take might contribute to orgasm difficulties. It's a long list.

- **Do you take an antidepressant?** The most popular class of antidepressants, the SSRIs (selective serotonin reuptake inhibitors), are notorious for causing sexual side effects, notably orgasm suppression. SSRIs include Prozac, Zoloft, Paxil, Celexa, Lexapro, Cipralex, Seroxat, Luvox, and Lustral. Ask your physician if you might switch to Wellbutrin (bupropion), an equally effective antidepressant with less risk of orgasm impairment.
- **Generalize your self-sexing.** The vast majority of people can masturbate to orgasm. Compare the stimulation you enjoy solo with what you receive during partner play. If they differ significantly, coach your lover to provide more of what you do for yourself.
- **Relax deeply.** Stress interferes with orgasm. Try hot baths or showers before sex. Embrace a regular stress management regimen: daily exercise, meditation, yoga, gardening, music, or anything else that leaves you feeling calm and refreshed.
- **During lovemaking, breathe deeply.** It's deeply relaxing. Emphasize slow, full exhalations.
- **Do it earlier.** With age, as the day progresses, orgasmic energy often ebbs. Many young lovers also enjoy daytime or early evening sex. Discuss playing earlier.
- **Got a vibrator?** These days, an estimated 10 percent of couples use vibrators in partner play. Most women with orgasm challenges can climax using them. Similar vibrating penis sleeves help many men. Discuss taking a vibe to bed with you. Ask your lover to hold you close as you vibrate yourself to orgasm, or teach your partner to use it on you.
- **Be supportive.** Reassure your lover that you're not watching the clock, that you enjoy pleasuring them, and are committed to their satisfaction, no matter how long it takes.

If it's your lover who takes "forever":

- **Implement all of the above.**
- **Encourage inward focus.** Some people lose their erotic focus imagining that their lovers must feel annoyed at how long they're taking. Provide reassurance that you're neither bored nor impatient. Encourage your partner to focus inward on experiencing pleasure—not on any fears of what you might be feeling.
- **Encourage hot fantasies.** Exciting erotic fantasies are key to many people's orgasms.
- If a woman takes a long time to climax, **try using a vibrator**. Be sure to ask for coaching beforehand. Pressing too hard may cause discomfort. It's usually best to hold the vibrator still and allow the woman to dance her vulva on it.
- If a man takes a long time, **see chapter 33.**

If these suggestions don't work, consider sex coaching or therapy.

Coaching Helps Relieve Women's Sexual Pain

Pain on intercourse (dyspareunia) afflicts 15 percent of American women. Coaching helps. In three trials, Canadian researchers surveyed 375 couples struggling with the women's sexual pain. Assertive coaching reduced the women's pain. However, women's sexual pain has many possible causes (chapter 39). If coaching doesn't help, consult a gynecologist or sexual medicine specialist.

CHAPTER 7:
The Magic of Lubricants:
Better Sex Quickly—Guaranteed

I T TAKES ONLY seconds to demonstrate that sexual lubricants enhance sex:

1. Close your mouth and dry your lips.
2. Run a finger lightly over them, focusing on how it feels.
3. Now, lick your lips.
4. Run a finger lightly over them.

If touching moist lips feels more sensual, lubricants can help you enjoy more pleasurable lovemaking—immediately.

Unfortunately, many sex resources underemphasize lube, mentioning it only in passing for older women suffering menopausal vaginal dryness (below). In addition, in porn, few people use anything other than saliva, so drugstore lubricants are off most men's radar. Actually, many women of all ages experience uncomfortable dryness.

Vaginal Dryness: Common in Women of All Ages

In porn stories, with any flirting, panties get soaked. *When he smiled, I got wet.* Actually, it's just as likely for women to feel aroused and *not* produce much lubrication.

During the 1960s, pioneering sex researchers William Masters, MD, and Virginia Johnson described vaginal lubrication as the first physiological sign of women's arousal. Usually, but not always. Many perfectly normal women of all ages are slow to produce natural lubrication. Even during extended loveplay, some don't produce much.

Vaginal dryness is more prevalent than many people believe. In surveys of several thousand women, University of Chicago researchers found that from age eighteen to fifty, around 20 percent of women—one in five—has trouble self-lubricating. With menopause, it's a problem for one-quarter of women in their fifties, one-third of women in their sixties, and more than 40 percent of women over seventy.

The Source of Vaginal Lubrication

Imagine pouring water on a dry sponge. It absorbs the fluid and expands until it's saturated. With additional water, the sponge drips. That's how vaginal lubrication works.

As women become aroused, the arteries in and around the vagina open (dilate) and extra blood flows into the clitoris, vaginal lips, and vaginal wall. In the clitoris, this blood causes erection. The little bump grows prominent. The vaginal lips part a bit, becoming more receptive to erections. The sponge-like vaginal wall soaks up a good deal of extra blood. Eventually, some of its fluid portion (plasma) gets pushed through the spaces between the cells, forming sweat-like beads on the inner vagina—vaginal lubrication.

Possible reasons for lubrication problems include:

- **Individual differences.** Some women just don't produce much.
- **Estrogen fluctuations.** In menstruating women, estrogen levels rise and fall cyclically, increasing lubrication during the fertile part of the month and decreasing it at other times. Breastfeeding, menopause, and conditions affecting the ovaries may also decrease lubrication.
- **Lack of desire or arousal.**
- **Lifestyle.** Smoking constricts the arteries, limiting blood flow into the vaginal wall. Dehydration reduces the amount of plasma available for lubrication. Alcohol is dehydrating. When women make love drunk, they may feel dry. Tampons may also contribute to dryness.
- **Medical conditions.** Diabetes, high blood pressure, pituitary problems, and other conditions may impair lubrication.
- **Medications.** Lubrication may decrease when taking drugs that cause dry mouth: antihistamines, decongestants, antidepressants, cannabis, and progesterone birth control pills.
- **Sex style.** Extended loveplay usually increases lubrication. Rushed intercourse may not allow time for it to appear.

Consequently, many women of all ages benefit from lube.

The Source of Pre-Ejaculatory Fluid

Like women, men also self-lubricate.

Semen is usually pearly white and viscous. But as men become sexually excited, the penis usually releases several drops of fluid that's watery, clear, colorless, and somewhat slippery—pre-ejaculatory fluid (pre-come). It's produced by the pea-size Cowper's gland, which sits below the prostate. Unfortunately, little research has focused on pre-ejaculatory fluid. To release enough to enhance intercourse, extend loveplay and avoid dehydration and medications that cause dry mouth (above).

Pre-ejaculatory fluid eases penile entry into the vagina. It also alters vaginal pH, which helps sperm survive as they swim toward eggs. But many perfectly normal men don't produce much. Lube to the rescue.

P.S. Pre-come may also contain sperm, one reason why contraceptive withdrawal (pulling out, coitus interruptus) is risky. If you use condoms for birth control, roll them on before pre-ejaculatory fluid appears.

More Popular Than Ever

Lubricants are nothing new. Since ancient times, saliva and vegetable oils have been used to prevent sexual discomfort.

During the 1940s, early sex researcher Alfred Kinsey interviewed thousands of Americans and found that more than half the women had used saliva and/or oils in solo or partner sex. But back then, discussions of lovemaking rarely mentioned lubricants.

During the 1980s, three things changed:

- AIDS arrived. Fear of AIDS drove millions of Americans to embrace condoms, which usually include a dusting of powdered silicone lubricant. Many new condom users liked the slickness and tried other lubes.
- Sex toys became popular. Sex toy marketers urge users to use lube in toy play.
- Surveys showed that vaginal dryness affected not only menopausal women, but at least one-quarter of all sexually active women.

These developments spurred lube sales. In 1991, lubricants grossed $23 million a year. By 2015, sales topped $200 million. Currently, an estimated fifty million Americans use lubricant regularly. Most consider it a quick, easy, inexpensive, erotic enhancement.

Wetter Is Better: Most Women Love Lube

Indiana University researchers asked 2,451 women, age eighteen to sixty-eight, if they agreed with these statements:

- Wet sex makes it easier to have orgasms—98 percent agreed.
- Lubricants make sex feel better—97 percent.
- Lubricants make sex feel more pleasurable—94 percent.
- My partner prefers lubricated sex—93 percent.
- I would feel offended if a lover suggested using lube—5 percent.
- If a woman needs lubricant, something is wrong with her—6 percent.
- Young women don't need lubricant—8 percent.
- Lubricants are mainly for menopausal women—10 percent.

How Lube Helps Men

Lubricants enhance the pleasure of self-sexing. They also reduce chafing of the penile shaft.

Want to earn points with the gal in your bed? Buy a selection of lubes and invite experimentation.

Many women complain that their lovers rush into intercourse before they feel receptive. Taking time to apply lubricant slows the pace a bit, giving women more time to warm up. And lubed erections slide more easily into lubricated vaginas, adding comfort and joy to intercourse.

Lubricant and Condoms

If you believe condoms dull sensitivity, lube restores it. Before donning condoms, place a drop on the head of your penis. Then roll it on and enjoy. But if you do this, someone should hold onto the base of the condom during intercourse and withdrawal. Lube under condoms increases risk of slip-offs.

Many popular songs tout sex that lasts "all night long." But extended intercourse may deplete women's natural lubrication and cause irritation. Sizzling sex may not last all night, but it goes on for a good while. Lube enhances extended play. Periodically add more or refresh it with a little water or saliva.

Older men face two sexual challenges: erection and arousal. Most focus on the former, but arousal difficulties are often equally problematic. Lube heightens pleasure and spurs arousal.

Four Kinds

In the finger-on-lips exercise, the lubricant was saliva, the world's most popular lube. It's effective and always available for free. But saliva is more watery than slippery, and it dries quickly. Many lovers prefer slipperier commercial lubricants that stay slick longer.

Don't squirt lubricant directly on lovers' genitals. It may feel cold and jarring. Apply a small amount to your hand, rub it with your fingers to warm it, then caress your lover with lubricated fingers.

Four types are available over the counter at pharmacies and some supermarkets. Each has advantages and disadvantages:

- **Water-based.** The vast majority of commercial lubricants. They're widely available, inexpensive, safe to use with latex contraceptives, don't stain bed linen, and are safe to ingest in small amounts during oral sex. But during extended lovemaking, they often dry out. Apply more or refresh them with water or saliva. They rinse off easily with water.

  Water-based lubricants come in liquids or gels. Liquids may feel runny. Gels may feel goopy. Experiment to see which you and your lover prefer.
- **Oil-based.** Your kitchen probably contains vegetable oils and Crisco. The former can be used on the vulva, clitoris, and penis during masturbation. But don't introduce vegetable oils into the vagina. They may upset the organ's delicate balance of microflora. The same goes for Crisco, which should be reserved for anal play. In addition, oil-based lubricants should not be used with latex contraceptives. They may damage condoms, diaphragms, and cervical caps. Oils may also feel greasy and might stain bed linens and clothing. They require soap and water to remove.
- **Petroleum-based.** These include Vaseline and baby oil. They work but can be problematic. They destroy latex and should *never* be used with condoms, diaphragms, or cervical caps. Don't use petroleum lubricants inside the vagina. They're difficult to wash out, may cause irritation, and change vaginal chemistry, increasing risk of infection. They should not be ingested and may stain bed linens.
- **Silicone-based.** A personal adaptation of WD-40, silicone lubricants dust many brands of condoms. They feel silky and remain slick longer than water-based lubes. They don't damage latex and are safe for use on and inside the genitals and anus. They do not stain bed linen or clothing. But they are incompatible with silicone sex toys. It's not clear how safe they are to ingest, so it's prudent not to. And not all pharmacies stock them.

If Women Get "Too Wet"

Some women self-lubricate so copiously that they have trouble feeling erections inside them. Erections may slip out. And someone might have to sleep on a wet spot.

For problems feeling erections inside vaginas, try intercourse in the man-on-top (missionary) position. When he inserts, she closes her legs, so he lies atop her thighs. With her thighs pressed together, she's better able to feel his erection, and he gets more friction.

If wet spots are an issue, make love with a towel beneath you.

CHAPTER 8:
Secrets of Sizzling Oral Sex

MANY PEOPLE RANK oral sex, fellatio and cunnilingus, among their top erotic pleasures. And not just receiving. Many people also love providing them.

Oral sex is key to many men's sexual fantasies and satisfaction. The best window into men's fantasies is porn, and almost all porn depicts fellatio.

Meanwhile, cunnilingus is crucial to many women's orgasms. At most, only 25 percent of women are reliably orgasmic from vaginal intercourse alone. Intercourse provides only indirect stimulation to women's orgasm trigger, the external clitoris, which sits outside the vagina, an inch or two above it beneath the top junction of the vaginal lips. To experience orgasms, 75 percent of women need direct clitoral caresses—hand massage, oral, or vibrators—and many women prefer cunnilingus.

Unfortunately, many men do not routinely provide genital kisses. Gentlemen, if you want your partner to feel sexually satisfied and sing your praises, what hangs between your legs is usually *less* important than how creatively you use your tongue.

What's Better? Intercourse? Or Oral?

It's a matter of personal preference. Intercourse is only "better" if you want to conceive. But procreation is rarely the goal of lovemaking. And intercourse can be problematic for older adults, those with disabilities, women with pain on intercourse, and those with no access to contraceptives. There's no "best" way to make love. Enjoy whatever pleases you both.

A Brief History of Head

The evolutionary imperative, reproduction, propels us into intercourse. Oral sex provides no survival advantage and might even be detrimental. It reduces baby-making intercourse. So why did it develop? No one knows, but it's not uniquely human. Lions, bears, and our closest evolutionary relatives, bonobos, have been observed going down on their mates.

Oral sex is as old as history:

- Ancient Chinese texts tout fellatio and cunnilingus.
- At Pompeii, destroyed by volcanic ash in AD 79, excavations have unearthed frescos that clearly depict fellatio and cunnilingus.
- The *Kama Sutra*, India's fourth-century sexual treatise, urges women to "suck the mango," and notes that some men enjoy returning the favor.
- The seventh-century Moche people of Peru left ceramics that depict fellatio.

- Medieval European church documents specify punishment for "abominable sex," including oral-genital contact.
- Studies of historical slang show that before the Civil War, Americans were very familiar with oral. They usually called it *cock sucking* and *cunt licking*.
- The first porn movies appeared around 1897. Much of it depicted oral sex. Ever since, fellatio has been nearly ubiquitous in porn, with cunnilingus fairly common.
- During the late 1940s, Alfred Kinsey was the first researcher to survey the popularity of oral sex. His team found that 70 percent of those they interviewed admitted giving or receiving head.
- Starting in 1975, videocassette players moved porn from seedy theaters into living rooms. The new, larger porn audience saw a great deal of fellatio and some cunnilingus. Many viewers decided that oral is routine and universal. Actually, it isn't.

How Popular Is Oral Sex?

Indiana University researchers asked a representative sample of 5,865 Americans age fourteen to ninety-four about their experiences with oral sex. Several findings leap out:

- For some, oral experimentation begins during the teen years. Around 10 percent of boys and girls age fourteen to fifteen have provided and received it.
- By age twenty-five, almost 90 percent of men and women have experienced fellatio and cunnilingus at least once.
- Oral sex remains fairly prevalent throughout the lifespan. But it's far from universal. During the previous month, averaging all age groups, only 27 percent of respondents said they'd participated in fellatio, 22 percent in cunnilingus.
- In almost every age group, men say they've received more oral than they've provided and women say they've provided more than they've received. This is a major reason why women's rate of orgasm is lower than men's.

Meanwhile, like self-sexing, many surveys have linked education and socioeconomic status with oral sex. As they increase, so does comfort with admitting oral. And compared with fundamentalists of any religion, religious liberals are more likely to say they engage in it.

In lovemaking, no one should ever feel obligated or pressured to do anything that makes them uncomfortable. But some people avoid oral, not because they object to it, but because they fear their technique may . . . suck.

A Man's Guide to Sizzling Cunnilingus

Most men call it *eating pussy*, but clinically it's "cunnilingus," from the Latin *cunnus* for vulva, and *lingere*, to lick. Some women don't care for cunnilingus—ask. But most enjoy it. For some, it's their favorite part of lovemaking.

Licking a vulva is similar to kissing women's top lips: the basics are pretty simple, but infinite creative variations keep it fresh, passionate, and fun. The myth is that men don't enjoy going down on women. In fact, many men love camping at the Y. Tongues are much softer than fingers and provide the gentlest clitoral and vulvar caresses. Many women say they enjoy gentle cunnilingus as much as intercourse—or more. And cunnilingus is much more likely than intercourse to bring women to orgasm, so men who go down frequently are likely to get kudos as lovers.

If men feel turned off by cunnilingus, they're under no obligation to provide it. No one should ever feel pressured to be sexual in ways they find objectionable. On the other hand, most women consider cunnilingus a precious erotic gift, and may feel deeply disappointed with men who decline to provide it.

Women's external genitals include the fleshy outer vaginal lips, the thinner inner lips, the visible clitoris nestled under the clitoral hood at the upper junction of the vaginal lips, the vaginal opening, and the erotically sensitive area between the clitoris and vagina. Basic cunnilingus involves licking the vulva from the vaginal opening to the clitoris. As women become sexually aroused, their outer vaginal lips fill with extra blood, which parts them somewhat, exposing the inner lips and the sensitive tissue between them.

Gentlemen, in new relationships, ask your partners about going down on them. Either say, *I'd like to. Is that okay?* Or kiss her as you slowly head south—her neck, breasts, belly, thighs—so she's clear where you're headed. Ask for coaching.

Cunnilingus may place men, particularly older men, in contorted positions. Lying prone between women's legs might strain necks or backs. Possible fixes: Slip a pillow under her hips to raise her vulva. Ask her to lie with her butt near the side of the bed and kneel on the floor. Or lie on your back and ask her to sit on your face.

Women's anticipation of cunnilingus can add to their arousal. Start by gently nuzzling, kissing, and licking her inner thighs and the area around her vulva. As you spiral toward her genitals, begin by licking her outer lips. Run your tongue up and down them. Work your tongue in between the outer lips to caress the inner lips. Then circle the vaginal opening and perhaps insert your tongue—and/or a finger or two—into her vagina. Eventually, focus tongue play around and on her clit.

Unless women request otherwise, lick *gently*. In porn, the men go at vulvas like parched dogs presented with bowls of water. Consequently, some men infer that intense, machine-gun tongue play is the way to go. Check in. *Is this okay?* Ask if she prefers more or less intensity. At first, many women prefer light oral caresses, then incrementally greater intensity as they approach orgasm. Inquire often until you're confident you understand her preferences. Over time, her preferences may change. Continue asking.

Some women enjoy a tongue directly on the little nub. Others find that too intense, even uncomfortable, and prefer being licked around it. And some enjoy having their visible clitorises sucked.

Some women feel reluctant to discuss their reactions to oral sex. Instead they use body language, squirming if they find certain licks uncomfortable. Unfortunately, men may misinterpret this, thinking that writhing in discomfort is actually delight. That's why it's crucial to ask: *Is this okay? Would you like more intensity? Or less?*

Finally, if women receiving cunnilingus take more than a few minutes to come, some decide that their men must be getting bored, weary, and resentful. Such doubts interfere with women's erotic focus and orgasms. If she takes a while to come, reassure her it's fine, that you enjoy muff diving and are happy to continue until she works up to climax.

The Fine Points

Gentlemen, ask if your partners enjoy these variations:

- As you lick around her vulva, alternate using the tip of your tongue, the flat of it, and your lips. Each provides subtly different sensations.
- Combine licking with gentle hand massage. After circling her vulva with your tongue, do the same with a finger or two, using light, moderate, or deep pressure as the woman prefers. Massage her inner thighs and use your fingers to gently part her vaginal lips.

- While focused on her vulva, massage her elsewhere. Some women enjoy having their breasts caressed. Others like nipple play—be sure to ask for coaching. Try slipping a finger or two into her mouth so she can suck them while you're licking her. Or combine oral sex with any sex toy(s) she enjoys.
- While licking the vulva, slip your tongue or a finger or two gently inside her vagina.
- When women feel highly aroused, try what's known as the "little lick trick." Instead of steady tongue pressure on the clitoris or swirling moves around it, use the tip of your tongue to tease the underside of the clit with light little licks every few seconds. This helps some women climax.
- Beyond technique, something else affects many women's enjoyment of cunnilingus— their lover's enthusiasm about providing it. If you enjoy giving head, say so and show it.
- Some women produce fluid on orgasm—female ejaculation. If so, they may feel concerned about "squirting" into men's mouths. Discuss your feelings about this. There's no right or wrong, just personal preferences. Many men enjoy being very close to the vulva as women ejaculate, and have no problem ingesting some liquid. It's not urine. It's chemically closer to semen, though it may contain traces of urine. It's not harmful.
- After orgasm, many women experience unusual clitoral sensitivity and can't tolerate additional touching or licking. This is normal. If you like "last licks" after she comes, check in about her postorgasm sensitivity. Or come up from between her legs and hold, kiss, and caress her any way she enjoys.
- Assuming you're both okay with it, cunnilingus during menstrual periods is fine. Menstruation may change women's aroma and taste. Discuss this. Some women insert tampons or diaphragms to catch the flow. If either lover feels turned off, the couple can refrain for a few days.
- Menopausal changes may also affect vaginal fragrance and taste. As vaginal lubrication subsides, normal vaginal microorganisms may not be flushed out as efficiently. Usually, soap, water, and lubricants eliminate any problem.

The Hazards of Douching

American women spend more than $150 million a year on douches. Trouble is, they're much less likely to prevent foul odors than to *cause* them.

Douches and other so-called feminine hygiene products change vaginal ecology and significantly increase risk of several malodorous infections, among them chlamydia, trichomoniasis, *Gardnerella*, bacterial vaginosis, and pelvic inflammatory disease. Douching also reduces women's fertility and increases risk of cervical cancer and ectopic (tubal) pregnancy.

For decades, women's health authorities have beseeched women not to douche, explaining that the vagina is self-cleansing, and that soap and water are all that's required for "freshness." Many women have listened. In 1988, 37 percent of reproductive-age American women douched regularly. Today, the figure is less than 12 percent (African Americans: 28 percent, Hispanics: 15 percent, whites: 9 percent).

Ladies, the vast majority of men feel fine about how your vagina smells and tastes.

Women's Greatest Sexual Insecurity

Data analyst Seth Stephens-Davidowitz uses web searches to investigate America's deepest anxieties. He analyzed one month of Google searches dealing with sex and discovered that women search "vagina" almost as often as men search "penis." Their top concern—odor. Women worry that their crotches smell like (in descending order) fish, vinegar, onions, ammonia, garlic, cheese, body odor, urine, bleach, feces, dirty feet, garbage, and rotten meat. Anxiety about this sends millions of women to pharmacies for douches.

Gentlemen, *never* joke about vaginal aroma. It takes only one quip about *smelly pussy* to make some women recoil from cunnilingus and possibly from you. Nasty comments may also reverberate in women's minds for years, making them self-conscious about sex, and preventing them from relaxing during lovemaking. If you enjoy providing oral, say so frequently. *I love eating you. I love how you smell and taste.*

Anal Fingering? Rimming?

Some couples combine cunnilingus with gentle anal sphincter massage, fingering, or oral-anal play (anilingus).

Before fingering, familiarize yourself with anal anatomy. There are two sphincters, one visible, the other an inch or so inside. The inner sphincter is more difficult to relax. Many lovers limit fingering to the depth of a fingernail, which avoids the often problematic inner sphincter. For anal massage or fingering, both the anus and finger should be well lubricated.

Some lovers enjoy oral-anal play (ass licking, rimming, anilingus). As long as the receiving anus has been washed beforehand with soap and water, there's nothing dirty or hazardous about licking it. For more on anal play, see chapter 42.

The Best Book on Cunnilingus

If you'd like to delve deeper into cunnilingus, the best book is *She Comes First: The Thinking Man's Guide to Pleasing Women* by sexologist Ian Kerner, PhD.

A Woman's Guide to Sizzling Fellatio

Many call it *cock sucking* or *sucking dick*, but the clinical term is *fellatio*, from the Latin *fellare*, to suck. Fellatio is an opportunity for men to lie back and just receive pleasure. Fellatio is wet, which increases penile sensitivity. And most women can be more creative with their lips and tongues than with their vaginas.

Many women enjoy sucking, but few relish what's frequently seen in porn—women's heads held firmly while men push erections down their throats (below). That makes most women gag and feel used. But with the man standing, seated, or on his back and the woman free to move, she can be playful and creative. Many women enjoy that—as well as seeing how much their lovers enjoy being sucked.

Many men feel self-conscious about their penises. The overwhelming majority are normal size, but most men believe they're too small. In addition, some men are born with penile birth defects, and might feel reluctant to have a lover's eyes close enough to notice. The two most prevalent are hypospadias (one in 200) and epispadias (one in 120,000). In hypospadias, the urethral opening is located not dead center at the tip of the head, but rather toward its underside. In epispadias, the opening is off-center on the upper side. Both are usually minor and left untreated. If major, surgical repair is usually possible. But hypospadias and epispadias make some men self-conscious about fellatio.

Some women worry that when giving head, men might accidentally urinate into their mouths. This is virtually impossible. A valve in the penis blocks one fluid—urine or semen—when the other flows. When men are erect, they can't urinate.

If women feel put off by fellatio, respect their feelings. But simple steps may allay their concerns.

One of the biggest turn-offs is poor hygiene. Men should wash their genitals with soap and water whenever they shower—and shortly before sex. Uncircumcised men should retract their foreskins and wash beneath them. Otherwise, dirt and bacteria build up that may make the penis look, smell, and taste foul—with increased risk of transmitting sexual infections.

Fellatio is as simple as eating a banana—without using your teeth. Start by kissing or licking the head. Next, lightly part your lips and lick around the head, the corona (the little ridge around the base of the head), and the frenulum (the part of the corona on the underside of the head). Then take the head into your mouth, using your lips and tongue to caress it. Eventually, move your head up and down so that your lips caress as much of the shaft as you can comfortably accommodate. Note: The shaft is less sensitive than the head, corona, and frenulum, so return frequently to these special places—unless men ask for something different.

The Fine Points

Ladies, consider these variations:

- Alternate sucking with licking the head and shaft.
- Flick your tongue rapidly around the head.
- Lick or nibble the scrotum.
- Stroke the shaft with one or both hands while sucking or licking the head.
- While sucking, cup and/or fondle the scrotum.
- Alternate sucking with gently squeezing the head or shaft between your thumb and index finger.
- Gently slap his erection against your lips or tongue.
- Try the "little lick trick." Lightly lick the underside of the head of the penis once every few seconds.
- While sucking, massage him elsewhere. Ask how he feels about anal massage.
- If you enjoy providing fellatio, say so. Most men get turned on knowing that their lovers like sucking them.
- Teeth? Most men prefer lips and tongue only. However, the erect penis is a tough little guy. Light nibbling with teeth is unlikely to cause injury, and some men enjoy this. Ask. If you use your teeth, request coaching: *Is this okay?*

Gentlemen, feel free to coach women's oral explorations to heighten your arousal. But unless you're into BDSM, gentle requests usually work better than terse commands. Remember, she's giving you a gift.

Deep Throat and Gagging

The 1972 porn movie *Deep Throat* invented a character whose clitoris was supposedly located at her vocal cords. To have orgasms, she had to take erections deep down by her throat. *Deep Throat* became the first—and only—porn film to play to mainstream audiences. Produced for less than $50,000, it grossed $100 million. Ever since, some men have wanted to push their erections down their lovers' throats, and many women have tried it. The problem is that deep throating—and for some women shallow fellatio—causes gagging.

Gagging is a defensive reflex that prevents choking. And some women have "short palates." They gag easily, which can make them reluctant to provide oral. To minimize gagging:

- Women should control fellatio. Gagging is partly triggered by anxiety. When men hold partners' heads and push erections down their throats, women are more likely to become stressed and gag. If men want deep throating, they should stay still and allow their lovers to control the speed and depth of insertion. When women feel in control, they're less likely to gag and better able to accept erections deeper.
- With self-training, some women can partly desensitize their gag reflexes. Start while brushing your teeth. Dentists recommend brushing the back of the tongue to prevent bad breath. Play with this. Breathe deeply and visualize yourself not gagging. Discover the point at which you gag. With practice, you may gag less.
- Another option is mock-deep-throating. Rub your hands together vigorously to warm them. Apply some lubricant. Suck him as deeply as you're comfortably able, then use your warm, lubricated hands to stroke the rest of his shaft. This approximates being deep-throated. Many men can't tell the difference.

Coming in Her Mouth? Swallowing?

Some women can't stand either. Others are happy to accept semen in their mouths but would rather not swallow. And some have no problem swallowing. Issues include:

- Some women fear injury from the force of ejaculation. Actually, it's not forceful. It feels more like biting down on a cherry tomato.
- Others fear gagging on huge mouthfuls of semen. Actually, typical volume is only around a tablespoon in young men and a teaspoon in older men.
- Some don't care for the taste of semen (below).
- Others fear contracting sexual infections. Gonorrhea of the throat is possible, but other infections are unlikely to spread orally. If you're concerned about sexual infections, get tested.
- Some women object to swallowing semen, preferring to spit it out. Gentlemen, try not to read ominous meanings into this. It's simply a personal preference and no reflection on her feelings for you. Respect women's sexual boundaries.

If women would rather not accept semen into their mouths, men can wear condoms during fellatio. That way they ejaculate *inside* women's mouths, but not *into* them.

In porn, few women swallow. They make a show of letting semen dribble out of their mouths and massaging it into their faces or breasts. Some men consider this a turn-on.

Semen is more than 95 percent water. It contains nothing hazardous—and it's not fattening, at only around twenty calories per ejaculation.

Here's a work-around for women who are willing to swallow but don't care for the taste of semen: suck on a Life Saver while sucking your man. The candy sweetens the taste. Internet discussions recommend peppermint and wintergreen.

Finally, surgery to treat advanced prostate enlargement eliminates natural ejaculation and offers some couples a possibly welcome benefit. No man should have surgery simply to prevent ejaculating into women's mouths, but if it is a big issue for a particular couple, urologists treat this condition surgically, which leaves most men with "retrograde ejaculation." Their semen gets redirected into the bladder and exits the body mixed with urine. The men still have orgasms, but no longer ejaculate out the penis, which eliminates any conflict about coming in women's mouths.

How to Improve the Taste of Semen

I've found no compelling research on this, but no shortage of opinions. Urologists generally say the taste can't be changed, that semen includes a fixed combination of constituents necessary to support sperm and if its composition is predetermined, its taste must be, too.

However, many women and gay men insist that diet and lifestyle affect the taste. One is former porn star Annie Sprinkle, who claims to have tasted the semen of one thousand men. She says vegetarians taste best; that drinking fruit juices improves the taste; and that smoking, alcohol, meats, and asparagus foul the taste.

Semen is mostly water, but it also contains:

- Sperm—about 2 percent by volume
- Fructose, fruit sugar, which nourishes sperm
- Vitamin C, which helps maintain sperm cells
- Sodium bicarbonate, an alkaline compound that helps protect sperm from the acidity of the vagina and uterus
- Minerals: magnesium, phosphorus, potassium, and zinc
- Proteins: amino acids and enzymes

In internet discussions, most women agree that fruit and fruit juices, especially apple and pineapple, sweeten semen, and that taste-spoiling foods include meats, alcohol, broccoli, cauliflower, Brussels sprouts, dairy, deep-fried foods, coffee, and asparagus, plus one nonfood item, cigarettes.

If men would rather not change their diets, or if diet changes don't work, women performing fellatio can try sucking on Life Savers at the same time to mask the taste of semen.

If disagreements about any aspect of oral sex drive you crazy, consider sex coaching or therapy.

Can't Come in Her Mouth?

Some men who are orgasmic during masturbation and intercourse have problems climaxing in women's mouths. Usually, the reason is that oral caresses don't provide enough of the stimulation they need to trigger orgasm. Show her how you stroke yourself. She can do that while sucking the head. It often helps.

CHAPTER 9:
Novelty: Sizzling Sex Feels New and Different

THE *NEW YORK Times* asked 2,903 subscribers: *If your entire sexual history were made public, would people find it shocking or boring?* Two-thirds said boring. Sexual boredom is quite common, especially in long-term relationships. It detracts from sizzling sex.

Most couples notice that compared with sex at home, doing it while traveling feels hotter. Travel brings new and different experiences—and novelty is a potent, reliable turn-on.

President Calvin Coolidge and his wife took separate tours of a chicken farm. The First Lady watched as a single rooster had sex many times. She asked the farmer to tell her husband. When the farmer did, the president asked if the rooster mated with the same hen every time. The farmer said no, new hens every time. Coolidge asked the farmer to tell his wife.

Desire and Arousal Issues: Surprisingly Prevalent

If the evolutionary purpose of life is to reproduce, everyone of reproductive age should feel horny much of the time, and everyone older should have no libido. But the interplay of evolution and culture can be confounding. Many reproductive-age folks feel little or no interest in sex, while many older adults retain strong desires. University of Chicago researchers asked 6,437 Americans age eighteen to eighty-five if they lacked interest in sex.

- Among men, from age eighteen to sixty, around 15 percent reported little or no libido; for men over sixty, around 25 percent.
- Among women up to age sixty, around one-third reported low libido; for older women, up to half.
- In every age group, compared with men, twice as many women reported little or no libido.

Many people with low libido make love anyway because they think they "should," or to appease their partners, but their hearts aren't into it. Sexual novelty can change that. Introducing anything new into the horizontal dance piques libido and arousal, and boosts pleasure and satisfaction.

Novelty, Dopamine, and Erotic Heat

You meet. You click. And suddenly, you're head over heels in love. You can't keep your hands off each other. The sex is fabulous. But not for long. After a year or so, most couples wonder, *What happened?*

If the relationship endures, time deepens mutual attachment—but almost always cools erotic heat. You feel as Abigail Adams did in 1793 when she wrote her husband, President

John Adams, "Years subdue the ardor of passion. But affection deep rooted persists." Yes, you still love, but no longer madly. The fireworks fizzle. The Fourth of July becomes Thanksgiving.

Almost everyone experiences this. You tell yourself, *That's what happens. Accept it.* But anthropologist Helen Fisher, PhD, couldn't accept it. She wondered why people fall so madly in love and why lust and sexual passion subside. On a message board at the State University of New York, Stony Brook, she posted, *Have you recently fallen madly in love?* Dozens of students replied. Fisher used MRIs to track their brain activity. She showed them two photographs—a face they didn't recognize and their new beloved. When looking at the former, their brains remained quiet. But pictures of their sweethearts made the MRIs light up like Christmas trees—and their brain levels of dopamine soared.

Dopamine is a neurotransmitter that enables communication among brain cells. When dopamine spikes, people become energized, exhilarated, and obsessed. Their hearts pound. They lose their appetites and have difficulty sleeping—all signs of falling in love.

Dopamine also governs cravings and dependency, two hallmarks of drug addiction. All addictions raise brain levels of dopamine. Those madly in love often compare it to intoxication. Falling in love has also been compared with addiction. It involves drug-like euphoria and dependency when new lovers are together, intense cravings when they're apart, and debilitating withdrawal reactions if they break up.

In addition, as dopamine rises, so does the testosterone family of hormones that fuels libido in all genders. Horniness is another feature of falling in love.

Finally, high dopamine suppresses another neurotransmitter, serotonin. Low serotonin is associated with obsession, another element of falling in love. Love obsession takes many forms. New lovers often daydream about their beloveds and communicate so frequently that they seem to have obsessive-compulsive disorder (OCD). Italian researchers tested serotonin in three groups: controls, some madly in love, and others with OCD. The controls showed normal serotonin levels, but levels were significantly lower in both the OCD and new-love groups. "Poets often call love madness or insanity," Fisher says. "In the brain, it really is."

Fisher asked her love-crazed volunteers to return for repeat MRIs. Their beloveds' faces continued to trigger sharp spikes in dopamine—but only for an average of seven months. Other researchers have found that what's often called the hot-and-heavy period lasts from six months to a year, two at most. Subsequently, dopamine returns to normal. New lovers may feel crazy in love, but it's temporary insanity.

If the relationship endures, it evolves into "married love," warm—but rarely hot—attachment that combines affection, security, trust, and contentment. Attachment also has a biochemical basis, the hormones oxytocin and vasopressin. Both are produced in two locations: the sex organs and the hypothalamus, headquarters of emotion in the brain. Levels of these hormones rise after orgasm. "They're 'cuddle compounds,'" Fisher explains. "They contribute to the closeness and connection lovers experience after sex."

From Embers to Flames

Many couples would like to pour kerosene on the embers of married love. Fisher's research points the way—boost dopamine. How? Novelty—doing new things or familiar things in new ways.

Psychologists surveyed long-term couples about relationship happiness. Then half the couples completed a dull task, while the others engaged in a new, exhilarating activity. Afterward, everyone retook the survey. Those who participated in the exciting, dopamine-raising activity said they felt more deeply in love and happier with their relationships.

These findings reinforce couple therapists' recommendations for keeping relationships fresh and exciting:

- **Have more fun together.** It's no coincidence we call weekend trips "romantic get-aways" or that sex often feels more passionate away from home. You're together enjoying yourselves in different settings. That's exciting, romantic, and arousing.
- **Laugh.** Humor is funny because the punch line is unexpected. Like other novel activities, laughter raises dopamine. In relationships that endure, spouses enjoy each other's senses of humor. When humor dies, relationships are often in trouble.
- **Keep 'em guessing.** Oscar Wilde said, "The essence of romance is uncertainty." An age-old strategy for winning new love is to play hard to get, which spurs anticipation but delays reward. Guess what surprise, uncertainty, and delayed gratification trigger in the brain? Release of dopamine.
- **Make love.** Sex boosts testosterone, which raises dopamine. To make sex hotter, include something new: a different time or place, new moves, new lingerie, a new sex toy—anything.

Did We Evolve to Cheat and Divorce?

In fairy tales, the prince and princess marry and live happily ever after. In real life, things are messier. Many marriages end in divorce. Clearly, neither love nor attachment is necessarily permanent.

Few mammalian species mate for life. They're much more likely to practice serial monogamy, one partner for a while then another. Most animals pair up only long enough to rear young. Then lust for novelty sends them to new mates.

People talk about a "seven-year itch," but when Fisher analyzed divorce data from fifty-eight cultures worldwide, she noticed that an unusually large proportion of breakups occur after about four years. That's how long most relationships last among the world's few remaining stone-age cultures. Fisher speculates that breakups after four years may echo an ancestral human pattern, coupling up only long enough to rear children through the period when they're neediest and most dependent.

With all due respect to happily ever after and the seventh commandment—*Thou shalt not commit adultery*—novelty cravings often lead to sex outside relationships. What proportion of supposedly committed lovers step out? That's controversial.

In face-to-face interviews, 15–25 percent of married folks admit affairs, though many don't confess to cheating. Studies with greater social distance, telephone and online surveys, show much more infidelity—around 55 percent of men and 45 percent of women. Several researchers estimate that up to 70 percent of spouses have cheated. Sometimes, clandestine affairs produce children. In a 1998 program that screened for genetic diseases, scientists were shocked to discover that 10 percent of the children tested were not the offspring of their legal fathers.

However, chemistry is not destiny. Many people remain monogamous for decades—but it's often a struggle. If you value monogamy, inject regular novelty into your relationship.

"You Want to Try *What?!*"

Desire for novelty impels many lovers to ask for new erotic moves: lingerie, vibrators, kink, whatever. Asking for changes in any aspect of a relationship involves risk. But when requests are sexual, the risks may feel paralyzing. How can you get what you want? It might be easier than you think.

Erotic freshness is a subset of novelty in general. As people become more willing to try new things out of bed, they often become more open to sexual experimentation as well. If you feel sexually bored, start promoting erotic novelty with new fun that's *nonsexual*—a new restaurant, a trail you haven't hiked, a trip to a first-time destination.

Keep things playful. Maintain your sense of humor. Novelty involves experimentation and many experiments fail. That's life. So what if that new bistro stinks? What's important is your willingness to share new experiences together.

When trying to persuade a lover to experiment with novelty, think small. Modest changes may be significant. Be patient. Look for reasons to laugh.

If your partner is a real stick-in-the-mud, that's frustrating, but ironically, you may be able to use it to your advantage. Many fuddy-duddies don't abhor change as much as they derive deep comfort from the familiar. But old habits feel cozier when you return to them from something else. To truly appreciate the tried and true, sample something exotic. One pleasure of vacations is returning home to familiar surroundings and your own bed. But to enjoy returning home, you have to get away. Try gently pointing out that novelty is the gateway to appreciating the familiar.

Surprise Dates, Birthdays, Anniversaries, Valentine's Day

Romance experts Barbara and Michael Jonas, coauthors of *The Book of Love, Laughter, and Romance*, urge couples to make regular "surprise dates." One plans an outing, but keeps it secret, telling the other only what to wear and what time to meet. Planners pledge not to arrange anything that might unnerve their partners. Followers agree to play along, even if surprise dates push their comfort zones.

Even without novelty that's overtly sexual, surprise dates carry an erotic charge. You're together anticipating something new and different. And demonstrating mutual trust. And you both know that next time, the tables turn.

During your first few surprise dates, don't introduce anything sexual. Give your lover time to warm up to the notion of regular novelty—and to trusting you not to overdo any surprises. When you introduce sexual novelty, don't venture very far out of the ordinary.

Say you're the planner and you take your reluctant-to-experiment partner to an old familiar bar, then on to an old favorite restaurant, and from there to a stroll along an old familiar route. By the time you've walked fifty yards, your spouse is bound to ask: *What's the surprise?* Your reply: *Wait till we get home.*

Once you've introduced the idea of ongoing experimentation, birthdays, anniversaries, Valentine's Day, and other special occasions offer opportunities. Again, don't expect great leaps beyond your lover's comfort level. But compared with the rest of the year, it's often easier to ask for experimentation on special days—and partners are more likely to grant such requests, especially in a new context, for example, a hotel room.

If you don't routinely use lubricant, for most lovers, lube enhances sex immediately. Your novelty-shy sweetie is likely to enjoy instant sexual benefits from lubricants—and possibly, down the road, welcome other erotic initiatives.

Half a Loaf Is Better Than None

Warming up to new moves often takes time. Give your lover the gift of that time. This is especially true when a lover says, *We're too old for that.* Advancing age may kill willingness to experiment. But it also opens doors to novelty. If your partner says, *You can't teach an old dog new tricks,* ask how your spouse plans to adjust to retirement, or if retired, review what's happened since. Retirement often includes travel, long-deferred activities, perhaps even relocating—all new tricks for old hounds. If your lover can consider a huge change like moving, why not a vibrator? Or other erotic novelties?

As you slowly transcend old routines, you may have some ultimate sexual goal in mind. If you reach it, great. But most lovers find that getting part of what they desire is almost as good. Half a loaf is better than none. In sex, half a loaf often feels good enough.

Courtship—for Life

As hot-and-heavy romance evolves into old married love, most couples make less special time for each other. Relationships become predictable . . . and maybe boring. Reintroducing novelty recreates some of the magic of falling in love. New shared experiences are a delightful, relationship-affirming way to say, *I love you.* Novelty is an essential nutrient that nourishes relationships and enables sizzling sex.

Novelty is what courtship is all about. Gentlemen, almost all women love to feel courted, no matter if it's your fifth date or fiftieth anniversary. Your willingness to invest time, energy, and enthusiasm in fun new activities together demonstrates that you value them, consider them special, and don't take them for granted. If you want sexual heat to endure, court your sweetie for life.

CHAPTER 10:
Sexual Fantasies: Revel in Your Erotic Imagination

SEXUAL NOVELTY INVOLVES activities—mussing the sheets in new ways in new settings. In addition to new *actions*, the sexual mind and body react similarly to new *thoughts*. An active erotic imagination contributes to sizzling sex by boosting libido, aiding arousal, and enhancing pleasure.

What Do Daydreams Mean?

Some people don't care for certain foods: beets, onions, bananas—anything. What does that mean? In almost all cases, nothing. Everyone has idiosyncrasies.

Meanwhile, we all daydream. Our little waking reveries cover a great deal of possible experiences: winning the lotto, a fairy tale wedding, exotic travel, smacking a grand slam in the bottom of the ninth, or seeing adversaries brought low. Do daydreams mean we hate our lives? Probably not.

The vast majority of daydreams don't mean anything. They simply exercise our imaginations. We may love our work, family, and friends, but who can't imagine something different? Mental health professionals urge people to accept their imaginations. Daydreams are normal, healthy, and no cause for alarm.

Having daydreams doesn't necessarily mean you want them to come true. Plenty of men fantasize being the hero, rescuing the damsel in distress—without the slightest wish to be caught in a fire on the twenty-ninth floor.

But inject s-e-x into daydreaming and in a culture as sexually apprehensive as ours, many reflexively assume the worst. If they fantasize other lovers, they may feel guilt and shame, question their relationships, or beat themselves up for being "mentally unfaithful." If they visualize risky sex—voyeurism, exhibitionism, playing in public—they may wonder if they're perverted. And if they picture anything kinky—BDSM, threesomes, swinging—they may wonder about their sanity. Relax. The vast majority of sexual fantasies are as natural and harmless as daydreams or food quirks.

Starting in 1973, journalist Nancy Friday (1933–2017) published several collections of women's—and later men's—erotic fantasies. Her first book, *My Secret Garden: Women's Sexual Fantasies*, caused a sensation. Friday documented the then-shocking fact that women not only have erotic fantasies, but that many successful, happily coupled, mentally healthy women admitted fantasies of rape, incest, and infidelity. The book crystallized two key truths: fantasies are no reflection on the fantasizer. And as long as people can distinguish fantasy from reality, in fantasy, everything is permitted and nothing is wrong.

Decades later, in 2009, psychotherapist Brett Kahr interviewed 3,000 people and collected 23,000 sexual fantasies for his book *Who's Been Sleeping in Your Head? The Secret World of Sexual Fantasies*. He found no relationship—none at all—between the content of even the wildest, most bizarre or abusive reveries and fantasizers' mental health. Your sexual fantasies are no reflection on you, your relationship, or your sanity.

Sexual fantasies are critical to sizzling sex. They boost dopamine, the neurotransmitter of arousal and pleasure. Conversely, fighting one's fantasies produces sex-killing anxiety, guilt, and shame that distract from the undivided attention the best sex deserves.

Welcome your fantasies. Accept them. Even if they seem abnormal, they're fine, and so are you—as long as you can tell the difference between fantasy and reality. If your sexual fantasies scare you, consult a sex therapist.

Lovemaking as Meditation

Sexual fantasies are best understood as a type of meditation. Meditation involves a time-out from daily routines. Meditators sit quietly and try to empty their minds. They breathe deeply or repeat a simple word or phrase (mantra). Eventually, they transcend selfhood and discover oneness with the world around them. After meditating, they emerge relaxed, refreshed, and resilient.

But emptying the mind isn't easy—random thoughts pop up constantly. Meditation teachers advise accepting these thoughts without judging them, no matter what their content. Teachers say: *Your thoughts are not you. They're like dreams. You can't control them and are not responsible for them. Don't judge your thoughts. Simply observe them, then let them go as you return to your breath or mantra.*

Lovemaking is similar. But instead of sitting quietly, it involves giving and receiving pleasure. Lovers take a break from their busy lives. They breathe deeply, relax, transcend their individual selves, and feel deeply connected. Afterward, they emerge relaxed, refreshed, and resilient. And just as random thoughts during meditation don't mean anything, neither do the vast majority of fantasies during sex.

The Most Popular Sexual Fantasy

It's sex with someone other than your regular lover. Several studies have shown that fantasizing about others is almost ubiquitous and totally normal.

University of Vermont researchers asked 349 coupled students and staff to keep diaries of their erotic fantasies. Over a period of two months, 87 percent reported fantasies of other lovers (98 percent of the men, 80 percent of the women). Their erotic reveries were independent of their demographics and anything having to do with their relationships or sexual inclinations.

For his book on sexual fantasies, Brett Kahr asked his more than one thousand coupled participants if they had fantasies of other lovers. Virtually everyone said yes.

Unfortunately, many people believe that thoughts of other lovers are the moral equivalent of cheating. A *New York Times* survey asked: "As long as you're faithful to your spouse, do you think it's okay to imagine sex with someone else?"

- Yes, it's okay—46 percent of respondents (52 percent of men, 40 percent of women)
- They're wrong—48 percent
- No opinion—6 percent

What a shame that almost half of these respondents disapproved of something as normal, healthy, and sex enhancing as fantasies of other lovers. Sizzling sex is a combination of friction and fantasy. Most lovers enjoy the friction. But many feel uncomfortable with their fantasies.

During lovemaking, it might be nice to empty the mind of all thoughts other than your lover. But that's usually impossible. Errant thoughts almost inevitably intrude—including fantasies of movie stars, old flames, new acquaintances, or friends' spouses. Even if your sexual fantasies disturb you, be kind to yourself. Accept them. They are no reflection on your morality, love, faithfulness, or sanity. Like meditation, in sexual fantasies, everything is permitted and nothing is wrong.

Guilt about sexual fantasies causes anxiety and stress—and interferes with erotic pleasure. The University of Vermont researchers just mentioned found that those who expressed the most guilt about their fantasies reported the most sex problems and the least erotic satisfaction. And in a study of 251 women, some orgasmic, others not, French researchers found that the orgasmic women felt more comfortable with their sexual fantasies and reported more of them.

The late comedian Rodney Dangerfield told a story about making love with his girlfriend. They're doing it, but neither can work up much enthusiasm. Finally, Dangerfield says: "What's the matter? Can't you think of anyone either?"

> ## Applied Fantasies: Simmering
>
> Many lovers, especially older adults, yearn to heat up quickly but actually become aroused slowly. To speed arousal, sex therapists recommend "simmering fantasies." Say you have a sex date some evening. Starting that morning, daydream something sexual every hour or so—anything involving anyone that excites you. Simmering beforehand boosts arousal and enjoyment later.

Should Couples Share Their Fantasies?

Many men have contacted me with variations on this story: For years, they'd fantasized arriving home and finding the wife wearing nothing but high heels and a smile. They'd shared it. Their wives had rolled their eyes. They coaxed. Eventually, their wives agreed. When their fantasies came true, the men were shocked to realize they felt little or nothing. Why? Simple. Sexual fantasies exist in their own psychological realm—and sometimes they're better left there.

The erotic imagination is a wonderful gift. But fantasies can feel so compelling that we may fool ourselves into believing that we really want them to come true. Just like *caveat emptor*, let the fantasizer beware. Plenty of men fantasize throwing the winning touchdown pass at the Super Bowl—without any actual desire to see a half dozen three-hundred-pounders charging at them, thirsty for blood.

Should couples share their sexual fantasies? There's no simple answer. If such discussions enhance your relationship—and for many, they do—then fine, share all you like. But I would urge caution.

Sharing fantasies offers two advantages. First, you might truly want your fantasies to come true, and how can they if you don't declare them? But the erotic imagination can be a trickster. You may *believe* you want a fantasy to become true, but when it happens, you just might realize you've been fooling yourself, like the men mentioned above.

Second, sharing promotes honesty. Many believe that committed couples should be completely honest with each other. Perhaps. But total honesty means no surprise parties and no little fibs that spare the other's feelings—*That dress makes you look fat.* Sometimes kindness trumps honesty.

Which brings me to the main disadvantage of sharing fantasies. Your lover might think you're weird, perverted, or worse. *You want WHAT? How could I be with someone who wants THAT?* Are you ready to take that risk?

I know of no credible research on this issue, but I've raised the subject with many sex therapists. Most have advised erring on the side of caution.

What if you have a fantasy that always has you reaching between your legs, and you really, truly, absolutely want it realized? Some suggestions:

- **Start small.** Instead of *I want to open the door and find you naked,* ask if she'd be willing to open the door clothed but braless.
- **Add on slowly.** If she's fine braless, down the road, you might request shedding other garments.
- **Pitch it as a minor elaboration of moves already in your repertoire.** If you fantasize him welcoming a vibrator into partner sex, you might couch it as an extension of the music and scented candles the two of you already enjoy—*just another enhancement . . .*
- **Take turns orchestrating little erotic surprises.** Quite often, intense fantasies signal a wish for *any* novelty that spices things up. Consider taking turns arranging surprise dates discussed in the previous chapter.
- **Most people don't need their fantasies completely realized.** Partial fulfillment is often enough. If not, over time you might ask for more.

What about sharing intense fantasies of unconventional sex: BDSM, swinging, sex parties, and so forth? Again, it's up to you. If you'd like to discuss anything kinky but are unsure how, you might accidentally leave this book open to chapter 43 or 44 where your partner will see it.

Hypnosis and Visualizations Can Enhance Erotic Fantasies

For most people, prerequisites for sizzling sex include deep relaxation and erotic fantasies. Hypnosis, also known as visualization, offers a quick, gentle path to both. Forget nightclub hypnotists who say "You're getting sleepy," and coax people to do silly things. Actual hypnosis and its medical application, hypnotherapy, are mind-body disciplines that foster deep, meditative relaxation and focus the imagination—which can enhance sexual fantasies. If you're interested, begin with self-hypnosis or do-it-yourself visualization exercises. Many recordings and books are available. If you'd like assistance, some sex coaches and therapists include hypnosis in their practices. For more, search hypnosis, self-hypnosis, and visualization therapy. Hypnosis can make erotic fantasies more vivid and exciting and add pleasure to solo or partner lovemaking.

Why Do So Many Women Have Fantasies of Being Forced/Raped?

Depending on the study, one-third to two-thirds of women admit having at least occasional fantasies of being coerced into sex. Sexual assault is a horrible, traumatic crime. Why would any sane woman fantasize about it, let alone the numbers who do?

Psychologists offer three possibilities:

- **Guilt avoidance.** This explanation posits that women's erotic desires may cause anxiety, guilt, and shame. How can women enjoy robust sexual fantasies without developing these feelings? Fantasize about being forced. That way, they aren't responsible for the sex and need not feel distressed about it. *I was forced. It wasn't my fault.*
- **Sexual desirability.** This explanation reflects the "bodice-ripper" subgenre of romance fiction. The handsome, powerful, dangerous cad becomes so infatuated with the irresistible heroine that he loses all control and *must* have her, even if she refuses. *I'm so hot. I drive men crazy.*
- **Sexual openness.** This explanation says women feel sufficiently comfortable with their sexuality to play with imaginary scenarios far beyond what they'd ever truly want to experience. *It's fantasy. I can fantasize anything.*

Many studies have explored this issue. The most illuminating have been conducted by psychologist Jenny Bivona, PhD, at the University of North Texas. Her team began by asking 355 college women to complete standard personality inventories. Next they asked: Have you ever been sexually assaulted? Fifteen percent said yes, in line with other research.

Then the researchers asked how often the women had fantasized men or women sexually overpowering/coercing/forcing/raping them. Sixty-two percent said they'd had such fantasies at least once.

Responses varied depending on the terminology. When asked about being "overpowered," 52 percent said they'd had that fantasy. But when the term was "rape," only 32 percent. These findings are in the same ballpark as other reports.

Fantasies of being forced into sex varied in frequency:

- I've never had them—38 percent
- Fewer than one a year—25 percent
- A few times a year—13 percent
- Once a month—11 percent
- Once a week—8 percent
- Several times a week—5 percent

Overall, 62 percent—almost two-thirds—admitted fantasies of being coerced. Thirteen percent reported having them weekly or more.

Next, Bivona's team asked if participants' fantasies were enjoyable or repulsive:

- Entirely enjoyable—45 percent
- Entirely repulsive—9 percent
- Mixed feelings—46 percent

Among those who admitted fantasies of being overpowered, 91 percent experienced some enjoyment.

Finally, the researchers explored the content of assault fantasies. They did not define "forced" or "rape," letting participants use their own understanding of the terms, with rape usually implying more violence:

- Forced by a man to have sex against my will—52 percent admitted this fantasy
- Forced by a woman to surrender sexually against my will—17 percent
- Forced into sex while I was incapacitated by alcohol, other drugs, or falling unconscious—24 percent
- Forced by a man into fellatio—28 percent
- Forced by a woman into cunnilingus—9 percent
- Forced into anal sex—16 percent
- Raped by a man—32 percent
- Raped by a woman—9 percent

The prevalence of these fantasies suggests they occupy a significant place in the imaginations of college-age women—and presumably older women as well (most of those who fantasized victimization by women assailants said they were heterosexual).

Bivona's team found no relationship between actually having been sexually assaulted and rape fantasies. Those who'd experienced sexual assault were no more or less likely to have them.

The most popular explanation for rape fantasies is guilt avoidance. *I was coerced. It wasn't my fault.* But the researchers found this the *least* supported explanation. The most sexually anxious and guilty women had the *fewest* rape fantasies. The most supported explanation was sexual openness. *I'm free to fantasize anything.*

The most sexually self-accepting women had the most fantasies of being forced. They also reported the most fantasies in general, the most arousal from their fantasies, and the greatest sexual satisfaction.

As sexual openness increases, so does willingness to daydream about sexual scenarios you'd never really want to experience. Women who have rape fantasies don't want to be assaulted. They feel comfortable with their own sexuality and are happy to embrace their erotic fantasies—wherever they may lead.

The Most Misunderstood Fantasies: Porn

Many men consider pornography a how-to manual. Meanwhile, 25 percent of women believe it's an abomination that turns men into "sex addicts."

Actually, porn's depictions of sex are fantasies, cartoons as realistic as Bugs Bunny. Porn is like the car chases in action movies—exciting and fun to watch, but *not* the way to drive. The vast majority of men use porn as a visual aid for self-soothing masturbation. In this context, it's usually as benign as other daydreams. Fewer than 1 percent of men have porn habits that threaten their relationships. Like other sexual fantasies, porn doesn't really mean anything (part VI).

Friction and Fantasy

Beyond the recommendations in chapters 1–9, sizzling sex requires imagination, creativity, and comfort with one's erotic imagination. Your fantasies are no reflection on you, your relationship, or your mental health. Try not to judge them. Instead, revel in the ways they make sex sizzle.

PART II:

From Infancy to Old Age: Sexual Issues Throughout the Lifespan

CHAPTER 11:
Does Circumcision Reduce Men's Sexual Sensitivity?

CIRCUMCISION INVOLVES SURGICAL removal of the foreskin, the skin that covers the head (glans) of the flaccid penis. Worldwide, one-third of men are circumcised. Judaism and Islam require it, so in Israel and across the Muslim world, the practice is virtually universal. Circumcision is also popular in the US and Asia, but less so in Europe, Latin America, and non-Muslim Africa.

Circumcision is sexually controversial. The foreskin contains touch-sensitive nerves. Opponents insist it's obvious that removing the foreskin *must* reduce the penis's sexual sensitivity and impair men's pleasure. Supporters counter that the vast majority of erotically sensitive nerve endings are located in the glans, not the foreskin, and that the procedure does not noticeably compromise pleasure.

Not Health, Faith

Jews and Muslims have circumcised boys since the founding of those faiths. During the nineteenth century, the practice spread to Christians who believed—mistakenly—that it prevented masturbation. Circumcision is not medically necessary, but offers several health benefits:

- **AIDS prevention.** The foreskin can trap dirt and pathogens. During the 1980s, as AIDS raged in Africa, World Health Organization studies showed that circumcising African men reduced their AIDS risk by 60 percent.
- **Phimosis.** Men with this condition have unusually tight foreskins that don't retract properly. Phimosis may interfere with urination and make erections painful. The treatment is circumcision.
- **Urinary tract infection.** Men's UTI risk is much lower than women's, but compared with circumcised men, those with intact foreskins face greater risk.
- **Penile cancer.** It's rare, but uncircumcised men are at increased risk.
- **Healthier women.** Compared with female lovers of uncircumcised men, those whose lovers are circumcised have lower rates of cervical cancer, herpes, trichomoniasis, chlamydia, bacterial vaginosis, and human papillomavirus infection (HPV, genital warts).

> ### Tastier Fellatio
>
> When bathing, intact men should retract their foreskins and wash thoroughly. If they don't, during fellatio, their penises may taste foul.

These findings have prompted some Jews and Muslims to claim their faiths were medically prescient and required circumcision for health reasons. But theologians of both religions insist that the practice has always been an act of faith and that its medical benefits, while welcome, are coincidental.

Surveys in Africa Showing No Sexual Impact: Questionable

Several studies of circumcision's impact on sex have involved before-and-after surveys of African men circumcised as adults to reduce AIDS risk:

- Researchers in Kenya surveyed the sexual function, pleasure, and satisfaction of 2,784 uncircumcised sexually active men. Then 1,391 got circumcised. The investigators resurveyed all 2,784 every six months for two years. The two groups showed no significant differences in sexual function, pleasure, or satisfaction. Far from decreasing penile sensitivity, 72 percent of the circumcised group said their sensitivity had *increased*.
- Researchers in Uganda conducted a similar trial involving 4,456 intact men, 2,210 of whom got circumcised. After two years, more than 98 percent of both groups said they felt "satisfied" or "very satisfied" with their sex lives.

But these studies are problematic. When they were conducted, millions of Africans were dying of AIDS, and many participants feared for their lives. Researchers reassured them that circumcision would not affect them sexually. Critics charge that circumcised subjects were so relieved to have their AIDS risk reduced that they parroted back what researchers had said—that circumcision caused no sexual impact.

Studies Showing Sexual Impairment: Also Questionable

Three studies suggest that circumcision impairs sexual function:

- Portuguese researchers surveyed adult men before and after circumcision for medical reasons. Postsurgically they all reported less pain during intercourse, but also experienced a significant increase in erectile dysfunction (ED) and difficulty working up to orgasm/ejaculation. However, those reporting sex problems were also very likely to have diabetes. The disease often causes ED and other sex problems. Using statistical techniques to eliminate the impact of diabetes, the sexual difference between circumcised and intact men disappeared.
- Michigan State researchers used a male-oriented website to solicit 300 men for an online survey—64 intact, 236 circumcised (192 as infants). The latter were 4.5 times more likely to report using erection drugs, suggesting that circumcision increases risk of ED. However, the participants were self-selected, and the survey site had links to sites that crusade against circumcision. Circumcision opponents are often quite zealous and look for opportunities to bash the procedure, for example by participating in surveys like this one. Most scientists would dismiss this trial as biased.
- Belgian researchers conducted a similar online survey that drew responses from 1,369 men (1,059 intact, 310 circumcised). The latter reported less sexual pleasure and weaker orgasms. Again, the participants were self-selected and judged their own sexual function subjectively. Credible studies use standard scales.

The Best Studies: No Discernible Difference

Instead of using potentially biased surveys, some researchers have wired men's penises with sensors that allowed measurement of their reactions to various types of touch on the glans, shaft, and, if men have them, the foreskin.

- Canadian investigators tested the penile perceptions of sixty-two adult men—thirty-two intact, thirty circumcised as infants. The two groups showed no differences in any measure of sensitivity.
- New Jersey researchers tested sixty-two men with foreskins and sixty-three circumcised as infants. Initially, the intact men showed better ability to sense touch and vibrations, but when the researchers corrected for age, diabetes, and high blood pressure, all of which reduce penile sensitivity, the difference disappeared.
- Turkish researchers timed how long it took twenty adult men to masturbate to orgasm/ejaculation before circumcision and after they had healed from it. If the procedure impaired erotic sensitivity, we would expect the men to take longer after. But this study showed no differences.
- Australian researchers surveyed 10,173 men, 41 percent intact, 59 percent circumcised, and British investigators surveyed 6,293 men, 79 percent with foreskins, 21 percent without. Participants' reports of sex problems did not differ based on circumcision status—except that the circumcised Australians reported slightly less ED, while the circumcised Brits reported slightly more. However, in both studies, the ED findings were barely statistically significant, so both may well have occurred by chance.
- Finally, European researchers surveyed the circumcision status of ten thousand adult male residents of Cottbus, Germany—93 percent intact, 7 percent circumcised. Then the investigators used standard scales to gauge participants' health and sexual function. Forty percent showed some level of ED. Age, smoking, diabetes, heart disease, and high blood pressure all increased ED risk—but circumcision status made no difference.

No compelling evidence shows that circumcision reduces men's sexual pleasure or raises their risk of sex problems.

Sizzling Sex Involves Much More Than Just the Penis—or Any Part of It

The body is remarkably redundant. Pet a cat using five fingers and focus on how it feels. Then pet the cat with four. Eliminating one finger means 20 percent fewer touch-sensitive nerves in contact with the fur. Does petting the cat with four fingers feel significantly less pleasurable?

Sizzling sex involves the whole body. Some men believe that sexual pleasure happens only in the penis. If that were true, circumcision might well impair sensitivity. But great sex excites every square inch of skin. The most pleasurable sex usually involves gentle, playful, extended mutual massage from head to toe.

Excessive preoccupation with the penis—or any part of it—substantially increases men's risk of premature ejaculation, orgasm/ejaculation difficulties, and erectile dysfunction. Resolving these problems involves de-emphasizing all parts of the penis and enjoying sex based on whole-body loveplay.

*   *   *

The controversy over circumcision and sexuality is usually moot. Men are either circumcised or not, and almost all have been sexual only that way. If you're intact and want to feel smug about greater sensitivity, feel free. But the weight of the evidence suggests that circumcision is much less important to men's sexual function and pleasure than their health and their appreciation of the ten ingredients of lovemaking (part I).

CHAPTER 12:
A Parents' Guide to Toddlers' and Preschoolers' Natural Sexual Curiosity

UNTIL THE 1700S, childhood as we understand it did not exist. Children were considered little adults—like their parents, just smaller. Their world was agricultural. As soon as they could, kids joined their parents in the fields, and when they fancied one another, they canoodled like adults as well.

Compared with today's children, the little adults of the preindustrial age witnessed a great deal more real live sex. I recall my third-grade class going wild when, on the playground, two dogs went at it. But back in Shakespeare's day, what bulls did with cows elicited no giggles. Family survival depended on livestock fecundity and farm families carefully managed breeding—with youngsters watching and helping.

In addition, the vast majority of people were peasants living in one- or two-room shacks. As John D'Emilio and Estelle B. Freedman relate in *Intimate Matters*, their classic history of American sexuality, "The small size of the vast majority of dwellings allowed children to witness adult sexuality with their ears or eyes. Curtains might have screened the parental bed, but all family members commonly slept in the same room, especially during winter, when a single fireplace provided heat." Furthermore, bed-sharing was common. One daughter recalled getting into bed with her mother and siblings, and when her father joined them, her mother instructed the kids to give the couple room to play "or she would kick us out of bed."

When I was eight, I played "show me" with a neighbor girl. At ten, I enjoyed my first kiss with the eight-year-old sister of a friend, who took my hand, led me to her basement, and puckered up. As far as I can tell, my childhood protosex caused no harm. For the 97 percent of men and 85 percent of women not burdened by childhood sex abuse, my experience turns out to be typical:

- UCLA researchers asked parents to keep diaries noting anything sexual in the lives of their two hundred sons and daughters from birth through age eighteen. Parents witness only a fraction of child sex play, but these parents saw three-quarters of their children masturbating and reported that half engaged in sex play with peers, typically touching each other's genitals. The researchers found zero correlation to later psychological distress.
- A University of Michigan researcher asked 132 young adults to recall their childhood sexual experiences, if any. "While some had negative memories—coercion or interruptions by adults who disapproved—most evaluated the large majority of their childhood sex experiences as positive. Childhood sex play is extremely widespread, hence normal."

- Researchers at Old Dominion University in Virginia surveyed 210 college students (77 men, 133 women) about their sexual functioning and recollections of seeing their parents and others naked during childhood. Compared with those who'd never seen naked adults as kids, those who had reported feeling more comfortable with their own bodies and sexuality.
- Swedish scientists asked 269 high school seniors if they'd been sexual before age thirteen. Eighty-three percent reported masturbating and 80 percent recalled sex play with a near-age friend. Compared with boys, girls reported more sex play—more "show me yours, I'll show you mine" and more genital touching and caressing.
- University of Georgia researchers surveyed the histories of 501 middle-class women age eighteen to sixty-one. Most recalled childhood sexual experiences. There were no significant psychological differences between those who had or didn't have such experiences. As long as early childhood sexual experiences were not abusive, they caused no harm later.
- Finally, in a classic anthropological study of 191 cultures worldwide, the researchers concluded, "If the adults of a society permit it, young children engage in practically every type of sexual behavior found in adults, including oral-genital play and attempted copulation."

From Permissiveness to Pushback

During the early twentieth century, Sigmund Freud (1856–1939) postulated that children were innately sexual and filled with Oedipal longings to do the deed with a parent. Freud found an ally in psychologist G. Stanley Hall (1846–1924), who coined the term *adolescence*. In 1904, Hall published a treatise on the developmental stage between childhood and adulthood. It was banned from many libraries for its frank discussion of turn-of-the-twentieth-century teen sex.

For a generation after World War II, Benjamin Spock, MD (1903–98), was the nation's most revered pediatrician. His landmark parenting guide, *Baby and Child Care* (1946, with dozens of later editions), sold more than fifty million copies. Earlier parenting manuals had admonished parents to put kids on strict feeding and sleep schedules and limit physical affection to kisses on the forehead. Spock argued that parents should jettison arbitrary timetables, trust their instincts, shower kids with affection, and grant them major behavioral leeway. He had no problem with childhood masturbation and sex play.

Social conservatives railed that Spock's "permissiveness" would produce a self-indulgent generation bent on anarchy. As the first children raised on the good doctor's advice came of age, Spock became an outspoken critic of the Vietnam War. Conservatives blamed the protests of the 1960s—against the war and in favor of the civil rights movement—in part on the parenting style he'd championed.

Spock was not alone in his acceptance of childhood sexuality. In *The Sex Handbook: Information and Help for Minors* (1974), coauthors Heidi Handman and Peter Brennan opined, "Sex is a natural appetite. If you're old enough to want sex, you're old enough to have it."

But during the late 1970s, the nation's sexual landscape abruptly shifted as videocassette players became must-have appliances. Suddenly, anyone with a VCR could watch porn at home. Social conservatives charged that the nation was awash in "kiddie porn," with thousands of children kidnapped, drugged, and raped by pedophile porn producers.

These allegations turned out to be wild hyperbole. In 1976, New York City hosted the Democratic National Convention. In preparation, the police "cleaned up" porn-filled Times Square by raiding its two dozen sex shops and seizing what they expected to be a mountain of kiddie porn. They grabbed thousands of videocassettes—but found next to none depicting children. The head of the NYPD Morals Division called kiddie porn "as rare as the Dead Sea Scrolls."

Now, *any* pornography depicting children is abhorrent. But contrary to the claims of anti-porn activists, porn actors have always been—and still are—virtually all adults. One notable exception was Traci Lords, a.k.a. Nora Kuzma (1968–), who showed producers a fake ID so she could cavort on camera—eagerly—at fifteen. When her real age came to light, distributors pulled her videos.

Despite the paucity of evidence for their claims, conservatives organized to crush media-driven sexualization of children. One was psychiatrist Judianne Densen-Gerber, founder of Odyssey House, a New York drug-rehabilitation program. In 1977 congressional testimony, Densen-Gerber asserted that 1.2 million American children had been coerced into sex work and kiddie porn. Eventually, Densen-Gerber was forced out of Odyssey House, accused of embezzlement. But before her disgrace, her lobbying contributed to congressional passage of the 1977 Protection of Children against Sexual Exploitation Act (P-CASE), which criminalized all erotic depictions of children under sixteen.

One of the law's first casualties was *Show Me!* by psychologist Helga Fleischhauer-Hardt, PhD, and photographer Will McBride, a sex education guide for children and parents that contained photos of smiling kids enjoying rudimentary sex play solo or with other children. When published in 1970, the book won awards. The *Los Angeles Times* called it "beautiful, charming, and elegant," but predicted it might "start an uproar." It did. Four state attorneys general indicted the publisher, St. Martin's Press, on obscenity charges. In all four cases, judges ruled the book not obscene. But the Justice Department targeted St. Martin's under P-CASE. In 1982, the US Supreme Court ruled that even though *Show Me!* was not obscene, it violated the new law. St. Martin's withdrew it.

Kiddie porn remains a daunting—but minuscule—problem. The 1996 federal Child Pornography Prevention Act made it a crime to receive, transport, or distribute sexual depictions of children. Convictions of those trading child-sex imagery on the internet jumped from a few dozen in the early 1990s to 1,886 in 2010 (0.0000061 percent of the US population). Law enforcement officials said the increase reflected more vigorous prosecutions, not any increase in kiddie porn production or consumption.

Adding to the nation's growing anxiety over child sexual abuse, in 1984, teachers at the McMartin Preschool in Manhattan Beach, California, were accused of sexually abusing their young charges. The case triggered a national media frenzy. *Daycare run by child molesters!*

Psychologists working with Los Angeles prosecutors interviewed the children on video. The recordings showed bewildered kids badgered into saying whatever their interrogators wanted to hear. The trial lasted seven years, the longest, costliest criminal proceeding in US history. It ended in 1990 with all defendants acquitted—and their lives destroyed.

Four years later in 1994, thirty-three-year-old paroled sex offender Jessie Timmendequas of Hamilton Township, New Jersey, raped and killed his seven-year-old neighbor, Megan Kanka. The case propelled the federal government and most states to enact "Megan's Laws" that require police registration of released sex offenders, whose addresses become public.

No other crime requires ex-convicts to register with police for life, but many Americans feel that for sex offenders who abuse children, it's justified. The public notification provision has turned released sex offenders into perpetual refugees, forced to move as soon as landlords or neighbors learn who they are.

Recidivism rates suggest that such hypersurveillance is an overreaction. Within five years of release from jail, police rearrest 82 percent of property-crime offenders, 77 percent of drug offenders, 71 percent of violent offenders—and 14 percent of sex offenders. But to most Americans, the comparatively low risk of sex-offender recidivism is irrelevant. Megan's Laws reflect a nation terrified of child sex abuse.

The threat, however small, has transformed American parenting. During the 1950s, I grew up in a Long Island suburb of New York City. When not in school, I roamed my neighborhood playing with friends—completely unsupervised by adults. I left home after breakfast and often didn't return until dinner. My parents, who were anything but permissive, had no problem with this.

Today few parents would leave kids as unsupervised as I was. While raising our son and daughter, my wife and I kept much closer tabs. They spent much more of their free time in adult-supervised activities: day care; Boys and Girls Club; summer camps; and music, art, and sports programs.

Many parents believe that dawn-to-dusk organized activities keep their children safe from sexual predators. Actually, organized activities may *increase* kids' risk.

Who Are the Pedophiles?

Don't take candy from strangers. Never get into a car with anyone you don't know. Nervous parents drill these admonitions into their children. My wife and I did.

Stranger-abduction child kidnappings do happen—but rarely. For a 2002 report based on more than 20,000 interviews, the US Justice Department analyzed the circumstances of the nation's 797,500 annual missing-children reports:

- Runaways or kids kicked out of their homes: 357,600 (45 percent)
- Benign explanations (at a friend's house): 340,500 (43 percent)
- Lost or injured: 61,900 (8 percent)
- Abductions by relatives (usually parents in custody disputes): 56,500 (7 percent)
- Stranger abductions: 12,100 (1.5 percent)

Of course, *any* abduction is abhorrent. But the threat posed by strangers is trivial compared with children's risk of sexual abuse by older kids and adults *they know.*

For example, priests. From media reports, one could infer that Catholic priests might be the nation's chief pedophiles. In fact, only a small fraction of child sex abusers are priests.

In 1996, researchers at the University of California, San Francisco, identified the extent of pedophilia in their National Sexual Health Survey (NSHS), a comprehensive study of American sexuality based on in-depth interviews with a representative sample of 8,400 Americans age eighteen to eighty-eight. The NSHS asked: "Have you ever felt forced or frightened into sex?" Fifteen percent of the women and 3 percent of the men said yes, figures that agree with similar surveys.

Young victims were asked at what age(s) they were molested. Abuse spanned all ages from two to seventeen, but victims clustered in two groups, six to ten and fourteen to seventeen.

Men accounted for 95 percent of abusers. Their ages ranged from ten to seventy, but half—48 percent—were in their twenties. Eighteen percent were in their thirties, 15 percent in their forties, and all other age groups accounted for 19 percent.

Who were the molesters? Dates, friends, and acquaintances comprised the largest groups (38 percent), followed by nonparent relatives (23 percent), others (15 percent), strangers (10 percent), parents (6 percent), and stepparents (4 percent).

Caregivers were the most frequent abusers of kids under age twelve: babysitters, camp or recreational-program staff, parents, stepparents, or other relatives. Friends or acquaintances were the top abusers of teens.

Under "other," the NSHS asked who. Some victims mentioned priests, but most were grandparents, neighbors, teachers, doctors, coaches, parents' friends or coworkers, or adults around the house—gardeners, cleaners, or repairmen—people like Dennis Hastert, former Speaker of the House of Representatives, imprisoned in 2016 for sexually abusing members of the high school wrestling team he'd coached in his twenties before entering politics.

No matter who they are, child sex abusers usually have two things in common—proximity to children and authority over them. Abuse is more likely to occur inside the child's home than outside it. This problem is much bigger than bad-apple priests. It's bad apples almost anywhere.

How to Keep Kids Safe

My two children attended day care, after-school programs, sports and music activities, and summer camps staffed by older kids and young adults—and thrived unmolested. I claim no special expertise in child sex abuse prevention. But I have three suggestions for anxious parents:

- Try not to become rattled by horrible headlines. Many studies show that 15 percent of girls and 3 percent of boys report feeling forced, frightened, or manipulated into sex. These numbers are tragic, but they mean that five out of six girls (85 percent) and twenty-nine out of thirty boys (97 percent) escape abuse. Most abuse episodes are one-time occurrences, and most kids are able to avoid subsequent manipulation. Only a small fraction of cases involve anything truly cringeworthy—2 percent of girls and 0.3 percent of boys.
- Even in worst-case molestations that leave enduring emotional scars—long-term parental incest—survivors *can* recover psychologically and enjoy happy, satisfying love and sex lives.
- Finally, from the day they're born, talk to your children about sex. Don't wait until they're some arbitrary age to have the Talk. Look for opportunities to discuss sexual issues and raise them.

Abusers' chief weapon is silence. *Don't tell anyone. This is our little secret. If you say anything, we'll both get in trouble.* These warnings make perfect sense to children raised in homes with parents who *don't* talk about sex. But kids raised in sex-positive homes are usually forthcoming about their sexual experiences, both positive and negative. If kids from sex-positive families find themselves in abusive situations, they're much more likely to tell their parents.

How to Talk with Young Children about Sex

It's not easy. When my wife and I had kids, I'd been a sex educator for more than a decade yet at times found myself at a loss for words.

That's why it's crucial to introduce the subject when kids are toddlers. You gain valuable experience—and confidence—when their questions are simple and you project an ask-me-anything tone that's sure to pay dividends as they become teens and the issues become more complicated:

- **Silence speaks volumes.** Kids look to their parents for guidance on values and behavior. Sex involves both, so they want to hear from you. Parents provide sex education *whether or not they raise the subject.* Parents who are silent or evasive declare loud and clear that the subject is unmentionable. So curious kids naturally turn to other sources:

uninformed peers or the internet, where sex searches may reveal good information, but are equally likely to provide nonsense and porn.

- **Answer kids' sex questions as forthrightly as possible.** Never say, "You're too young for that" or "That's for grown-ups." Kids are curious about sex. Sex education never hurt anyone. What causes problems is its *absence*.
- **Try.** To discuss sex productively, you don't have to feel comfortable with the subject. You don't need training in biology or psychology. And you don't have to be articulate. All you have to do is *try*. And keep trying. With practice, the task usually becomes easier. You don't have to get it perfect the first time. Conversations evolve, including sex talks. If you want to amend previous statements or add additional information, feel free.
- **Be brief.** There's no need for convoluted dissertations. Most young kids are happy with brief, matter-of-fact answers.
- **Keep talking.** Many parents say little if anything about sex until children reach some arbitrary age and then stumble through the Talk, often just once. But one-and-done is unrealistic. Sex is everywhere. Talk about it whenever the subject arises: on TV, after movies, in song lyrics, in the news, anywhere and everywhere.
- **Answer kids' questions with a loving tone and a big smile.** Your manner and grin communicate as much as your words. Information delivered with a smile shows that sex is just another aspect of daily life.

Sperm-and-Egg and Welcome-to-Puberty Books: Seriously Flawed

When I was seven, my mother read me a book called *How I Was Born*, which explained sperm and eggs and how they meet. I recall being astonished. *Really? Something comes out besides pee? Men stick it into women?* I also recall feeling delighted. I knew nothing about sex, but understood it was a grown-up subject. My parents shared it, which showed they trusted me with adult information. I felt a bit more grown-up myself.

How I Was Born is long gone, but today's parents can choose among two dozen sperm-and-egg and welcome-to-puberty guides. To the extent that they help nervous parents deal with challenging subjects, they're valuable. But they're also problematic. Billed as providing "sex" education, all but one of the books I reviewed focus almost exclusively on procreation, mentioning erotic pleasure only in passing, if at all.

That's a shame. Recall that making babies has little to do with why people make love. Conceiving children usually requires intercourse, but the vast majority of partner rock 'n' roll is about mutual attraction and pleasure. Unfortunately, most sex education resources for children and teens largely ignore erotic pleasure. Even in books for children and adolescents, pleasure deserves more ink. I urge parents to correct a few key points that even the best of these books mangle.

Most books say: "Boys have penises. Girls have vaginas."

Actually, girls have *vaginas, vulvas, and clitorises*. The female equivalent of the penis is *not* the vagina. During the first months of gestation, the genders' fetal genitalia are indistinguishable. Then boys' embryonic genital cells develop into the penis while girls' become the clitoris and vulva. Biologically, the penis and vagina are not analogous.

Ever since the late 1940s when Alfred Kinsey launched modern sex research, one finding has been reconfirmed repeatedly. Compared with men, women are considerably less likely to have orgasms. Why? Often because many men (and some women) are unaware of the clitoris and the key role it plays in women's pleasure and orgasm. From day one, parents should tell both boys and girls that boys have penises for making babies and sexual pleasure, while girls have vaginas for babies and vulvas and clitorises for pleasure.

This downplaying—or ignoring—of the clitoris leaves most boys (and some girls) in the dark about women's sexuality. The same misinformation gets repeated in welcome-to-puberty books. Then, during young adulthood and beyond, many men get ridiculed for their ignorance of women's sexuality. But when raised on consistently repeated misinformation, how are boys, young men, and many older men supposed to know any different?

"Masturbation is perfectly normal. Some people think it's wrong or harmful, and some religions call it a sin. But masturbating cannot hurt you. Many people masturbate. Others don't. It's your choice."
My suggestion: you're free to masturbate or not. But we, your parents, encourage it—in private. Masturbation is the foundation of a healthy, happy sex life. It allows us to learn what kinds of touch provide erotic pleasure. Parents should teach their children that masturbation is not only harmless and almost universal, but *beneficial*. Left alone, children are enthusiastic masturbators. Why not? It's such fun. But while encouraging solo sex, parents should also say that, like going to the bathroom, masturbation is a private pursuit. When you want to play with yourself, do it behind closed doors.

"Sexual intercourse is often called making love."
Actually, there are many ways to make love: kissing, cuddling, hugging, gentle massage from head to toe, hand jobs, fellatio, cunnilingus, penis-vagina intercourse, anal play, and kink. For those so inclined, they all provide great pleasure.

There's no "right way" to make love or "correct" gender to bed. Making babies usually requires intercourse with penises ejaculating in vaginas. But lovemaking is not limited to intercourse and need not include it. Plenty of people enjoy marvelous sex and earthquake orgasms *without* penis-vagina intercourse: gay men, lesbian women, elders, and lovers with many disabilities. Even when heterosexual couples are fully capable of intercourse, some *prefer* to make love in other ways.

"As the penis moves inside the vagina, both people grow increasingly excited. When excitement reaches a climax, the penis releases semen and the muscles in the vagina contract in waves, then relax. That's orgasm."
My revision: after you masturbate for a while, you notice feeling increasingly excited. At a certain point, you feel muscle contractions between your legs accompanied by a wave of pleasure followed by a few minutes of dreamy contentment. That's orgasm. Lovers can also help each other have orgasms by caressing each other's genitals.

Unfortunately, the books almost always say that penis-vagina intercourse produces orgasm. This is usually true for men, but not for women. To climax, three-quarters of women need direct clitoral caresses by hand, mouth, or vibrator.

Many men and women believe that women "should" come during intercourse. This belief causes tremendous misery: women who think they're defective, men critical of "frigid" lovers, and women who fake orgasm to spare men's supposedly fragile egos while keeping men in the dark about what they actually need to feel satisfied. The notion that intercourse produces orgasm in women is a toxic distortion.

Finally, none of the parent-child books I reviewed and few books for teens mentioned oral sex.

This is a major oversight. Most lovers delight in receiving fellatio or cunnilingus and almost as many enjoy providing them. Many say it's their favorite part of lovemaking, their preferred way to climax.

When the books ignore oral sex, parents rarely discuss it. The subject remains unmentioned and by implication unmentionable. Failure to discuss oral sex, particularly cunnilingus, causes real problems. Both boys and girls continue to believe that "sex" equals vaginal intercourse. They remain in the dark about a wonderful way to give and receive pleasure. Girls grow into young women unlikely to have orgasms with partners—and decide something must be wrong with them. And boys grow into young men unaware of how most women experience pleasure and orgasm.

When I told my kids about the erotic primacy of the clitoris for women, they absorbed it just as they had sperm-and-egg information. After we emphasized that they could masturbate as much as they liked—in private—I found their bedroom doors closed more often. When I told them that intercourse isn't the only way to do it, that many couples prefer oral sex and that cunnilingus is much more likely than intercourse to bring women to orgasm, they said, *Really? Eeww!* Yes, I replied, it's hard to imagine, but that's what happens in grown-up sex. And when you grow up, try it. You'll probably like it.

Don't "Protect" Children from Sex. Guide Them to Enjoy It.

No matter what parents say or don't say, kids are sponges for sex information. Even if they don't look for it, they're exposed to a great deal. The only questions are: What do they learn? And from whom?

Kids naturally explore their bodies and discover the pleasure provided by self-touch, being touched, and touching others. Childhood sex play is near universal. Absent coercion, there is no credible evidence that childhood genital displays or protosex play cause any harm. The main problem is adult disapproval that may engender guilt and shame and take years—and possibly therapy—to overcome.

Parent-child sex education has one modest disadvantage and many big advantages. The disadvantage: It makes parents uncomfortable. The advantages:

- Children learn that sex is normal and healthy, a topic of everyday conversation.
- They gain adult acknowledgment that they are sexual, which contributes to self-esteem.
- They're more likely to develop firm foundations for giving and receiving lifelong sexual pleasure.
- Children are more likely to tell their parents about sexual abuse.
- They're more likely to grow into adolescents open to information about contraception and sexual infection prevention.
- They're more likely to appreciate the clitoris in girls' pleasure.
- Girls are more likely to grow into young women who assert their sexual needs, including the caresses that bring them to orgasm.
- Boys and girls are less likely to go all the way as young teens. They're more likely to wait until they're over sixteen.
- Children are less likely to become adults with sex problems.

I hope parents weigh the pros and cons of sex-negative silence vs. sex-positive erotic education, and then decide for themselves how they want to approach this important aspect of parenting.

Sex and Children with Disabilities

All the advice in this chapter goes double for parents of children with disabilities. Our society generally assumes that disabled people are not sexual. This is false and cruel. Except for the asexual 1 percent, *everyone* is sexual, including those with disabilities. Differently abled lovers may not be able to accomplish vaginal intercourse, but they can—and have every right to—experience loving touch to whatever extent they're able: kissing, cuddling, massage, masturbation, partner play, sex toys, and, if they feel so inclined, kink. My suggestions for parents of children with disabilities:

- Your children are sexual. Don't deny their sexuality.
- Discuss sexuality with them at every opportunity.
- All disabled children can experience sensual pleasure. Look for ways to encourage this.
- Some children with severe disabilities require a great deal of care and may not have much opportunity for private self-exploration and masturbation, let alone partner play. To whatever extent possible, grant them privacy and opportunities to explore their sexuality by themselves and with special friends.

CHAPTER 13:
Childhood Sex Abuse: Recovery and Sizzling Sex Are Possible

CHILD SEX ABUSE involves a spectrum of victimization from unwelcome fondling once by the boy next door to years of nightly rape by one's father. Many people believe serious abuse is so devastating that survivors never fully recover and can never enjoy lovemaking. Actually, recovery is quite possible, and so is a sizzling sex life.

Recovery isn't easy. It typically takes years and requires professional help. During the recovery process, there may be times when survivors can't focus on anything but their own experiences. This may leave their families, friends, and lovers feeling ignored or shut out. But survivors eventually emerge from the dark tunnel of abuse and recovery into the light of healing. They often report sex lives transformed from horrible to deeply fulfilling.

What Proportion of Children Suffer Sexual Abuse?
The extent of child sexual abuse provokes heated controversy. Definitions differ and academics, law enforcement agencies, and victim-advocacy organizations have produced wildly different estimates. The following come from three national victim-advocacy nonprofits:

- Rape, Abuse, and Incest National Network (RAINN): One girl in nine (11 percent), one boy in fifty-three (2 percent)
- Darkness to Light: One girl in seven (14 percent), one boy in twenty-five (4 percent)
- National Association of Adult Survivors of Child Abuse: One girl in four (25 percent), one boy in six (17 percent)

That's quite a range, especially for boys: one girl in four to nine, one boy in six to fifty-three. Advocacy organizations' disparate findings raise questions about their estimates' credibility.

Meanwhile, investigators with the Crimes Against Children Research Center at the University of New Hampshire (UNH) insist the rate is much lower than even the lowest of these estimates, around one-tenth of 1 percent (0.11 percent) of children. Using data from the National Child Abuse and Neglect Data System, David Finkelhor and Lisa Jones found that from 1975 through 1990, child sex abuse steadily increased to approximately twenty-three children per ten thousand population—around two-tenths of 1 percent of US children. But from 1990 to 2004, they say the rate fell by half to eleven per ten thousand— one-tenth of 1 percent, or a small fraction of the lowest advocacy-group figure. The Justice Department's authoritative National Crime Victimization Survey corroborates the Finkelhor/ Jones estimate.

Finkelhor and Jones can't explain precisely why child sexual abuse has declined, but they point to:

- Greater public awareness; better, faster reporting helps spare younger siblings
- More funding for child-protection agencies
- Better training of police; better, faster recognition of abuse
- Demographic changes; fewer children as a proportion of the population
- Legal abortion; fewer unwanted children
- The end of the crack cocaine epidemic
- More effective treatment of emotional disorders, possibly deterring potential perpetrators

Of course, even one sexually abused child is one too many, but if the UNH researchers are correct, we've made significant progress against this horrible crime.

Healing Is Possible

Girls experience the vast majority of child sexual abuse, so this discussion largely focuses on them.

Laura Davis, of Santa Cruz, California, is the coauthor of *The Courage to Heal: A Guide for Women Survivors of Child Sexual Abuse*. The book reflects her struggle to recover from her grandfather's abuse—and the joy she discovered in recovery: "When I had my first memories of the incest, I went from being a very sexual person to being totally erotically shut down. I had flashbacks every time I was touched, couldn't bear to be touched, and changed my mind

Male Survivors Face Special Recovery Challenges

Childhood sex abuse is horrible for everyone who endures it, but our culture stereo-types the genders differently and these generalizations have profound implications for survivors. Girls are supposedly passive and submissive, boys dominant and in control. Whether or not children or the adults they become actually act that way, as people grow up, they internalize gender stereotyping.

As horrible as child sex abuse is for girls and the women they become, it meshes with the stereotype. Girls are seen—and often see themselves—as passive and submissive, therefore powerless to stop abuse. In contrast, boys and the men they become may buy into the myth of the indomitable man and feel like "failures" for not being "real men" and stopping their abuse.

Many male survivors see themselves as less than men and go to great lengths to prove their masculinity with foolish daredevil activities, law breaking, and violence, including possibly perpetrating sexual abuse themselves. Many also develop profound emotional problems, including confusion about their sexuality and problems maintain-ing intimate relationships.

Unfortunately, compared with most women, most men are less willing to seek help, feeling that real men put the past behind them and move on. Actually, male abuse sur-vivors need therapy just as much as their female counterparts, if not more. I urge male survivors and those who love them to begin the recovery process by reading *Victims No Longer* by Mike Lew and by visiting MaleSurvivor.org.

constantly: *Yes, I want sex. No, I don't.*" After six months, this proved too much for Davis's relationship.

After her recovery, Davis built another relationship. She says most of the time she "enjoys being touched and considers partner sex a way to connect, heal, express love, and have fun."

Staci Haines is another survivor and author of *Healing Sex: A Mind-Body Approach to Healing Sexual Trauma.* After years devoted to her own recovery, she now enjoys a pleasurable, fulfilling sex life and has become a psychotherapist specializing in helping abuse survivors rediscover erotic pleasure. "Healing is possible," she explains, "emotional and sexual healing. I tell survivors: you survived. You're more powerful than what happened to you. Victimization is terrible. Surviving it is very hard. So is recovery. But now that you're an adult, you have the capacity to recover and to build the life—and the sex life—you choose."

The Impact of Childhood Sex Abuse

It usually depends on the type and duration of the abuse and the familial closeness of the abuser. Occasional fondling by a babysitter is much less likely to produce chronic trauma than frequent rape by close relatives. But any survivor may experience long-term consequences. Compared with nonabused women, survivors show significantly greater risk of anxiety, depression, insomnia, obesity, chronic pain, chronic illnesses, eating disorders, suicide attempts, borderline personality disorder, addictions to alcohol and other drugs, and, for those with children, profound insecurities about parenting.

Consequently, it's not surprising that many people, both survivors and the public, believe child sexual abuse ruins survivors for life—which is possible. Some survivors commit suicide or become disabled by addictions or mental illness. But in most cases, with time, professional therapy, and loving emotional support, survivors of childhood sexual abuse *can* recover.

One key issue is trust. Someone who should have been nurturing, honorable, and trustworthy was the opposite. Sex is based on trust. Survivors have a hard time with trust, which is why they have difficulty with sex.

Another important issue involves survivors' loss of control. Their desires and personal integrity were ignored. They had no control over what happened to them. Many survivors feel a deep need to assert total control over every aspect of their lives, relationships, and sexuality. This, too, complicates lovemaking. Sizzling sex involves a combination of control and letting go—setting limits others respect while feeling sufficiently safe to surrender to erotic enjoyment and orgasm. Survivors' need for control often interferes with letting go, which complicates lovemaking and orgasm.

A third issue is "dissociation," a natural defense against trauma. Survivors' minds block what happened to their bodies. Dissociation is not unique to child sexual abuse. Survivors of any trauma—war, torture, car wrecks, and so forth—do whatever it takes to escape their memories. When children face trauma before developing other coping skills, dissociation may be their only option. Many survivors of child sex abuse withdraw physically and emotionally. They may grow into numb, dissociated adults. Survivor-author Laura Davis once asked a survivor how she felt about her body. Her reply: "What body?"

Dissociation often includes an inability to experience physical pleasure. One survivor explains: "I was afraid to feel pleasure. My body could contain lots of pain, but no pleasure." Another confesses: "Physical pleasure repelled me. I wanted to throw up every time I had an orgasm. All I could think about was my uncle."

Some survivors feel repulsed by sex. Others become sexually reckless—seeking wild, drunk, unprotected sex with strangers. And some swing back and forth, one moment craving physical closeness, the next freezing or fleeing. All these reactions reflect dissociation.

In addition, even if lovemaking is tender, nurturing, and consensual, it may trigger flashbacks, vivid memories of the abuse that make sex difficult, if not impossible. One survivor's description: "My lover was standing over me about to join me in bed. I knew he was the man I loved, a gentle, wonderful person. But all I could see was my father. He'd been dead a dozen years. But I saw my father."

Another survivor: "My memories of abuse and my erotic passion live in the same place. If I refrain from sex, I don't relive the abuse, but I don't experience the passion either. Whenever I open myself to passion, horrible memories come flooding back."

The Rocky Road to Sexual Healing

Therapeutic approaches vary, but survivor-therapist Staci Haines combines traditional talk therapy with hands-on efforts aimed at reintroducing survivors to their bodies. A focus on the body, somatic therapy, helps survivors inhabit their own skins, a process that eventually empowers erotic pleasure.

A key goal of the talk therapy is to overcome guilt and shame. Many survivors believe the abuse was their fault. Over time, they realize that as children they were powerless in the abusive relationship and not responsible for what happened. Eventually, they forgive themselves—and get angry at their abusers, a key step in healing. Talk therapy also explores survivors' dissociations and tendency to fake pleasure and orgasm.

On the body side of somatic therapy, the goal is to overcome dissociation and learn to enjoy sensual touch. "To feel is to heal," Haines insists. "It can feel very intense for survivors to relive their abuse deep in their bodies. But this is critical. Body awareness allows them to move beyond dissociation, and eventually experience genuine sexual pleasure."

However, before sexual healing, most survivors require a period of celibacy, or perhaps loving touch without genital play: hand holding, kissing, cuddling, hugging, and massage. For some, the sexual time-out lasts months, for others, years.

"When I entered therapy," one survivor recalls, "I couldn't stand being touched. For a time, my lover and I had no physical contact. Then I wanted to be in his arms, to feel close, but all I could tolerate was being hugged. Eventually, we became more sexual."

To gain comfort with physical pleasure and sexual sensations, a key tool is masturbation. "Know thyself," Haines explains. "Masturbation is the foundation of sexual self-education. During self-sexing, survivors relearn how to feel fully present in the moment, how not to disappear while having sexual feelings—without all the complications of partner sex. Masturbation allows survivors to experience sexual pleasure on their own terms in their own ways. It provides the gift of sexual self-knowledge, which forms a healthy foundation for coupled sex."

Haines's program of guided masturbation is similar to the program sex therapists use to teach nonabused preorgasmic women how to have orgasms. Both put the women in control and encourage them to discover their own sexuality at their own pace. Many survivors have difficulty with orgasm. For them, the solo sex program is even more crucial.

Unfortunately, self-pleasuring may trigger flashbacks. When they strike, Davis advises, "Open your eyes. Ground yourself in the present. Understand that even if it conjures up painful memories, touching yourself or being touched by a lover is not abuse. Tell yourself it's your right to receive loving touch, that it's pleasurable, and you deserve pleasure."

Ten Steps to Healing Masturbation

(Adapted from *Healing Sex: A Mind-Body Approach to Healing Sexual Trauma* by Staci Haines)

1. **Schedule it.** Compared with most men, most women engage in less solo sex, particularly abuse survivors. If necessary, work with a therapist to overcome any reluctance. Then mark your calendar. Schedule regular self-sexing. How often? Discuss it with your therapist.

2. **Create a nurturing setting.** Arrange flowers. Play music. Light candles. Set the thermostat so the room is warm. To enhance nongenital touch, use a massage lotion. To enrich genital play, keep lubricant handy. And if you enjoy erotica and sex toys, have them close by.

3. **Breathe slowly and deeply.** Deep breathing is profoundly relaxing and fundamental to satisfying sex. When erotically aroused, breathing naturally deepens. But many abuse survivors feel uncomfortable with breathing deeply. Give yourself permission. Inhale and exhale slowly and fully. Focus on exhaling each breath completely. If you feel yourself tensing, continue to breathe deeply, focusing on extended exhalations.

4. **Make some noise.** Let yourself moan and groan. Vocalizing fosters deep diaphragmatic breathing. It also reinforces arousal. If walls are thin and you feel constrained, turn up the music.

5. **Move your whole body.** Don't just lie still and move your hand. Move your hips. Rock your pelvis. Arch your back. Curl your toes. For survivors who were pinned down during abuse, moving helps loosen the hold of those memories.

6. **Touch your whole body.** Mention self-sexing, and many people envision only genital play. But the entire body—every square inch—can become sensually aroused. Start by caressing your scalp and work all the way down to your toes, saving your genitals for last. Whole-body caressing feels marvelous and prepares the mind and body to enjoy genital touch.

7. **Stay present.** Fight dissociation. Work to remain present. One effective tool is self-talk: *I'm touching my neck. My neck feels soft and warm and a little ticklish. . . .* Describe your feelings as you explore your whole body. If you start to dissociate, refocus on steps 3–6.

8. **Vary self-touch.** Don't fall into self-touching ruts. Mix it up. Vary your strokes from light to firm. Change the order of what you caress and vary what touches you: fingers (with and without lubricant), your palm, a feather, silk, a vibrator.

9. **Enjoy erotic fantasies.** The most popular involve sex with someone other than your regular partner. In fantasy everything is permitted and nothing is wrong, even fantasies of being forced.

10. **Consider audiovisual aids.** Men often masturbate to porn. Women may prefer music or female-produced erotic stories, podcasts, or videos. Search "women's erotica."

Rediscovering Partner Lovemaking

Self-sexing begins the process of sexual self-rediscovery, but survivors' biggest challenge is returning to partner play. One key, at least for a while, is for survivors to control it. That way they know they're not victimized. However, this can be very difficult for survivors' lovers, who may not feel comfortable surrendering all control. Be patient. Over time, survivors' need for total control subsides and sex usually becomes more reciprocal.

Flashbacks may feel frightening. So may the situational triggers that pull survivors back into the dark well of past abuse. Haines advises using flashbacks as tools in healing: "Suppose the abuse involved the survivor's father on top of her. Having her husband in the same position might trigger flashbacks. Some survivors tell the husband: 'I can't have you on top of me—ever.' But most survivors have lots of triggers. If they orchestrate their sex lives to avoid every one they can't have sex at all."

Instead of avoiding triggers, Haines urges survivors to *embrace* them: "Don't shut down when they bubble up. Think: *Okay, my husband is on top of me. I'm triggered, thinking about my uncle. I'm slipping back into the past. I'm not present here and now. But instead of avoiding this type of sex, I'm going to turn into this trigger and really feel it.*"

Embracing flashback triggers is emotionally similar to confronting any fear: The more you face it, the easier it becomes. Over time, triggers lose their ability to traumatize. "Eventually," Haines explains, "survivors arrive at a place where their abuse-related emotions no longer control them or limit their sex lives. It's a place where survivors can honestly say: 'In the past, I was a victim, but I'm not anymore. In the past, sex was used against me. It isn't anymore. Today, sex can feel pleasurable.'"

University of British Columbia researchers enrolled twenty survivors in a cognitive behavioral therapy (CBT) program that helped them reframe their stories away from abuse toward recovery and personal empowerment. Half the group also learned mindfulness meditation (MM), which focuses on nonjudgmental awareness of the present moment. At the end of the month-long study, both groups reported less sexual distress, but those who learned MM reported greater relief.

The Stages of Recovery

(Adapted from *The Courage to Heal* by Ellen Bass and Laura Davis)

Individual survivors may not traverse all stages of recovery, but this list summarizes the process:

- **Realization.** Emotional turmoil as suppressed abuse memories surface.
- **Recalling.** For those who did not suppress their memories, recalling involves getting in touch with how it felt. For those who suppressed their memories, it involves facing both the past and their feelings about it.
- **Believing it happened.** Survivors often doubt their own memories, especially when family members say, *You're crazy. He wouldn't.*
- **Speaking up.** The beginning of healing often involves discussing the abuse with friends, family, therapists, and lovers.
- **Not your fault.** Children often believe they bring sexual abuse on themselves. Actually, the abuser is to blame.
- **Grief.** Grieving is part of healing. It allows survivors to experience what they've lost: innocence, trust of others, trust in themselves.
- **Anger.** A key element in healing is the ability to get angry at the abuser.

- **Confronting the abuser.** This is not for everyone. But for some survivors, it can be a powerful healer.
- **Self-forgiveness.** Some survivors never forgive their abusers. Others eventually do. Whichever survivors choose, it's crucial for them to forgive themselves for any role they feel they played in the abuse and anything they regret they did to survive it.
- **Resolution.** Over time, with emotional work and professional therapy, feelings of victimization eventually subside. Survivors come to terms with their abuse and with those on its periphery, usually family members. Survivors can't change what happened, but ultimately, they arrive at a place where it neither controls nor haunts them. They feel healed.

How Men Can Help Survivors Recover
(Based on *Allies in Healing* by Laura Davis)

If 15 percent of women experience childhood sexual abuse, men have one chance in seven of involvement with survivors. It's challenging and those relationships may not last, but men can help survivors recover.

Expect a period of sexual rejection. Survivors often can't stand the thought of sex or just go through the motions without joy, connection, or orgasm. Laura Davis, author of *Allies in Healing: When the Person You Love Was Sexually Abused as a Child*, explains, "Partners always tell me they can't stand being sexually rejected when they had nothing to do with the abuse. I ask them: 'Do you want to make love with someone who isn't there? Someone totally disconnected from you?' They always say, 'I guess not.'"

When men support survivors' recovery with love, understanding, and patience—boatloads of patience—relationship intimacy deepens and eventually lovemaking feels more fulfilling:

- **Control yourself.** Abuse teaches women that men are sexually out of control. Stay in control. If abusers are still in survivors' lives, don't even mention revenge. Survivors should make all decisions about contact with their abusers.
- **Learn about it.** Read the books mentioned in this chapter. Try a support group or therapy.
- **Understand the risks.** As survivors struggle through recovery, it may be difficult to deal with them. Your relationship may not survive. That's sad, but fairly common.
- **Go slow.** Understand that for a while, survivors must be in total control of their sexual frequency and repertoire. This may last longer than you'd like.
- **You can't heal survivors or "make" them enjoy sex.** They must heal themselves. Your job is to provide encouragement and emotional support. Ask how they feel, then really listen. You can't manage their recovery. All you can do is get out of their way.
- **The sex versus the woman.** Survivors need to know you care about *them* more than you care about sex with them. Say that often.
- **Brace yourself.** Survivors often become maddeningly self-absorbed with recovery. This is part of the process. It can also be hard to live with.
- **Be honest about your feelings.** No doubt during survivors' recovery process, you'll feel impatient, frustrated, and rejected. It's okay to feel that way and say so. But never blame survivors. Always blame the abuse.
- **Their call.** It's fine for you to want sex and ask for it. But during recovery, survivors need to be in control.
- **You may become the target of rage.** You're not to blame, but survivors often explode at whoever is handy. Try not to take it personally. Of course, that's very difficult.

- **Offer to explore nonsexual sensuality.** If survivors can't deal with genital sex, experiment with the many other ways you can be physically close: kissing, cuddling, massage, bathing her, showering together.
- **Gently encourage masturbation.** Self-sexing is central to recovery. Don't order survivors into solo sex. Instead, remind them that you support it. If they don't feel comfortable with partner sex, you might each stroke yourselves while watching one another. You might also suggest vibrator shopping, or buy your survivor a vibe or two.
- **Develop signals for flashbacks and dissociation.** Survivors are likely to experience both. Either can derail lovemaking. When you return to partner sex, develop signals so survivors can communicate feeling triggered. If they signal stop, suspend sex and ask how they want to proceed. They may need to get out of bed or continue but with nongenital caresses or just being held—whatever. Honor their wishes.
- **Stop!** Survivors may feel they have to end sex right in the middle of it. Let them. Say: "I'm listening. What do you need?"
- **Who? What?** When survivors have flashbacks, ask: "Who are you seeing? What are you feeling? You're safe here with me. I won't do anything you don't want."
- **Help them stay in the present.** Flashbacks happen. Provide reassurance that survivors' memories are real, but they're not what's happening now, that you're not *him*.
- **Check in frequently.** Ask: "Is this okay? Do you want to continue? Or do you need a break?"
- **Get support yourself.** It's not easy being a survivor's boyfriend, fiancé, or husband. Even if you rarely ask for help, in this situation, you may need it. Talk with family and/or friends. Join a support group. Try therapy yourself.
- **Ask for time off from dealing with the abuse.** Initially, many survivors obsess about their abuse and recovery. That's natural but maddening. Ask for periods when they don't discuss it—one day a week, on vacation, whatever works for the two of you.
- **Your tool kit.** To aid survivors, your best tools include information, compassion, flexibility, resourcefulness, humor, knowledge of your own needs and limits, and patience— mountains of patience.

CHAPTER 14:
Age of Consent:
How Old Is Old Enough?

WITHOUT GENUINE CONSENT, any sex is sexual assault, or rape. Lovers must consent freely without pressure, coercion, or incapacitation, and without fear of shaming or retaliation for refusing. Chapter 4 discusses affirmative consent as a key ingredient of sizzling sex. This chapter deals with the long and winding historical road to current age-of-consent legislation and its implications for contemporary sexuality.

Statutory Rape Laws: Exceptions to the Exceptions

In 1970 at age twenty, I fell in love with a wonderful young woman of seventeen. More than four decades later, we're still together, with two adult children and a grandson. Anne and I were lucky our paths crossed in Michigan, where the age of consent, the minimum age for legal lovemaking, was sixteen. Had we lived in any of the dozen states where it was eighteen, I might have landed in prison for statutory rape.

If you think this never happens, think again. The FBI estimates that US law enforcement agencies process fifteen thousand statutory rape complaints annually. More than 95 percent involve cases like Anne's and mine, adult men and minor women. A few involve abuse or assault, but the vast majority are consensual. In some, the underage girls are the initiators and pursuers. And some men go to prison:

- In 2015, an Idaho judge sentenced twenty-one-year-old John Polomo to fourteen years for consensual sex with a friend who was seventeen.
- In 2008 in Florida, twenty-two-year-old Morris Williams was imprisoned for having consensual sex with Alisha Dean, whose Facebook page said she was nineteen. He didn't know she was actually thirteen.
- In 1997, a Rhode Island judge sentenced twenty-one-year-old Dylan Healy to twelve years for having consensual sex with thirteen-year-old Heather Kowalski, who ran away from home to live with him, testified in his defense, railed at his sentencing, and swore that upon his release, she would marry him.

The girls never contacted police. It was always their parents.

Examples like these have disturbed state legislatures, which have tempered most age-of-consent laws with exceptions. Here's one that lasted until after World War II. For statutory rape to stick, victims had to be "chaste." If defendants, overwhelmingly men, could produce witnesses swearing that girls were promiscuous, charges could be dismissed. The last state to repeal this exception only did so in 1998.

Currently, most states have "close-in-age" exceptions that allow two minors or a minor and an adult to have legal sex if their ages are within four years of each other. Anne and I are three years apart. Had Michigan's age of consent been eighteen, this exception would have saved me.

But in most states, there's an exception to the close-in-age exception. If the older lover has authority over the younger—teacher-student, coach-player, military officer-recruit—sex is verboten. Age-of-consent laws show that society considers some people "too young" for sex. But the exceptions—and the exceptions to the exceptions—show how convoluted this issue can be.

Romeo's Juliet Was Thirteen

How old is old enough? Scripture says sex is all about procreation. If we embrace the biblical view, people are "too young" if they can't produce viable sperm or eggs.

Boys start making sperm at puberty, typically age eleven to thirteen. Biblically speaking, they may consent to sex around twelve.

Procreation readiness is more complicated for girls. They don't reliably release eggs until a year or so after their first menstrual periods (menarche). In 1800 in the US and Western Europe, that occurred around sixteen, so their biblical age of consent would have been around seventeen.

However, over the past 150 years, for reasons not entirely understood, age at menarche has fallen. Today, around 7 percent of American girls begin menstruating by eleven and more than 90 percent have periods by fourteen. Median menarche occurs around twelve, so biblically speaking, girls are "too young" until after around thirteen.

But throughout history, religious dictums have played only a minor role in governing sexual initiation. The Roman emperor Flavius Augustus (AD 359–83) decreed that children could legally consent to marriage, and therefore sex, at seven. The first age-of-consent law, the English Statute of Westminster (1275), declared it a misdemeanor to "ravish" a maiden with or without her consent until she was twelve. The law's intent was not to safeguard girls, but rather to protect their fathers from losing valuable property: their daughters' virginity.

In *Romeo and Juliet* (1594), the young heroine was all of thirteen years old. The play never specifies Romeo's age, but scholars generally peg it at sixteen. Juliet can't wait to bed her guy. "Romeo . . . leap to these arms . . . and learn me how to lose a winning match." Translation: *By losing my virginity, I win you.*

By the eighteenth century the European age of consent was twelve, except in France, where it was eleven. In 1875, England raised it to thirteen.

The "White-Slavery" Panic

In the medieval world, a tiny minority of nobles exerted near-absolute power over their many peasant farm workers. Fieldwork was backbreaking, but in addition, many peasant girls and women (and some boys and men) also toiled on their backs.

This was droit du seigneur, "the right of the lord," the feudal custom that gave the nobility the right to have their way with their peasant subjects, notably brides on their wedding nights. It's not clear how often the gentry crashed wedding parties, but throughout history, rich, powerful men have generally considered subordinate women their sexual playthings with full legal impunity. In colonial America, an estimated 20 percent of maidservants gave birth to children fathered by their employers, either by rape or voluntarily to improve the women's social positions or some combination of the two.

During the mid-1700s, England spearheaded the Industrial Revolution. Within a century, tens of thousands of peasants had migrated to England's burgeoning factory cities. Like Oliver

Twist, they labored under deplorable conditions that for many girls and women (and some boys and men) included sex with their employers—rape or voluntarily or mixed circumstances.

The Industrial Revolution caused social upheaval. Traditional agricultural norms lost their hold and as factory cities absorbed hordes of new residents, urban sex work surged and became more visible. Poverty or pimps coerced some girls and women into selling sex. Others faced more complex choices. They could toil away twelve hours a day in hellish factories for next to nothing while contending with employers' sexual demands. Or they could quit factory work for sex work. Prostitution was degrading and dangerous, but to some young women, it was preferable, providing a modicum of self-determination unavailable in the few other occupations open to women.

Meanwhile, partly in reaction to the woes of the Industrial Revolution, the period from 1800 to 1850 saw the rise of Romanticism in philosophy and the arts. Romantics held that children were not junior adults, but innocents who lived "natural" lives until contact with the adult world corrupted them. By the 1870s, English Romantic social reformers had become appalled by the prevalence of child prostitution and agitated to stop it.

Their efforts bore fruit—in 1885, the *Pall Mall Gazette*, a London tabloid, published one of the most influential exposés in journalism history, W. T. Stead's "The Maiden Tribute of Modern Babylon," an investigation of English child prostitution. The series alleged that myriad virgin girls had become "white slaves," kidnapped by pimps or sold by desperate parents, then forced into sexual slavery that few survived. The allegations triggered one of the greatest moral panics in history.

The series contained a germ of truth. Some young girls were, indeed, trafficked for sex. But as Eric Berkowitz explains in his authoritative *Sex and Punishment: Four Thousand Years of Judging Desire*, crusaders against "white slavery" vastly exaggerated the number of sex-trafficked girls.

Despite the exposé's questionable figures, reformers demanded that England raise its age of consent from thirteen to sixteen. In Parliament, the battle was hard fought. Many aristocratic members objected to what they called misguided usurpation of men's traditional sexual prerogatives over pubescent girls. But eventually, England raised its age of consent to sixteen.

Across the Atlantic, American newspapermen learned that "The Maiden Tribute" had been a circulation and advertising bonanza. Looking around their own rapidly industrializing cities, they discovered a plague of child sex work. Their similar exposés prodded state legislatures to raise the age of consent throughout the US from around twelve (in Delaware, seven) to sixteen. As of 2020:

- Thirty-one states and the District of Columbia peg age of consent at sixteen.
- In eight states, it's seventeen—Colorado, Illinois, Louisiana, Missouri, New Mexico, New York, Texas, and Wyoming.
- And in eleven, it's eighteen—Arizona, California, Delaware, Florida, Idaho, North Dakota, Oregon, Tennessee, Utah, Virginia, and Wisconsin.

The Detour around Age of Consent: Child Marriage

Raising the age of consent left one big loophole: wedding rings legally entitled husbands to consummate their marriages no matter their brides' ages. As of 2020, more than half the states have no statutory minimum age for marriage. However, most require parental and/or judicial consent for marriages before sixteen:

- **No statutory minimum**: Arizona, Arkansas, California, Colorado, Connecticut, Delaware, Florida, Idaho, Kentucky, Louisiana, Maine, Michigan, Mississippi, Missouri, Nevada, New Jersey, New Mexico, Ohio, Oklahoma, Pennsylvania, Rhode Island, Tennessee, Texas, Washington, West Virginia, Wyoming
- **Thirteen**: New Hampshire (for girls)
- **Fourteen**: Alaska, New Hampshire (for boys), North Carolina
- **Fifteen**: Hawaii, Indiana, Kansas, Maryland, Utah
- **Sixteen**: Alabama, DC, Georgia, Illinois, Iowa, Massachusetts, Minnesota, Montana, North Dakota, South Carolina, South Dakota, Vermont, Virginia, Wisconsin
- **Seventeen**: Nebraska, New York, Oregon

If you think child marriages are a thing of the past, think again. From 2000 to 2010, before New York raised its minimum age from fourteen to seventeen, 3,900 minors married. Most of these nuptials were arranged by parents whose religions or cultural traditions embraced the practice. Forty percent of these child marriages involved someone, usually the woman, who was fourteen or fifteen.

Currently, several states are reconsidering their age-at-marriage laws in an effort to bring them in line with their age-of-consent statutes.

Cougar-Cub Sex: Is It Child Abuse?

If thirty-year-old men bed twelve-year-old girls, the former are pedophiles, the latter are victims, and most Americans would happily lock the men up. But if thirty-year-old women (cougars) dance prone with twelve-year-old boys (cubs), are they pedophiles?

Legally, yes. Women involved sexually with minor boys are pedophiles, felons. But the vast majority of men with histories of cougar-cub relationships believe there's nothing wrong with them. In one study, almost two-thirds of adult men who, as minors, had sex with significantly older adult women felt fine about it. Many expressed *gratitude* for their sexual initiation and the erotic lessons they'd learned. Of those who felt less than positive, 33 percent felt neutral. Only 5 percent said they'd been abused.

Despite how former cubs feel, judges feel differently. In 1996, Mary Kay Letourneau was a married, thirty-four-year-old elementary school teacher in Burien, Washington, when she began a consensual sexual relationship with her then twelve-year-old student, Vili Fualaau. The following year, she gave birth to their daughter.

Letourneau's husband divorced her over the affair. A relative of his called the police. In a plea bargain, she was sentenced to six months in jail on the condition she never see Fualaau again. A month after her release, police caught them together, and Letourneau was sentenced to seven years in prison.

In 2004 when she was released, Fualaau was a legal adult. He petitioned the court to rescind the no-contact order. His request was granted. The couple married in 2005 and had another child. They divorced in 2019. Letourneau died in 2020.

Until the late 1970s, the legal system typically ignored cougar-cub sexual relationships based on the belief that they caused no harm. Since then, things have changed, but slowly. Compared with adult men, when women get busted for sex with minors, they're much less likely to go to prison and if imprisoned, serve shorter sentences.

How Old Is Old Enough?

Ideally, everyone would share the same sexual values. No one would exploit anyone. Parents would provide children with supportive, practical sex information and young people would take it to heart. All children would mature at the same rate and intoxicants, poverty, racism, surging hormones, thrill seeking, and peer pressure would not affect their sexual decision-making.

Alas, our world is quite different. Consequently, age of consent is certain to remain controversial.

CHAPTER 15:
Teen Pregnancies Have Plummeted, But School Sex Education Doesn't Work—Huh?

I SPENT MUCH OF the 1970s working in family planning, often speaking to middle and high school students. I focused on the boys, urging them to use condoms, which, when used intelligently, reliably prevent both pregnancy and sexually transmitted infections (STIs). It was a tough sell. This was years before AIDS made condoms a household term, long before pharmacies displayed them openly. The boys parroted the myth that "rubbers" destroy men's pleasure—*like showering in a raincoat.*

"Really?" I asked. "Imagine you and your girlfriend are at the movies. She leans over and starts rubbing your crotch . . ." Nervous titters. "Then she unzips you . . ." Laughter. "I bet you're getting tangled up in your shorts *right now.*" Guffaws.

"Your pants and underwear are *five hundred times* thicker than any condom. No one has even touched you and you're getting hard. Really, guys, how much sensation can condoms block?"

Eyes widened.

"In great sex, you touch each other all over. If you touch everything, covering one little part with something as thin as a rubber hardly matters. Condoms aren't like showering in a raincoat. They're like showering *with a ring on one finger.* And if you carry condoms and offer to use them, you'll impress your girlfriend—and just might get lucky."

Then I produced a box of condoms and offered them for free. The boys cleaned me out. I believed I'd made an impression.

But I accomplished little, if anything.

Forced to Reconsider

Fast-forward forty years, and dozens of studies with hundreds of thousands of adolescent participants show that school-based sex education programs do not work. They have no impact on teen sexual activity. That goes for both conservatives' insistence on abstinence until marriage and liberals' so-called "comprehensive" agenda—what I taught. Neither significantly reduces teen sexual frequency, pregnancies, or STIs.

Wet Dreams: Totally Normal

Many teen boys are surprised to awaken from erotic dreams with sticky goo in their pajamas. They've had wet dreams, nocturnal emissions. Wet dreams typically occur periodically from young men's teens through their twenties. Then they fade. Wet dreams are a normal part of male adolescence and young adulthood, and nothing to worry about.

Now, over the past several decades, a few programs have shown modest pregnancy reductions. They're outliers. The vast majority show no delay in sexual initiation and no impact on pregnancies or STIs. When the few promising pilot programs have been rolled out to more teens, replication efforts have failed.

Meanwhile, I spent much of the 1990s into the 2000s parenting two teens, a boy and a girl. I discussed sex and contraception with them—until they rolled their eyes and fled.

Around this time, I became aware of the substantial research literature showing that adolescents' most effective sex educators are their *parents*. I found this hard to believe. My kids seemed to ignore me. Actually, they were sponges.

The research is quite consistent. When parents speak up about their sexual values, whatever they may be, teens feel acknowledged as sexual beings and don't feel they have to prove it by being reckless. They become more likely to delay first intercourse. In addition, when they finally go all the way, they're more likely to use condoms the first time and ever after. Teens want to hear about sex from their parents, and most listen.

> ### "Don't Think About It"
> Many social and religious conservatives admonish their children not to think about sex. This often backfires. An Israeli researcher surveyed the frequency of sexual thoughts among 1,500 Israeli adolescents, some secular, others ultra-Orthodox Jews. The latter reported thinking about sex significantly more.

Surprise! Today's Teens Are Sexually Conservative
Social liberals and conservatives both rail about the "teen sex crisis." If there ever was one, it has abated:

- According to the National Center for Health Statistics, as of 2018, births to teens have dropped 55 percent since 2007 and 70 percent since 1991. Over the past few years, births to teens have inched back up a bit, but the rate is still substantially below a generation ago, when today's parents were horny teens.
- In 1991, 54 percent of teens age fifteen to nineteen said they'd had intercourse. Today, it's 41 percent, a drop of 13 percent.

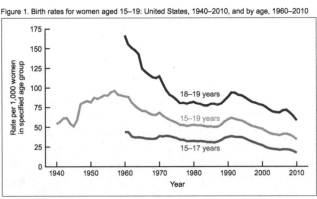
Figure 1. Birth rates for women aged 15–19: United States, 1940–2010, and by age, 1960–2010

NOTE: Data for 2010 are preliminary.
SOURCE: CDC/NCHS, National Vital Statistics System.

- In 1991, 10 percent of thirteen-year-olds reported intercourse. Today, it's 3 percent, down by two-thirds.
- In 1991, 46 percent of sexually active teens said they'd used condoms the last time they had intercourse. Today, it's 59 percent, up 13 percent.
- Since 1991, the teen gonorrhea rate has dropped 69 percent.

Today's teens are *less* sexually active than their parents and grandparents were as teens. Who deserves credit? Both conservatives and liberals have rushed to claim it. Both are mistaken.

What Sexually Active Teens Actually Do

For all the hand-wringing about teen sex, surprisingly few studies have explored what "sexually active" really means. Fortunately, Indiana University researchers surveyed 932 teens age fourteen to nineteen (482 girls, 450 boys):

Among boys, by age fifteen:
- 68 percent admitted masturbating.
- 6 percent said they'd received or provided genital hand massage.
- 13 percent reported having received fellatio.
- 8 percent stated they'd provided cunnilingus.
- 10 percent said they'd had vaginal intercourse.
- 4 percent claimed participation in anal play.

Among boys, by age nineteen:
- 86 percent admitted self-sexing.
- 49 percent said they'd received or provided hand jobs.
- 59 percent reported having received fellatio.
- 61 percent stated they'd provided cunnilingus.
- 63 percent said they'd participated in vaginal intercourse.
- 10 percent reported experience with anal play.

Among girls, by age fifteen:
- 43 percent admitted solo sex.
- 9 percent said they'd received or provided genital hand massage.
- 10 percent reported having received cunnilingus.
- 13 percent stated they'd provided fellatio.
- 12 percent said they'd experienced vaginal intercourse.
- 4 percent claimed they'd played anally.

Among girls, by age nineteen:
- 66 percent admitted masturbating.
- 39 percent said they'd received or provided hand jobs.
- 62 percent reported having received cunnilingus.
- 61 percent stated they'd provided fellatio.
- 64 percent said they'd had vaginal intercourse.
- 20 percent claimed experience with anal sex.

Many people, both liberals and conservatives, see calamity in these numbers. *Fourteen-year-old girls having anal sex!* Some do, but very few. Like children for millennia, many of today's teens have histories of childhood sex play, and some have been abused. It's no surprise that as puberty unfolds and hormones rage, many teens proceed to closer approximations of adult sex. While some adults fret that 11 percent of fifteen-year-olds have joined genitals, this means that 89 percent have not.

Compared with men, women of all ages are considerably less likely to receive oral sex. Lack of clitoral kisses is the main reason why fewer women than men have orgasms. The findings above show one welcome development. While fifteen-year-old boys continue to receive more oral sex than they provide, nineteen-year-old boys now provide as much as they receive. Let's hope it's a trend.

Sexual Individuation Continues . . .

Individuation, the process of creating one's own unique identity, begins in childhood. More than half of kids engage in childhood sex play, but somewhat less than half don't. Sexual individuation continues during the teen years as young people ponder their sexual orientation (exclusively heterosexual or not) and their erotic sensibilities (conventional or not). By the end of high school around half have shed their virginity.

Teen sexuality may or may not predict their adult sex. Some wild teens become sexually conservative adults. And some prudish teens become highly sexual adults who embrace unconventional play.

The Failure of Abstinence-Only Sex Education

Since the 1990s, Congress has allocated more than $1 billion to abstinence-only school sex education, which exhorts young people to just say no until their wedding nights. Social conservatives claim that abstinence-only has been a huge success—proven by plummeting teen pregnancies. However:

- Abstinence-only programs began in earnest in 1998. But teen pregnancies began to fall in 1992, six years earlier.
- Abstinence-only is most deeply entrenched in the South. It's less popular elsewhere. Figures from the Centers for Disease Control and Prevention (CDC) show that the teen birth rate is highest in the South.
- Many abstinence-only programs ask teens to sign pledges swearing to remain virgins until marriage. But a CDC study shows that only 12 percent of those who take virginity vows keep them—a failure rate of 88 percent.
- Researchers at McMaster University in Hamilton, Ontario, analyzed twenty-six studies of school-based pregnancy-prevention efforts. With abstinence-only, pregnancies often *increased*.
- University of Georgia researchers analyzed trends in teen pregnancies in all fifty states and found that as states increased their emphasis on abstinence-only sex education, their teen pregnancy rates *rose*. "Abstinence-only sex education is ineffective in preventing teen pregnancy and may actually contribute to it."

The Failure of "Comprehensive" Sex Education

Liberals claim comprehensive sex education is the reason teen pregnancies and STIs have fallen so dramatically. Actually:

- The just-mentioned McMaster University analysis of twenty-six studies included many comprehensive programs. They had zero impact on teens: no delay of first intercourse, no increased use of contraceptives, and no fewer pregnancies or STIs.
- British researchers analyzed eight studies of comprehensive school-based pregnancy- and STI-prevention programs involving 55,157 teens. Before-and-after statistics showed no reductions in pregnancies or STIs.
- Italian researchers surveyed 559 high school students before and after school sex education courses. Afterward, they knew more about contraception and STIs—but did not curtail risky sexual practices.
- In 2016, the *American Journal of Public Health* published a supplement devoted to rigorous evaluations of US comprehensive teen pregnancy-prevention programs, most school based, with some at Boys and Girls Clubs. The fifteen studies involved more than sixty thousand teens at 250 sites in two hundred cities and evaluated large-scale rollouts of pilot programs that had appeared promising. The results were, at best, poor:
  - Only two programs (13 percent) showed any decline in teen sex, pregnancies, or STIs—and those decreases were a trivial 2 percent.
  - Two programs (13 percent) showed no less sex and no fewer pregnancies and STIs among white and African American teens, but a slight decrease in Hispanic teens.
  - The large majority of studies (74 percent) showed that comprehensive programs have no impact on teen sex, pregnancies, or STIs.
  - Comprehensive school-based sex education has contributed little, if anything, to the huge drop in teen pregnancies over the past generation.

Do Condom Giveaways Spur Teen Promiscuity?

Many conservatives believe so, but a University of Washington study shows differently. The researchers tracked 4,018 sexually active teens over nine years. Compared with non-users, condom users had virtually the same number of partners. The main difference— the condom users contracted fewer STIs.

Success! Parents Discussing Sex with Teens

AIDS was identified in 1981 and by the end of that decade had become a nightmare as the disease, then almost always fatal, became a significant public health threat. Parents feared for their children's lives, and many who'd never uttered a peep about sex and condoms spoke up. These discussions had major impact. Teen pregnancies peaked in 1991 and have declined 70 percent since.

In the current century, AIDS has largely dropped from the headlines, and some parents have stopped talking. Consequently, the teen pregnancy rate has inched up a bit, but it's still more than two-thirds below where it was during the late twentieth century.

A mountain of research confirms the effectiveness of parental sex education. It shows that mothers have tremendous impact on girls' sexuality. Fathers have considerable effect on boys. And when fathers are absent or silent, mothers also have significant impact on their sons:

- University of Oklahoma scientists surveyed 1,083 teens (half girls, half boys). When parents discussed sex and contraception, "Teens were much less likely to have intercourse, and if youth were sexually active, they were significantly more likely to use birth control."
- University of Minnesota researchers interviewed 2,006 teens, age fourteen and fifteen, who said they were virgins. One year later, 16 percent of the girls and 11 percent of the boys reported intercourse. Among the 84 and 89 percent who didn't, the strongest predictor was frequent discussion of sex and birth control with their mothers.
- Atlanta scientists interviewed 522 sexually active African American teens age fourteen to eighteen. Compared with those whose parent(s) did not discuss sex, teens whose parent(s) did were twice as likely to use condoms and/or other contraceptives. They were also three times more likely to raise the issue with their partners.
- Columbia University investigators surveyed 130 sexually active teen girls. "Among our most striking findings—open, positive, parent-teen sexuality communication is a strong predictor of regular contraceptive use." And the discussions did not spur promiscuity.
- CDC researchers interviewed 372 teens, age fourteen to seventeen, in New York, Alabama, and Puerto Rico. Some talked with their mothers about sex, STIs, and contraception, others did not. The former were three times more likely to use condoms during first intercourse and *three times* more likely to use condoms regularly. Those using them their first time were *ten times* more likely to have used them during their most recent partner sex, and *twenty times* more likely to become regular users.
- Finally, researchers at North Carolina State University analyzed fifty-two studies of home sex education involving more than twenty-five thousand teens over thirty-two years (1982–2014). Eleven reports (21 percent) showed little benefit, but in forty-one (79 percent), when parents discussed sex, teens remained virgins significantly longer. When they became sexually active, they had less sex and were much more likely to use condoms. "Parent-adolescent sexual communication increases adolescents' use of contraceptives regardless of how parents deliver their messages."

Note the final phrase, "regardless of how parents deliver their messages." As mentioned in chapter 12, to discuss sexuality, parents need not be sex experts, psychologists, or health professionals. And they don't have to be articulate. They just have to *try*—and keep trying.

From "Dangers-of-Sex" Education to Sex Education Based on Pleasure

Social liberals and conservatives appear to hold polar opposite views of sex education. Actually, they're Romeo and Juliet, from clashing clans but in bed together. The two sides share a core belief that unites them more than anything divides them—the idea that for teens, sex is *dangerous*.

It certainly can be. During the 1980s and '90s, my hometown, San Francisco, lost more than twenty thousand residents to AIDS, including my letter carrier, barber, next-door neighbor's

Almost All Americans Have Sex before Marriage

A researcher with the Planned Parenthood–affiliated Guttmacher Institute analyzed 2003 data from the CDC's ongoing National Survey of Family Growth, which combines face-to-face interviews with anonymous surveys. Americans reporting intercourse before marriage—more than 95 percent.

brother, and more than a dozen acquaintances and friends of friends. For a while, it seemed every social event was a funeral.

In response, San Francisco instituted one of the nation's most comprehensive, no-nonsense sex-education programs in grades five, six, and seven. My children were taught the curriculum. It included frank discussion of all contraceptives, with a big emphasis on condoms. It also included a parade of guest speakers, young adult women who'd had children as teens. They minced no words about the magnitude of their mistakes.

Still, one day my son announced there was only one 100 percent effective contraceptive—abstinence.

Nonsense, I replied. Another method is 100 percent effective, absolutely free, available to everyone, and fun—lovemaking without intercourse: hand jobs and oral sex.

But even in San Francisco, with one of the nation's most comprehensive sex-education programs, the curriculum never mentioned it. Doing so would have acknowledged sexual pleasure, undermining the core message of school sex education—that doing it is *perilous*.

Liberal or conservative, abstinence only or comprehensive, schools don't offer "sex education," but "dangers-of-sex" education. So-called "comprehensive" programs are inclusive only in that they discuss all contraceptives, not just abstinence.

School programs completely ignore what really interests teens—how to get it on. There's no mention of kissing, caressing, mutual massage, negotiating erotic escalation (other than saying "no"), and tragically, rarely a word about the clitoris's importance to women's sexual pleasure and satisfaction. Imagine if driver education ignored driving and just taught students how to fasten seat belts—then put them behind the wheel. That's school sex education in a nutshell.

Of course, even woefully inadequate school sex education is a political hot potato. No public schools could get away with teaching actual lovemaking skills (part I). Many, if not most, liberals and virtually all conservatives would oppose it.

Welcome to Sex Ed Class—For *Parents*

Recent federal budgets have allocated hundreds of millions of dollars to school-based sex education—both abstinence-only and comprehensive. What a waste.

It would be much more cost-effective to abolish school sex education and invest the money in evening and weekend classes *for parents*—to help them crystallize their own sexual values, whatever they may be, and discuss them more effectively with their children.

Conservatives have long argued that, because it involves values, sex education belongs in the home. They're right—not just because parents control the message, but because home-based sex education is the only approach that actually works:

- Penn State researchers gauged family sex conversations by surveying fifty eleven- to fifteen-year-olds and their mothers. Then the mothers took two brief classes on discussing sexual issues. Afterward, both mothers and children said it was easier to talk about sex.
- Scientists at Emory University in Atlanta recruited 582 mothers, average age thirty-eight, mostly single African Americans, into a program that encouraged sex discussions with their adolescent children. The researchers tracked the families for two years. Compared with controls, the mothers in the program "showed substantial increases in comfort talking about sex, and surveys of their children showed increased use of condoms."

The Best Book to Give Teens

Welcome-to-puberty books are usually lame. Most repeat all the errors found in sperm-and-egg books (chapter 12). They generally focus on mollifying parents (who buy them) rather than empowering adolescents to discover—and enjoy—their emerging sexuality, whatever it may involve.

Older adolescents with decent reading comprehension should have no problem with this book. Parents, if you can't bring yourself to give it to your teens, *hide it* where they'll find it. But this book may prove daunting to younger or less literate teens.

Fortunately, one book written expressly for teens stands head and shoulders above the rest—*S.E.X.: The All-You-Need-To-Know Sexuality Guide to Get You through Your Teens and Twenties* by Heather Corinna, founder of Scarleteen.com, which has provided accessible, accurate, inclusive, sex-positive sex and relationship information to young people since 1998. *S.E.X.* is by far the best sex book written expressly for adolescents.

What I Told My Two Teens

Conservatives have every right to tell their children to abstain from sex until marriage. Their kids are almost certain to ignore that message, but when parents discuss sex with adolescents, the message matters less than the discussions. By raising the issue, parents acknowledge their children's sexuality, which boosts kids' self-esteem, helps them feel grown up, and reduces the temptation to prove they're sexual by involvement in pregnancies. As a social liberal, I exhort conservative parents to share their sexual values with their children. Say whatever you like, just please speak up.

It wasn't *easy*, but I spoke up. I told my kids it was entirely up to them to decide when and how they became sexual. I said I hoped they'd wait until they were at least sixteen, but the decision was theirs. Then I explained that when they crossed that bridge, I hoped their play included four elements: consent, condoms, lubrication, and pleasure.

- **Consent.** No shaming, pressure, or coercion *ever* at any step up the erotic ladder. I said if you ever feel uncomfortably pressed, do whatever it takes to extricate yourself. Feel free to call me any time, twenty-four seven. I'll move heaven and earth to help you.
- **Condoms.** I offered to supply as many condoms as my kids wanted. When used carefully, condoms virtually eliminate risk of pregnancy and STIs.
- **Lubrication.** Vaginal lubrication reduces risk of condom breakage and increases comfort during intercourse, especially for girls. Commercial lubes are inexpensive, take only seconds to apply, and enhance comfort. I offered to supply it.
- **Pleasure.** Sizzling sex depends not only on mutual desire, but on pleasure. Who can enjoy getting it on with a lover who ignores the real risks of pregnancy and STIs? Safe sex involves more than public health. It's crucial to the deep relaxation necessary for erotic pleasure.

Advertisers sell everything with sexual sizzle. Why not use sizzling sex to sell sexual responsibility? It's one of the few instances where a "sex sell" is actually appropriate.

I told my two teens, "When you feel ready for partner sex, embrace sexual responsibility because it leads to the best sex." My approach might sound radical. But I believe it would further reduce teen pregnancies and STIs. It would also help teens grow up to be something they all want to become—good lovers.

CHAPTER 16:
Men Who Want Sizzling Sex *Must* Participate Fully in Birth Control

SIZZLING SEX REQUIRES deep relaxation. If you're not trying to conceive a child, it's impossible for the vast majority of reproductive-age women—and many men—to relax when they feel anxious about pregnancy.

Sizzling sex also requires trust. The vast majority of women—and many men—can't trust a lover who doesn't care enough about unplanned pregnancy to discuss contraception.

Finally, sizzling sex requires leisurely, playful, whole-body massage, which allows plenty of time to discuss contraception—and do something about it.

Contraception is not the woman's responsibility. It's the *couple's*. Want to get laid, dude? Raise the issue as soon as things heat up. Visit a family planning clinic. Discuss each method's advantages and disadvantages. Decide which one best suits your needs. Then use your chosen method every time.

Most people consider condoms the only "men's" method and all the others "women's." In fact, many contraceptives can be shared—and they work better when both lovers are involved. Women can roll condoms onto men's erections. Men can buy spermicide for diaphragms and fill them. And men can check for IUD strings and help women chart their menstrual cycles. Finally, "outercourse," sex without intercourse, is a completely shared method based on whole-body loveplay, hand jobs, oral sex, toys, and perhaps some kink.

Birth control is not the easiest subject to discuss, particularly for new lovers. But it's easier than talking about sexual frequency or the moves you want in bed. Discussing contraceptives can be excellent practice for negotiating more intimate issues.

Considering contraception doesn't interfere with sexual pleasure any more than slowing down for a turn interferes with enjoyment of driving. It reduces stress, encourages deep relaxation, fosters intimate communication, and builds trust—all of which enhance sex.

This chapter presents a brief overview. For individual counseling and methods, visit a family planning clinic. Most county health departments provide contraceptive services. In addition, Planned Parenthood operates more than six hundred clinics around the US—plannedparenthood.org.

More Effective Than You Might Think
If a method is 90 percent effective, some people believe they are fated to get pregnant one out every ten times they use it during sex. No.

Effectiveness rates are based on "100 couple-years." A "couple-year" is one couple using the method exclusively for one year. If a method is 90 percent effective, ten pregnancies can be expected among 100 couples who use it for twelve months. Assuming sex once a week,

100 couples would make love 5,200 times per year, and experience ten pregnancies, or one pregnancy every 520 times (0.0019 percent). Ninety percent effectiveness isn't perfect, but it's quite effective.

The chart summarizes effectiveness. The high end of the range assumes perfect use. The low end reflects studies of actual use. Methods are listed from least to most technological.

Contraceptive Effectiveness (in 100 couple-years)

Method	Effectiveness
No contraception	15% effective
Calendar rhythm	Not well researched, estimated at 70%–85%.
Outercourse (sex without intercourse)	100%
Withdrawal	78%–96%
Male condom	82%–98%
Female condom	79%–95%
Spermicides	Alone, 72%–94%. With condoms, up to 98%.
Vaginal contraceptive film	Alone, 75%–94%. With condoms, up to 97%.
Diaphragm	88%–94%
Cervical cap	Childless women, 80%–90%. Mothers, 60%–80%.
Sponge	70%–90%
Fertility awareness	80%–99%
Birth control pills	95%–99+%
IUD	99%–99+%
Injected Depo-Provera	94%–99+%
NuvaRing	91%–99%
Evra patch	98%–99%
Nexplanon	99+%
Emergency contraception	First 24 hours, 95%. After 72 hours, 89%.
Male sterilization	99+%
Female sterilization	99+%

Hatcher, R.A., et al. *Contraceptive Technology*. 20th edition. New York: Ardent Media, 2015.

Outercourse (Sex without Vaginal Intercourse)

Couples using outercourse can enjoy kissing, cuddling, mutual whole-body massage, hand jobs, oral sex, anal play, sex toys, and kink—just not vaginal intercourse.

- Effectiveness: 100 percent
- Availability: Anytime, anywhere, for free
- Side Effects: None
- Advantages:
  ○ 100 percent effective
  ○ Available anytime, anywhere
  ○ Free
  ○ No devices
  ○ No doctor or clinic visits
  ○ No side effects
- Disadvantages:
  ○ No vaginal intercourse
  ○ No protection against sexually transmitted infections (STIs) of the throat or anus

Withdrawal (Pulling Out)

The man removes his erection from the vagina before ejaculation. No sperm in the vagina, no risk of pregnancy—*almost*. Pre-ejaculatory fluid may contain sperm. Even if the man withdraws before ejaculating, pregnancy might still occur.

Keep an emergency (morning-after) contraceptive handy just in case (page 121). If the woman gets a copper IUD inserted within five days after unprotected intercourse, her pregnancy risk drops 99 percent (page 117).

- Effectiveness: 78–96 percent
- Availability: Anywhere, anytime, for free
- Side Effects: None
- Advantages:
  ○ Reasonably effective if men have ejaculatory control
  ○ Available anytime, anywhere
  ○ Free
  ○ No devices
  ○ No doctor or clinic visits
  ○ No side effects
- Disadvantages:
  ○ Considerable risk of pregnancy. Pre-ejaculatory fluid may contain sperm.
  ○ The man must pull out before ejaculation
  ○ Requires excellent ejaculatory control
  ○ No protection against STIs

Condoms for Men

Condoms cover erections during intercourse, preventing sperm from entering the vagina.

Three materials are available: latex rubber, lamb intestine, and polyurethane. Latex is cheapest and most widely available.

Many brands have nipples at the tip to catch ejaculate. Some people think the nipples help prevent breakage. Actually, even the most powerful ejaculation can't rupture condoms. Nipples catch ejaculate to keep it from leaking out the base of the condom—and possibly into the vagina.

Condoms are available straight-sided or contoured like erections. Most come dusted with silicone powder lubricant—but not enough to guarantee women's comfort. Consider a water- or silicone-based lubricant. Do not used oil- or petroleum-based lubricants—they eat holes in latex.

Several myths still surround condoms:

Showering in a raincoat. The myth that condoms reduce enjoyment flows from the idea that men's sexual pleasure happens only in the penis during intercourse. But sizzling sex involves whole-body play. In fact, preoccupation with the penis is a major reason why men develop sex problems.

Men who accuse condoms of reducing sensitivity tend to be teens and young adults inexperienced in lovemaking. Indiana University researchers gave a dozen condoms to each of 1,875 men age eighteen or older and asked them to keep daily sex diaries for a month. Those least comfortable were the youngest. As age increased, so did comfort with condoms and enjoyment of sex while using them.

Condom manufacturers claim their brands "deliver" the most sensitivity. Actually, all condoms are about the same. Personal preferences are possible, but condoms don't *deliver* pleasure, lovers *create* it.

Some condoms have ribbed sides that supposedly excite women. But the ribs are virtually imperceptible and don't touch the clitoris.

They interrupt. Some lovers dislike the moment required to unroll condoms. While fiddling with them, some men's erections subside.

Condoms need not interrupt lovemaking. Open the package beforehand. If women roll them on while continuing to caress men's erections, there's no interruption. If erection subsides, relax, breathe deeply, fantasize, and ask your lover for the stimulation you find most arousing. Your erection should return.

They break. That's possible but unlikely and easily prevented. Never store condoms near heat sources—a wallet, pants pocket, or glove box. Heat degrades latex. Open the wrapper before you're in the throes. Roll the condom on slowly. And keep spermicide handy. If condoms break, women should immediately insert spermicide, then obtain emergency contraception (page 121) and follow package directions. Women should *not* douche. Follow these steps and pregnancy is highly unlikely.

Men won't use them. Many young women believe this, often erroneously. Australian researchers surveyed 819 sexually active young adults. The women consistently underestimated the men's willingness to use condoms.

Some women dislike the taste of condoms during fellatio. If you like, try sucking on a Life Saver while sucking your condom-covered man.

Among contraceptives, condoms provide the best protection against STIs. Many couples in new or nonmonogamous relationships who use other methods for contraception also use condoms to prevent STIs.

- Never use a condom whose wrapper has come unsealed.
- Slip it on before you slip it in. Pre-ejaculatory fluid may contain sperm.
- Use condoms with spermicide. This boosts effectiveness.
- Avoid "pull-offs." It's possible for the vaginal lips to pull a condom off the penis. To prevent this, gentleman, don't pump in and out. Press in and use a circular motion. During withdrawal, hold the base of the condom to prevent leaving it—and semen—inside the vagina.
- Discard condoms after one use.
- Effectiveness: 82–98 percent. More effective with spermicide.
- Availability: Over the counter at pharmacies and some convenience stores and supermarkets.
- Side Effects: Possible latex allergy causing redness and irritation. If you notice this, try more lubricant. If irritation persists, you may be allergic. Look for non-latex condoms or use another method.
- Advantages:
  ○ Highly effective when used properly.
  ○ Modest cost.
  ○ Widely available.
  ○ Best protection against STIs.
  ○ No doctor or clinic visits.
  ○ Used only when making love.
  ○ Placement can be incorporated into lovemaking.
  ○ Some men last longer when using condoms.
- Disadvantages:
  ○ If used improperly, significant risk of pregnancy.
  ○ Possible latex allergy.

Both Men and Women Overestimate Their Condom Use

The ongoing General Social Survey (GSS) provides some of the best information about Americans' behavior. In recent GSS surveys, women have said they use condoms during 16 percent of partner lovemaking, which would require 1.1 billion condoms a year. Men tell the GSS that they use 1.6 billion condoms a year. But actual annual US condom sales total only 600 million—well below what both men and woman claim.

Internal Condoms

Internal condoms keep sperm out of the vagina, and may also be used anally to prevent transmissions of sexual infections. Previously called the female condom, internal condoms are disposable polyurethane or nitrile pouches with plastic rings on each end. When inserted into the vagina, one ring covers the cervix. The other rests on the vulva to keep the device from slipping into the vagina. Anal use is similar—one ring inside while the other remains external.

Problems inserting? Consult your family planning provider. Discard them after one use.

- Effectiveness: 79–95 percent. Less effective than male condoms, and some find them harder to use.
- Availability: Over the counter at pharmacies and on the internet

- Side Effects: Allergy and genital irritation are possible.
- Advantages:
  - Highly effective if used properly
  - Modest cost, though more expensive than male condoms
  - Easily available
  - Protects against penis-vagina STI transmission
  - No doctor or clinic visits
  - Used only when making love
  - Placement can be incorporated into lovemaking
  - May be used by those allergic to latex
  - No serious side effects
  - The external plastic ring may provide some clitoral stimulation and heighten the woman's arousal
- Disadvantages:
  - If used improperly, significant risk of pregnancy
  - Possible genital irritation

Spermicides (Foam, Gel, Cream, Film, Suppositories)

Spermicides kill sperm in the vagina. Marketed for use with diaphragms and cervical caps (page 113), they may also be used alone or with condoms (page 109).

Foams come in aerosol containers with plunger applicators. Either lover loads the applicator, inserts it deep into the vagina, then pushes the plunger. To be effective, foam must be inserted no more than one hour before sperm enters the vagina.

Gels and creams should be inserted with fingers or applicator as deep as possible.

Film and suppositories should be placed inside the vagina at least ten to fifteen minutes before intercourse—but no more than two hours—to allow time for dissolving.

Women should not douche after using spermicides. They should not douche at all.

Some couples wonder about spermicides and cunnilingus. With careful use, it's rarely a problem. Spermicides go deep inside the vagina. Men lick the vulva and clitoris, both outside it. However, some spermicide may leak and affect the taste and aroma of the woman's genitals, a possible issue for some men. Ingesting small amounts of spermicide causes no harm.

In addition to killing sperm, spermicides also kill gonorrhea and chlamydia. However, one spermicide, nonoxynol-9, may cause vaginal irritation and minor bleeding, possibly allowing the AIDS/HIV virus into the bloodstream. Few spermicides still contain nonoxynol-9. Check labels.

- Effectiveness: By itself, 72–94 percent. With condoms, up to 98 percent
- Availability: Over the counter at pharmacies and some supermarkets
- Side Effects: If irritation or rash develop, use another method.
- Advantages:
  - Modest cost
  - Available over the counter
  - No doctor or clinic visits
  - Offer some lubrication
  - Used only when making love
  - No serious side effects
  - Reduces risk of some STIs

- Disadvantages:
  - Less effective than many other methods.
  - Some people consider spermicides messy.
  - May irritate genitals.
  - Some men object to the aroma and taste during cunnilingus.

Barrier Contraceptives: Diaphragm, Cervical Cap, and Sponge

Diaphragms are round, dome-shaped, plastic or rubber cups with metal spring rims. They hold spermicide and cover the cervix. Cervical caps are similar but smaller. Sponges are pillow-shaped and preloaded with spermicide.

The diaphragm's spring-like rim allows it to be folded in half for insertion. Once inside the vagina, it covers the cervix, blocking sperm and holding spermicide.

Diaphragms and caps must be professionally fitted. Consult a family planning provider. Childbirth or significant weight gain or loss may necessitate refitting.

Sponges don't require professional fitting. They include spermicide. Diaphragm and cap users must add spermicide every time.

Diaphragms should be left in for at least eight hours after intercourse, but no longer than a day. Extended wear may cause cramping, and increase risk of toxic shock syndrome (TSS, below). Caps may be worn for up to forty-eight hours, but extended wear increases risk of TSS. Sponges should not be worn for more than twenty-four hours.

Before insertion, women should wash hands with soap. Men or women can add the spermicide. During insertion, women should confirm proper placement over the cervix.

Insertion may interrupt lovemaking. Insert the device beforehand.

Men may feel diaphragms or caps during fingering or intercourse.

During deep intercourse, particularly rear entry (doggie style), penises may dislodge caps. Women should check their caps after. If dislodging occurs, men should not insert so deeply.

Diaphragms can last up to several years. Caps should be replaced annually. In doubt about their integrity? Consult your family planning provider. Sponges should be used once, then discarded.

The spermicide used with these devices kills gonorrhea and chlamydia.

- Effectiveness: Diaphragm: 88–94 percent. Cap: childless women, 80–90 percent, mothers, 60–80 percent. Caps do not form tight seals around cervixes that have been stretched during delivery. Sponge: 70–90 percent.
- Availability: Diaphragms and caps, by prescription. Sponges over the counter at pharmacies.
- Side Effects: Possible increased risk of UTI. Slightly increased risk of TSS (below). Women with TSS histories should not use diaphragms or caps.
- Advantages:
  - Modest cost
  - Durable
  - Can be used after forty, when the Pill is generally not recommended
  - Used only when making love
  - Help prevent several STIs
- Disadvantages:
  - Less effective than some other methods

- ◦ Insertion might interrupt lovemaking.
- ◦ Some couples find spermicide messy.
- ◦ Some women have trouble inserting or removing diaphragms and caps.
- ◦ Possible vaginal irritation.
- ◦ Possible allergic reactions to latex or spermicide.
- ◦ Some men dislike feeling the device during fingering or intercourse.
- ◦ Some increased risk of UTI and TSS.

Toxic Shock Syndrome (TSS)

TSS is a sudden, potentially fatal condition caused by the release of toxins from an overgrowth of *Staphylococcus* ("staph") bacteria that live inside many women. During the 1970s, TSS killed several young women who'd used superabsorbent tampons (no longer sold).

Diaphragms and cervical caps pose a small risk of TSS. Women who use them should recognize the signs of TSS and call 911 immediately if they develop:

- Fever and chills
- Vomiting
- Diarrhea
- Dizziness, faintness, and/or weakness
- Sore throat with aching muscles and joints
- Sunburn-like rash

Fertility Awareness

Fertility awareness, also known as natural family planning, the symptom-thermal method, or the Billings ovulation method, is a scientific—and much more reliable—version of the traditional calendar rhythm method. Fertility awareness teaches couples how to recognize the subtle but distinct signs of women's fertile and infertile days each menstrual cycle. This method can be used to prevent—or facilitate—pregnancy.

Women are fertile for only part of each cycle. About midway between periods, they release eggs (ovulation), triggering hormonal changes that increase vaginal receptiveness for sperm. Fertilization can occur only from seven days before ovulation to three days after (based on the survival time of sperm and eggs). During infertile days, couples don't need contraception. During fertile days, they can abstain or use outercourse, condoms, or barrier methods.

Charting women's fertility involves three elements: the calendar, basal body temperature, and the consistency of cervical mucus. The calendar is the only element in the calendar rhythm method. It attempts to predict fertile days based on women's menstrual history. It assumes that women's cycles are regular enough to distinguish between fertile and infertile days.

To use fertility awareness, for six to eight cycles, women track the start of their periods. Each cycle begins on the first day of one period and ends on the first day of the next. Ovulation occurs about midway between periods. While tracking, women should use other contraceptives—but not the Pill, which chemically controls women's cycles. Tracking allows women to calculate when they're most likely to ovulate and estimate fertile and infertile days.

However, few women's cycles are consistently regular, and many factors can affect cycle length and ovulation: travel, illness, drugs, fatigue, and stress—including worries about this method's reliability.

With fertility awareness, women observe not only the calendar, but also their bodies. Basal body temperature (BBT) is temperature on waking, typically a few degrees below 98.6. It's measured using a special thermometer with an expanded scale in the normal range. Once women become familiar with their BBTs, they can recognize the sudden, approximately one-half-degree increase that signals ovulation.

Cervical mucus changes also predict ovulation. The cervix secretes mucus continually, but its texture changes. During safe days, it's scant, white, and thick; while fertile, it's copious, clear, and thinner.

Fertility awareness works best in monogamous relationships, when men understand and support it. Those interested should take a class or read a book, then invest six to eight months to learn the woman's fertility pattern. For classes, consult family planning providers.

- Effectiveness: 80–99 percent
- Availability: Requires training and months of observation before it can be used reliably
- Side Effects: None
- Advantages:
  - After training, it's free
  - When used carefully, highly effective
  - No need for contraception for up to ten days each month
  - Sex can be spontaneous during infertile times
  - Can prevent or facilitate pregnancy
  - Increases men's familiarity with women's menstrual cycles
- Disadvantages:
  - When used improperly, considerable risk of pregnancy
  - Takes six to eight months to master
  - Other contraceptives are necessary during fertile times
  - No protection against STIs
  - Vaginal infections and douching may change cervical mucus

Birth Control Pills: Combination Estrogen-Progestin Pills and Progestin-Only Pills

All birth control pills—oral contraceptives or the Pill—use one or two female sex hormones to prevent ovulation. They also thicken cervical mucus, deterring sperm from entering the uterus.

Two types are available. Monophasic and multiphasic pills combine estrogen and progestin. Minipills contain only progestin.

Women must take one pill a day every day. If they miss one pill, they may take two the next day. If they forget two pills, they can take two a day for two days. Women who miss one or two pills should also use a backup method until their next period. If women miss three or more days in a row, they should stop taking the Pill and use another method until their next period, when they may return to taking one pill a day.

Some women should not take the Pill—those who might be pregnant, and women with:

- Liver disease—hepatitis, cirrhosis
- History of heart disease, stroke, breast cancer, or internal blood clotting (venous thromboembolism)

Physicians may also advise against the Pill if women are:
- Over thirty-five with risk factors for cardiovascular disease
- Smokers
- Overweight
- Breastfeeding

Or if women have:
- Varicose veins
- Migraines
- High blood pressure
- High cholesterol
- Gallbladder disease
- Diabetes
- Uterine fibroids
- Sickle cell anemia
- High risk of breast cancer
- Family history of death from heart disease before age fifty

Women who get pregnant while taking the Pill tend to be overweight. While taking the Pill, some women gain weight. Others notice breast tenderness. Some experience increased breast size.

- Effectiveness: 95–99+ percent
- Availability: By prescription
- Side Effects: Birth control pills decrease many women's libidos. Multiphasic pills are least likely to do this. Other common effects include nausea, headaches, breast tenderness, depression, fatigue, irritability, weight gain, dry eyes, and bleeding between periods (spotting).

Pill users should contact physicians immediately if they develop:
- Severe abdominal pain
- Chest pain
- Shortness of breath
- Severe headaches
- Blurred vision or vision loss
- Severe leg pain

Estrogen stimulates growth of breast cancer. Some studies have shown increased risk among Pill users. The current medical consensus is that combination pills increase breast cancer risk somewhat, but also reduce risk of uterine (endometrial) cancer and ovarian cancer.

If women feel comfortable taking one pill every day and can afford this relatively costly method, the Pill is convenient and effective.

Women who stop using birth control pills typically return to normal ovulation within three to six months.

Women taking birth control pills should never share them or use other women's pills.

The Pill offers no protection against STIs.
- Advantages:
  - With proper use, highly effective
  - Convenient
  - No interruption of lovemaking
  - Allows spontaneous sex
  - Regularizes irregular menstrual periods
  - Shorter periods
  - Decreases menstrual flow and cramping
  - Helps prevent or relieve acne, premenstrual syndrome, endometriosis, ovarian cysts, osteoporosis, ovarian and endometrial cancer, ectopic pregnancy, and pelvic inflammatory disease
  - May increase breast size
- Disadvantages:
  - Without insurance, comparatively expensive
  - Requires regular physician visits
  - Many women can't use it
  - Often discouraged for women over thirty-five
  - May increase breast size
  - May depress libido
  - Possible nausea, headaches, breast tenderness, depression, fatigue, irritability, weight gain, and spotting
  - Increased risk of breast cancer, stroke, heart attack, high blood pressure, and abnormal blood clotting
  - When stopped, fertility takes months to return
  - No protection against STIs
  - May be incompatible with contact lenses

Intrauterine Devices (IUDs)

Some release hormones, others do not. All are small T-shaped objects professionally inserted into the uterus. IUDs cause uterine changes that disable sperm. A string attached to the device protrudes through the cervix, allowing removal.

Women should not use IUDs if they:
- Are pregnant or suspect pregnancy
- Have had pelvic inflammatory disease
- Have recently had gonorrhea or chlamydia

Physicians may not prescribe IUDs for women who had problems with previous IUDs or have:
- Histories of tubal (ectopic) pregnancy
- Anemia, heavy periods, or painful periods
- Uterine fibroids

IUDs' main advantage is convenience. Once inserted, they remain in place until removal, usually every few years. However, women must check for their IUD strings regularly by reaching into their vaginas. No string? Contact your provider immediately.

IUDs increase risk of spotting. The IUD insertion requires two office visits. The first includes counseling, medical history, physical exam, blood tests, Pap test, and tests for pregnancy and STIs. If all's well, on the second visit, clinicians insert the device. Women should be instructed how to feel for the string. After insertion, women may experience transient cramping or bleeding.

IUDs may not provide reliable contraception immediately. Discuss this with your provider and, if necessary, use a backup method for a few weeks.

IUD insertion provides effective emergency contraception—if insertion takes place within five days of unprotected intercourse.

- Effectiveness: 97–99+ percent
- Availability: By prescription
- Side Effects: Contact your provider immediately if you:
  - Cannot feel the string
  - Feel any part of the IUD itself in the cervix or vagina
  - Develop fever, lower abdominal pain, heavy discharge, or abnormal bleeding
- Advantages:
  - With insurance, modest cost
  - Highly effective
  - Convenient
  - Long lasting
  - No interruption of lovemaking
  - Allows spontaneous sex
  - No pills to take or devices to use
  - Levonorgestrel may reduce or eliminate menstrual flow
  - After removal, fertility returns quickly
  - Protection against endometrial and cervical cancer
- Disadvantages:
  - Without insurance, expensive
  - Requires insertion by a physician
  - Must check for strings regularly
  - Possible menstrual disturbances
  - Increased risk of pelvic inflammatory disease
  - No protection against STIs

Injected Contraception (Depo-Provera)

Depo-Provera is the female sex hormone progestin injected four times annually. The hormone prevents ovulation and thickens cervical mucus, deterring sperm from entering the uterus.

After stopping injections, it may take many months for fertility to return.

- Effectiveness: 94–99+ percent
- Availability: By prescription
- Side Effects: Menstrual disturbances, weight gain, depression, bone density loss, headache, nervousness, libido loss, breast discomfort
- Advantages:
  - Modest cost. Most health insurers cover it.
  - Highly effective
  - Reasonably convenient; quarterly injections
  - No interruption of lovemaking

- ◦ May be used by women who can't take estrogen
- ◦ Allows spontaneous sex
- ◦ Often reduces menstrual flow
- ◦ Reduced risk of endometrial cancer, and pelvic inflammatory disease
- • Disadvantages:
  - ◦ Quarterly medical visits
  - ◦ Side effects
  - ◦ No protection from STIs
  - ◦ After stopping, fertility may not return for many months

NuvaRing

NuvaRing is a small circle of flexible plastic. Women insert one deep in the vagina monthly and remove it after three weeks. The ring releases hormones that prevent ovulation and thicken cervical mucus.

- • Effectiveness: 96–99 percent
- • Availability: By prescription
- • Side Effects: Similar to combination birth control pills (page 115)
- • Advantages:
  - ◦ Highly effective, assuming monthly replacement
  - ◦ One size fits all
  - ◦ No interruption of lovemaking
  - ◦ Allows spontaneous sex
  - ◦ Regularizes irregular menstrual periods
  - ◦ Shorter periods
  - ◦ Typically decreases menstrual flow and cramping
  - ◦ Noncontraceptive benefits similar to birth control pills
  - ◦ Rapidly reversible
- • Disadvantages:
  - ◦ Must be replaced regularly
  - ◦ Possible confusion about use schedule
  - ◦ May depress libido
  - ◦ Possible increased vaginal discharge
  - ◦ Possible nausea, breast tenderness
  - ◦ Rarely, increased risk of stroke, heart attack, gallbladder disease, blood clots
  - ◦ No protection against STIs

Contraceptive Patch (Ortho Evra)

Ortho Evra is an adhesive skin patch impregnated with estrogen and progestin. Women place one weekly—for three weeks per month—on the upper arm, abdomen, or buttocks. The hormones prevent ovulation and thicken cervical mucus.

- • Effectiveness: 98–99 percent
- • Availability: By prescription
- • Side Effects: Similar to birth control pills (page 115)
- • Advantages:
  - ◦ Highly effective, assuming proper use

- ◦ One size fits all
- ◦ Convenient
- ◦ No interruption of lovemaking
- ◦ Allows spontaneous sex
- ◦ Regularizes irregular menstrual periods
- ◦ Shorter periods
- ◦ Typically decreases menstrual flow and cramping
- ◦ Helps prevent or relieve acne, premenstrual syndrome, endometriosis, ovarian cysts, osteoporosis, ovarian and uterine (endometrial) cancer, ectopic pregnancy, and pelvic inflammatory disease
- • Disadvantages:
  - ◦ Possible confusion about use schedule
  - ◦ Possible irritation at placement site
  - ◦ May be incompatible with contact lenses
  - ◦ Less effective in obese women
  - ◦ May depress libido
  - ◦ Possible nausea, headaches, breast tenderness, depression, fatigue, irritability, and spotting
  - ◦ Rarely, increased risk of stroke, heart attack, high blood pressure, and abnormal blood clotting (thromboembolism)
  - ◦ When stopped, fertility may take several months to return
  - ◦ No protection against STIs

Implant

One is available in the US, Nexplanon, a matchstick-size rod implanted in women's upper arm that releases hormones that suppress ovulation and thicken cervical mucus.

- • Effectiveness: 99+ percent
- • Availability: Must be placed and removed by a trained clinician
- • Side effects: Similar to the Pill (page 115)
- • Advantages:
  - ◦ Highly effective, assuming replacement every three years
  - ◦ Can be used by women who can't take estrogen
  - ◦ May reduce acne, menstrual cramps, endometriosis pain
  - ◦ Rapidly reversible
- • Disadvantages:
  - ◦ Irregular menstrual bleeding
  - ◦ Possible weight gain
  - ◦ Possible libido loss
  - ◦ Possible loss of bone density
  - ◦ Headache, breast pain, nausea, vaginal dryness
  - ◦ No protection against STIs

Emergency Contraception

Often called the "morning-after Pill," emergency contraception is actually effective for up to five days. And users need not wait until the morning after. Three brands are available in the US: Plan B, Next Choice, and ella.

This method is a major reason why the abortion rate has fallen to a record low.

Plan B and ella involve one high-dose birth control pill. Next Choice requires two pills. All three prevent ovulation and thicken cervical mucus.

Women can use emergency contraception if:

- They didn't use another method
- They missed three birth control pills in a row
- They forgot to insert NuvaRing or apply a patch
- They can't feel the IUD string
- The condom broke
- The diaphragm or cap slipped out of place
- Couples using fertility awareness miscalculated infertile days
- The man didn't withdraw
- After sexual assault

Women should not use emergency contraception if they:

- Know or suspect they're pregnant
- Experience abnormal vaginal bleeding that has not been medically evaluated

Women know this method worked if their next period arrives as expected. If it's more than a week late, pregnancy is possible. Take a pregnancy test and consult a physician or family planning clinic.

Women who cannot take birth control pills also cannot use this method.

- Effectiveness: 95 percent if taken within twenty-four hours. Eighty-nine percent if taken within seventy-two hours.
- Availability: Over the counter at pharmacies. Thirty-five to fifty dollars. Anyone of any age may purchase it.
- Side Effects: Possible nausea, vomiting, fatigue, breast tenderness, and diarrhea. Women who vomit within two hours of taking emergency contraception must take another dose.
- Advantages:
  ○ Emergency pregnancy protection
  ○ Easily available
  ○ Effective for up to several days after unprotected intercourse
- Disadvantages:
  ○ For emergency use only
  ○ Side effects
  ○ No protection against STIs

Male Sterilization: Vasectomy

Around 500,000 American men have vasectomies annually. It involves minor, twenty-minute surgery under local anesthesia. The surgeon makes two tiny incisions in the upper scrotum, finds the tubes that carry sperm out of the testicles (vas deferens), cuts them, and seals their ends. After vasectomy, sperm cannot leave the testicles and semen eventually becomes sterile.

Men are not sterile immediately after vasectomy. Sperm remain in the tubes above incision sites. It takes two dozen ejaculations to eliminate them. During that time, couples must use another method. Weeks after vasectomy, men return for follow-up semen analyses. When it's sperm-free, couples no longer need to use contraception.

After vasectomy, men ejaculate normally. Sperm account for only 2 percent of semen volume, so men notice no difference.

Urologists perform most vasectomies on Fridays. Over the weekend, men should avoid heavy lifting. Most feel fine by Monday.

After vasectomy, the testicles continue making sperm, but the body reabsorbs them.

Vasectomy is cheaper and less traumatic than women's sterilization.

After vasectomy, some studies show an increase in couple's sexual frequency and satisfaction lasting up to one year.

Sterilization decisions should never be made impulsively. Postvasectomy surveys show that men happiest with sterilization ponder it for at least a year. Consider these questions: Suppose you divorced or became widowed and remarried. Would you or your new wife want more children? Suppose your children died. Would you want a new family?

Vasectomy should be considered permanent. If you think *I can get it reversed*, think again. Reversal attempts are costly. Few insurers cover them. And success cannot be guaranteed. Most men who seek reversals have new wives who want children. If you're certain you want a vasectomy, ask your doctor for a referral to a urologist.

- Effectiveness: Virtually 100 percent. Failures are extremely rare but have been documented.
- Availability: Surgery
- Side Effects: After vasectomy, men usually feel sore and see some discoloration around incision sites. Around 1 percent of men develop postsurgical wound infections or anesthesia reactions. Vasectomy does not increase risk of prostate cancer, heart disease, stroke, or other serious conditions.
- Advantages:
  - No need for contraception ever again
  - Modest cost. Most insurers cover it
  - After sterilization, some couples experience temporarily increased libido and sexual frequency
- Disadvantages:
  - Possible incision site soreness
  - Possible wound infection
  - It takes two dozen ejaculations to become sterile
  - No protection against STIs
  - Permanent. Reversals are possible, but costly and can't be guaranteed

Female Sterilization: Tubal Ligation

Some 700,000 American women get sterilized annually. It involves cutting the tubes that connect the ovaries to the uterus (fallopian tubes).

Tubal ligation involves an abdominal incision and requires hospitalization and anesthesia.
Scarring is possible. Recovery typically takes several days.

Tubal ligation is more traumatic and costly than vasectomy.

After women become sterile, some studies show an increase in sexual frequency and satisfaction lasting up to one year.

Sterilization decisions should never be made impulsively. Suppose you divorced or became
widowed and then remarried. Would you want more children? What if your new husband
wanted more children? Suppose your children died. Would you want a new family?

Tubal ligation can be reversed but it's costly. Insurers don't cover it. And there's no guarantee of success.

Women certain they want to be sterilized should ask their physicians for surgical referrals.

- Effectiveness: Tubal ligation is virtually 100 percent effective immediately after surgery.
- Availability: Requires surgery
- Side Effects: Complications include wound infection, anesthesia reactions, abdominal
  pain, extended recovery, and very rarely, sterilization failure.
- Advantages:
  - No need for contraception ever again.
  - Modest cost. Most insurers cover it.
  - After sterilization, many couples experience temporarily increased libido and sex-
    ual frequency.
- Disadvantages:
  - Tubal ligation requires hospitalization and anesthesia.
  - No protection against STIs.

Abortion

Abortion involves surgical removal or drug-induced destruction of embryos before independent survival is possible.

Abortion was legalized in the US in 1973. Legal abortions peaked in 1982 at twenty-nine
women per thousand. By 2014, the rate had fallen to fifteen per thousand, a drop of 48 percent. Why? Most couples became more committed to contraception, and emergency contraception (page 121) became available over the counter.

- Teens account for 15 percent of abortions, women in their twenties account for 60
  percent, and women in their thirties for 25 percent. From 2008 to 2014, the proportion of teens obtaining abortions decreased 32 percent—largely because emergency
  contraception became available over the counter.
- Ninety percent of abortions take place during the first trimester, 60 percent during the
  first eight weeks. Only 1 percent of women who get abortions are more than twenty
  weeks along.
- White women account for 36 percent of abortions; African Americans, 29 percent;
  Hispanics, 25 percent; others, 9 percent.
- Abortion recipients tend to be low income.

- Catholic women account for 24 percent of abortions; mainline Protestants, 17 percent; Evangelical Christians, 13 percent; other religions, 8 percent; no religious affiliation or unstated, 38 percent.

Many women—and their lovers—have mixed feelings about aborting. For some, the main feeling is relief. For others, it's profound loss. Studies show that first-trimester abortions cause the fewest psychological ramifications.

Most women realize they are pregnant from week three to eight. First-trimester abortions can be obtained until the end of week twelve, so most women can consider their decisions for several weeks and still obtain the simplest, safest procedure.

Abortions absolutely require experienced doctors. Never attempt self-abortion or take herbs to trigger it. Several plant oils cause abortive uterine contractions, but the effective doses may be lethal. Women have *died* shortly after swallowing as little as a teaspoon of abortifacient plant oils.

Several types of abortion are currently available. Women who are interested should discuss them with providers.

Afterward, some women experience cramping and/or nausea. With local anesthetic, most women are able to leave the medical facility within two hours. General anesthesia requires longer recovery.

After abortions, women should:

- Rest for at least one day
- Avoid strenuous activity for three days
- Take any antibiotics as directed
- Abstain from intercourse for at least two weeks
- Not use tampons for three weeks
- Have a follow-up exam after two weeks
- Start using an effective birth control method

Consult a physician immediately for:

- Fever
- Chills
- Muscle aches
- Persistent fatigue
- Severe abdominal pain, cramping, or backache
- Abdominal tenderness
- Prolonged or heavy vaginal bleeding
- Any unusual vaginal discharge
- No menstrual period within six weeks, especially if you still feel pregnant

CHAPTER 17:
Men Who Want Sizzling Sex *Must* Prevent Sexually Transmitted Infections

SIZZLING SEX REQUIRES deep relaxation. It's difficult—often impossible—to relax when anxious about the possibility of contracting sexually transmitted infections (STIs). That risk is substantial. Americans develop twenty million STIs annually, and half of sexually active teens and young adults contract one by age twenty-five.

Sizzling sex also requires trust. It's difficult—or impossible—to trust lovers who don't care about the possibility of passing STIs or don't mention they have one.

Finally, sizzling sex requires leisurely, playful, whole-body massage. This allows plenty of time to discuss STIs and their prevention.

Having an STI *does not* mean you're toxic or condemned to a sexless life. Most STIs can be cured fairly easily. Even if you have one that persists—notably herpes, genital warts, or HIV— you can still enjoy sizzling sex as long as you take the simple steps that prevent transmission.

Speak Up!

It's difficult to admit you suspect an STI or that you're being treated for one. Nonetheless, speak up. Men who don't inform women about the possibility of two common STIs—chlamydia and gonorrhea—*risk women's lives*. These infections rarely cause symptoms in women but may progress to pelvic inflammatory disease (PID), a serious condition that can cause infertility, serious illness, and possibly even death. Women have *died* because their lovers were too embarrassed or unconcerned to inform them about infections that could have been cured if treated.

Did Your Lover Cheat? Maybe . . . Maybe Not

Some people assume that if lovers develop STIs, they've been unfaithful. That's possible, but several STIs can be contracted without infidelity, without sex.

Only three STIs are transmitted *exclusively* sexually: gonorrhea, syphilis, and genital warts (HPV). Herpes and chlamydia are almost always passed sexually, though nonsexual transmission is theoretically possible. All other STIs may be contracted nonsexually.

In addition, several STIs—trichomoniasis, chlamydia, herpes, gonorrhea, genital warts, and HIV—may cause no symptoms for quite a while after infection. HIV, herpes, and warts may not cause symptoms for *years*. It's quite possible to become infected in one relationship yet show no symptoms until a subsequent relationship that's completely monogamous.

Age and STIs

The greatest STI risk occurs during adolescence and young adulthood. As age increases, risk declines but does not disappear. Age-related risk for gonorrhea and chlamydia are typical of STIs in general:

Age group	Gonorrhea diagnoses	Chlamydia diagnoses
0–14	1% of all diagnoses	1%
15–19	18%	26%
20–24	32%	39%
25–29	21%	18%
30–39	18%	12%
40+	10%	4%

CDC figures

Getting Treated

Some feel reluctant to consult their doctors, especially residents of small towns. Even if physicians respect confidentiality, support staff may read medical records and gossip. If you're reluctant to consult your doctor, most public health departments treat STIs, often for free.

Here are brief discussions of the major STIs. For more information, visit the Centers for Disease Control and Prevention: cdc.gov, or call the CDC's National STI Hotline: 1-800-232-4636 (twenty-four seven, English and Spanish).

Urinary Tract Infection in Women

(UTI, cystitis, bladder infection)

Half of US women become infected at least once. Millions suffer recurrent infections.

- **Transmission prevention.** Careful sexual hygiene. Nothing that touches either lover's anal area should come in contact with the woman's vulva or vagina.
- **Cause.** Intestinal bacteria introduced into the urethra, which opens in the middle of the vulva.
  - ○ **Transmission.** Careless lovemaking accounts for most, but not all, risk.
  - ○ **Symptoms.** Burning on urination, an urgent need to urinate frequently, possible blood in urine, itching, foul odor.
  - ○ **Diagnosis.** By symptoms and identification of the bacteria.
  - ○ **Treatment.** At the first sign of symptoms, drink lots of water. This may flush bacteria from the bladder before full-blown infection. If infection develops, take antibiotics.
  - ○ **In addition.** Complications are rare, but kidney infection is possible.

Treatment often involves sulfa drugs. African Americans should be cautious about taking them. Fifteen percent cannot metabolize sulfa drugs and ingesting them may prove *fatal*. Before taking sulfa, African Americans should be tested for G6PD enzyme deficiency. Anyone with this condition should take other antibiotics.

To prevent UTIs:

- **Make love hygienically.** Fingers, tongues, penises, and toys that touch either lover's anal area should not touch the woman's vulva or vagina.
- **Less sex.** As intercourse frequency increases, so does risk. Before premarital sex became near universal, many virgin women had honeymoon sex so frequently they developed "honeymoon cystitis."
- **Less vigorously.** Pounding intercourse may irritate women's urethras, making them more susceptible.
- **Lube?** Some women find that commercial lubricants help prevent UTIs. Others notice the opposite.
- **Outercourse.** Some women have gentle intercourse with excellent hygiene—and still develop UTIs. If so, consider outercourse: hand jobs, oral sex, and toys.

In addition, women should:

- **Wipe from front to back after urinating.** This keeps anal bacteria away from the urethra.
- **Urinate before and after lovemaking.** This helps flush bacteria out of the urinary tract.
- **Consume cranberries.** Drink cranberry juice. Eat dried cranberries and use them in cooking. Cranberries are a centuries-old folk preventive for urinary problems. Many studies show that cranberry products reduce risk of UTI by preventing bacterial adhesion to the bladder wall. Boston University researchers asked 373 women with recurrent UTIs to drink a placebo beverage or cranberry juice daily. Six months later, the cranberry group reported significantly fewer UTIs. Auburn University researchers analyzed eight studies and confirmed cranberries' effectiveness.
- **When you feel the urge, go.** Studies of women with recurrent UTIs show they have a tendency to hold their urine. Don't. Physicians urge women troubled by recurrent UTIs to go every hour or two even if they *don't* feel the urge.
- **Eliminate urinary irritants.** They include cigarettes, spicy foods, alcohol, coffee (including decaf), and tea.
- **Don't irritate the vulva.** Perfumed deodorant soaps may cause irritation. Use mild unscented soap. Wear cotton underwear—less irritating than synthetics. Stay away from restrictive, tight-fitting clothing, for example, leotards, which may move anal area bacteria forward.
- **Change tampons or pads frequently.** Blood is a bacterial growth medium.

Men may also develop UTIs, but compared with women, they're at much lower risk. Women's urethras are only around two inches long, while men's are about eight. Bacteria are more likely to reach women's bladders. In addition, the female urethra opens closer to the anus.

Trichomoniasis
("Trick")
More than three million infections annually.

- **Transmission Prevention.** Condoms
- **Cause.** A parasite, *Trichomonas vaginalis*
- **Transmission.** The parasite can pass from penis to vagina or vagina to penis. It can also spread from vagina to vagina.
- **Symptoms.** Only 30 percent of infected individuals show symptoms. If symptoms develop, they usually appear from a week to a month after exposure. However, symptoms may not appear until much later. Symptoms include genital irritation, itching or burning, vaginal redness, pain on urination or ejaculation, penile discharge, or vaginal discharge with a fishy odor.
- **Diagnosis.** A lab test identifies the parasite.
- **Treatment.** Antiparasitic medication
- **In addition.** The genital irritation increases susceptibility to other STIs, notably HIV. Pregnant women should be screened. Trichomoniasis is associated with preterm delivery and low birth weight.

Chlamydia
1.5 million diagnoses annually.

- **Transmission Prevention.** Condoms work best. Diaphragms and cervical caps also help prevent transmission, but not as reliably.
- **Cause.** Bacteria, *Chlamydia trachomatis*
- **Transmission.** Usually by direct contact during vaginal or anal intercourse. After exposure, it takes a week to a month to develop infection.
- **Symptoms.** Half of men and 75 percent of women notice none. If men develop symptoms, they typically include mild burning on urination and a pus discharge from the penis. Women's symptoms include unusual vaginal discharge, lower abdominal pain, pain during intercourse, or spotting between periods. Rectal chlamydia may cause anal itching, cramping, a watery discharge, or diarrhea.
- **Diagnosis.** Urine test or analysis of any discharge
- **Treatment.** Antibiotics
- **In addition.** Peak prevalence occurs from age eighteen to twenty-four. The vast majority don't know they're infected. Because women rarely show symptoms, they should be screened periodically during pelvic exams.

Chlamydia infection triples women's risk of contracting HIV if exposed.

Birth control pills and IUDs increase susceptibility. All pregnant women should be screened. Mothers can pass chlamydia to fetuses. Infected newborns may develop potentially serious problems.

Genital Warts (HPV)
465,000 diagnoses annually. Among Americans age eighteen to fifty-nine, 25 percent of men and 20 percent of women are infected.

- **Transmission Prevention.** Male condoms provide the best protection. However, HPV can be transmitted from skin-to-skin contact in areas not covered by condoms. Female condoms prevent spread in and around the vagina, but not the anus.
- **Cause.** Human papillomavirus (HPV). One type causes warts on the genitals. Others cause warts on the hands or feet.
- **Transmission.** Sexually through genital skin-to-skin contact during vaginal, anal, or (rarely) oral sex. Warts of the hands and feet *cannot* spread to the genitals and vice versa.
- **Symptoms.** After exposure, those with robust immune function may never develop warts. Or they may erupt after weeks, months, or even years with infected lovers. Consequently, it's often impossible to know when you contracted the virus and from whom.

  Genital warts appear as small persistent bumps on the penis, vaginal lips, cervix, or anus. They may be raised or flat, single or multiple, large or small. Many look like warts of the hand. Others resemble miniature cauliflowers. Some cause itching, pain, or bleeding. Anal warts may be mistaken for hemorrhoids.
- **Diagnosis.** By appearance. When in doubt, physicians apply vinegar (acetic acid) to suspect areas. It turns warts white and makes them more visible. Or after abnormal Pap tests, physician submit cervical cells for analysis that can identify HPV.
- **Treatment.** Over-the-counter treatments for warts of the hands or feet are ineffective. Genital warts must be treated by physicians. Caustic chemicals may be applied. Or warts may be frozen off with liquid nitrogen. Or zapped with lasers. Repeat treatments are often necessary, especially for anal warts, which tend to persist.

  During treatment, two medicinal herbs, echinacea and astragalus, may help the immune system control the virus. Both are safe when used as directed. They're available at health food stores and supplement shops. Follow package directions.

  Medical treatment suppresses warts, but does not eradicate the virus, which remains in the body. If the person's immune system becomes compromised by injury or illness, warts may reappear.

  Physicians treat cervical HPV that has caused precancerous cell changes by destroying abnormal cells. Methods include cell removal (cone biopsy), freezing (cryosurgery), and laser treatment.
- **In addition.** In women, HPV infection causes cervical cancer. In 2016, thirteen thousand American women developed the disease and four thousand died. HPV vaccine prevents infection and cancer. Cervical cancer can almost always be cured if caught early by Pap testing. Women with active warts or a history of HPV infection should have Pap tests at least annually.

Gonorrhea (Clap)
395,000 diagnoses annually.

- **Transmission prevention.** Male condoms are most reliable. Female condoms protect against vaginal gonorrhea, but not against infection of the throat or anus. Diaphragms and cervical caps offer some protection against vaginal gonorrhea.
- **Cause.** Bacteria, *Neisseria gonorrhoeae*
- **Transmission.** Gonorrhea spreads only during vaginal or anal intercourse or oral sex. When exposed to air, the bacteria die almost immediately. It's impossible to catch gonorrhea from toilet seats, towels, sex toys, or showers.

- **Symptoms.** In men: pain or burning on urination and a white, green, or yellow pus discharge from the penis. Oral gonorrhea may cause a sore throat. Anal gonorrhea may cause pain on defecation. Women with vaginal gonorrhea usually show no symptoms, but may develop an unusual vaginal discharge, pain or burning on urination, and bleeding between periods.
- **Diagnosis.** In men, by symptoms and laboratory identification of the bacteria. In women, usually by an infected lover's referral, then by laboratory analysis of cervical mucus. Or by screening during pelvic exams or contraceptive medical visits. Every possibly infected orifice should be tested.
- **Treatment.** Antibiotics. However, some strains are resistant. Take all prescribed pills, even if symptoms clear quickly. Then schedule a follow-up test a few weeks after treatment to make sure the infection has been cured.
- **In addition.** In women, untreated gonorrhea may progress to pelvic inflammatory disease (PID), a fertility- and life-threatening condition. Women should be screened for gonorrhea periodically. If diagnosed with gonorrhea, everyone *must* inform all recent sex partners of their infection risk and urge them to get tested. Babies born to women with gonorrhea are at risk for blindness. Pregnant women should be tested before delivery.

Herpes
776,000 diagnoses annually.

- **Transmission prevention.** Male condoms are most reliable. However, herpes may be transmitted from skin-to-skin contact in uncovered areas. Female condoms protect against vaginal infection, but not infection of the lips or anus. Herpes sores are painful. Few herpes sufferers feel like making love when they have them.
- **Cause.** Either of two viruses, herpes simplex 1 or 2. Either may infect the penis, vagina, or anal area (genital herpes) or the lips (cold sores, fever blisters).
- **Transmission.** Usually by skin-to-skin contact with an infected individual who has a visible sore or during the day or two *before* one erupts (prodrome). It's also possible to transmit the virus without showing any symptoms (asymptomatic shedding). It's not clear how often this occurs. Many people with herpes don't develop symptoms and don't know they're infected—but may still transmit the virus.

  Oral herpes is usually spread by kissing or oral sex, genital herpes by oral sex, or vaginal or anal intercourse. However, the virus can survive up to a few hours outside the body, so transmission might conceivably occur by sharing towels (genital herpes) or lipstick (oral herpes). However, to survive, the virus requires warmth and moisture and most environments outside the body—notably toilet seats—do not provide them.
- **Symptoms.** Twenty-five percent of infected individuals do not develop symptoms—for years—but may still transmit the infection. When symptoms develop, the virus causes an open, red, itchy, painful sore or blister (lesion) or a group of lesions surrounded by red, irritated skin. In men, lesions can appear anywhere on the penis, scrotum, thighs, buttocks, anus, or perineum (between the genitals and anus). In women, genital sores typically develop on the vaginal lips, vulva, anal area, buttocks, thighs, or perineum. Sores may also develop inside the vagina or on the cervix.

  Initial eruptions are worst. Without antiviral drugs, they typically last seven to ten days, then clear. With treatment, they resolve faster. First lesions may also cause fever, swollen glands, and feeling ill (malaise). Depending on health and immune function, the immune system usually suppresses the virus—quickly or slowly. Some suffer only one outbreak. Others have one recurrence. Some experience several. Only a small proportion of people suffer multiple recurrences. Some suffer no recurrences for years—until they develop other illnesses that preoccupy their immune systems. Recurrences tend to be mild and last only a few days.

- **Diagnosis.** Usually by appearance of a painful sore. (A painless sore suggests syphilis, below.) A lab test definitively identifies the virus.
- **Treatment.** Antiviral medication. But no drug eradicates the virus. It remains in the body. If the immune system becomes compromised by injury or illness, new sores may erupt. Topical salves containing the medicinal herb lemon balm (*Melissa officinalis*) have shown benefit:
  - German researchers asked 116 people with new sores to apply either a placebo compress or one containing strong lemon balm tea. Herbal treatment was significantly more effective.
  - Another German team gave sixty-six people with recurrent herpes either a placebo cream or one containing 1 percent lemon balm extract. Sores treated with the herbal cream healed significantly faster. Lemon balm ointment is available in the US—Herpalieve. Follow package directions.

    During treatment, two other medicinal herbs, echinacea and astragalus, may help the immune system fight the virus. Both are safe when used as directed. They are available at health food stores and supplement shops. Follow package directions.
- **In addition.** Everyone with herpes should inform new lovers before the relationship becomes sexual. During lovemaking, use condoms.

Don't touch herpes sores. Fingers can become contaminated and spread the virus.

Recurrences usually develop in the same spots as original eruptions. Sores may develop when you're stressed, fatigued, or sick. That's why herpes of the lips, cold sores, appear during colds and flu.

A day or two before recurrent sores erupt, they cause itching or tingling in the area(s) where previous sores formed (prodrome). You're contagious from the moment the prodrome begins until sores heal.

Claims that herpes is "incurable" are mistaken. While the virus remains in the body for life, the immune system is usually able to suppress it after the initial episode or a recurrence or two. Once it's contained, those with herpes are unlikely to infect lovers, though transmission is still possible.

Recurrences can be suppressed with daily low-dose prescription antiviral drugs. After stopping antivirals, rebound outbreaks are possible.

Herpes is not life threatening to healthy adults, but it can be to those with impaired immune function and to newborns infected at birth. Active herpes in a woman entering labor is an indication for cesarean section.

An amino acid, lysine, inhibits herpes replication. Some—but not all—studies show that lysine supplementation reduces recurrences. Indiana University researchers gave fifty-two people with recurrent herpes either a placebo or lysine (1,000 mg three times a day). After six months, the placebo group averaged 4.2 outbreaks with moderate symptoms, the lysine group 3.1 outbreaks with mild symptoms.

Syphilis

75,000 diagnoses annually.

- **Transmission prevention.** Male condoms. However, syphilis may be transmitted by skin-to-skin contact in uncovered areas. Female condoms offer no protection against transmission during oral and anal intercourse.
- **Cause.** A bacteria-like microorganism, *Treponema pallidum*
- **Transmission.** Vaginal, oral, or anal intercourse
- **Symptoms.** First, a painless open sore appears. On the penis, sores are easily visible. Sores in the vagina, throat, or anus may not be. The sore heals by itself in a few weeks. Soon after, a rash develops somewhere on the body, often accompanied by fatigue and malaise. The rash disappears in a few weeks. Syphilis then goes dormant for many years, after which it may cause severe, life-threatening complications.
- **Diagnosis.** A blood test or microscopic examination of material from sores.
- **Treatment.** Antibiotics. While being treated and for one month after, abstain from sex.
- **In addition.** Because women are often unaware of syphilis sores, men diagnosed with syphilis *must* inform all their lovers.

Babies born to women with syphilis are at risk for birth defects and death. Pregnant women should be tested.

HIV/AIDS

39,500 diagnoses and 7,000 deaths in 2015.

- **Transmission prevention.** Select lovers carefully. Avoid those who have ever used IV drugs. Male condoms provide substantial, but not absolute protection. Female condoms prevent penis-vagina transmission but do not protect against transmission during anal intercourse.
- **Cause.** Human immunodeficiency virus (HIV)
- **Transmission.** Three ways: semen-to-blood contact during vaginal, oral, or anal intercourse; blood-to-blood contact during use of contaminated syringes; or from infected mothers to fetuses.

  Recipients in anal intercourse are at highest risk.

  Transmission during oral sex is possible but rare.

  Other STIs increase risk of sexual transmission.
- **Symptoms.** The most insidious aspect of HIV is its long incubation period, the time from infection to symptoms. Infected individuals may not know they're infected for years—yet spread the infection to others.

  Eventually, symptoms include chronic fever, night sweats, chills, swollen glands, weakness, appetite and weight loss, and other infections that develop because those with HIV lose immune function to combat them. Common HIV-related opportunistic infections include pneumocystis carinii pneumonia (PCP), herpes, tuberculosis, yeast infections, non-Hodgkins lymphoma, dementia, cryptococcal meningitis, and others.
- **Diagnosis.** A blood test
- **Treatment.** Antiviral medications

- **In addition.** In the US AIDS was first identified in gay men, but *anyone* can become infected and *everyone* is potentially at risk. The CDC recommends testing at least once for all those who are sexually active.

In new or nonmonogamous relationships, discuss your AIDS risk—particularly any history of IV drug use—*before* you become sexual.

CHAPTER 18:
The Virgin's Guide to Happily Losing It

THE TEEN YEARS usually extend childhood protosex into more adult lovemaking. This is normal and natural.

But many parents feel conflicted about teens' emerging sexuality. Some insist on abstinence until marriage, but most believe teen sex is inevitable. They just hope their children postpone penis-vagina intercourse (PVI) until at least sixteen, and the later the better. The best way to encourage this is to discuss sex proactively at home starting when kids are toddlers. Ultimately, teens decide for themselves when they go all the way.

"Am I Still a Virgin?"

On the question-answer site I publish, GreatSexGuidance.com, many young people have voiced confusion about virginity. *My boyfriend fingered me. We dry-humped on the sofa. My girlfriend gave me a hand job (or blowjob). Am I still a virgin?*

Conventionally, a virgin has not had PVI. Losing one's virginity may be a rite of passage, but the term is virtually meaningless. Some young people who commit to virginity until marriage have no problem with hand jobs, oral, and even anal play while insisting that no PVI means they're still "technically" virgins.

Some who embrace PVI as the standard still find wiggle room based on orgasm/ejaculation. *I didn't come.* And depth of insertion. *It only went in an inch.* Finally, if PVI is the benchmark, those exclusively lesbian or gay would be lifelong virgins, even if they enjoyed same-gender lovemaking daily.

The notion of losing virginity misrepresents the continuum of unfolding sexuality. It implies an either/or situation—virgin or not. Most sexual initiation involves gradual escalation of erotic play that, for able-bodied heterosexuals, culminates in PVI. But just as a driver's license doesn't confer instant competence behind the wheel, first PVI—or second or tenth or hundredth—does not necessarily confer sexual expertise.

Would You Say You "Had Sex" If . . . ?

Confusion about virginity reflects a larger issue—what constitutes "sex"? This issue made headlines in 1998, when White House intern Monica Lewinsky fellated President Bill Clinton, who said it wasn't PVI, so it wasn't "sex."

Then there's the definition proposed in *Seinfeld*. George fools around with a woman and asks Jerry if they had sex. Seinfeld asks if she bared her breasts. George nods. "When the breasts come out of the bra, it's sex."

Is it? Indiana University researchers asked 599 college students what they considered "sex."

Activity	Women calling it "sex"	Men calling it "sex"
Kissing with tongue play	1%	3%
Your nipples touched or sucked	2%	5%
You touch or suck nipples	2%	6%
You touch the other's genitals	12%	17%
Your genitals touched	12%	19%
You provide fellatio/cunnilingus	37%	44%
You receive fellatio/cunnilingus	38%	44%
Penis-anus intercourse	82%	79%
Penis-vagina intercourse	100%	99%

Sanders, S. A., and J. M. Reinisch. "Would You Say You 'Had Sex' If...?" *Journal of the American Medical Association* 281 (1999): 275.

The Original Virgins: Just Women

Until the nineteenth century, only women were "virgins." The term derives from the Latin, *virgo*, meaning "maiden." It was coined around 1200 when a Catholic manuscript mentioned "consecrated virgins," cloistered celibate nuns. By 1300, the definition included the Virgin Mary. By 1400, the term meant women who had not had PVI. No one cared about boys. Virginity was only an issue for girls.

Historically, female virginity was all about property and paternity. Most human societies have been patriarchal. In them, until recent centuries, fathers owned their daughters as property including their virginity, a valuable asset that boosted girls' bridal value.

When girls married, their ownership passed to their husbands, who wanted to be sure their children were theirs. The only way to be certain was to marry a virgin. But how could they know? Some brides spent months sequestered from men (except eunuchs) until any premarital impregnation showed. But usually, male physicians examined young women's hymens. If they were intact, girls were virgins. If not, they weren't—and some suffered severe consequences.

Actually, the condition of the hymen has no bearing on women's experience with PVI. Virginity exams still take place in some cultures—including in the US, which came under speculation when Atlanta rapper T.I. openly discussed subjecting his teenaged daughter to virginity exams. The World Health Organization condemns this as violence against women.

The Hymen: A Membrane Misunderstood

Hymen derives from the Greek for membrane. Hymen was also the Greek god of marriage. These two facts crystallize the conventional wisdom about the fabled tissue, that it covers the vaginal opening and gets "pierced," "torn," or "broken" when women wed and have PVI, presumably for the first time.

For millennia, many cultures have believed that "tearing" the hymen inevitably causes pain, hence the belief, still current, that women experience—*should* experience—pain on first PVI.

Many cultures have also believed that "piercing" the hymen causes bleeding. Shortly after weddings, many new husbands were expected to produce bloody sheets to prove they'd married virgins and had consummated the marriage.

During first PVI, some women do, indeed, feel pain and bleed—but much of this folklore is mistaken. Here's the truth about the hymen.

For reasons that remain unclear, girls are born with membranes partially surrounding their vaginal openings. Anatomists now call it the "vaginal corona," but the conventional term remains *hymen.*

Hymens differ widely. Some are thin, others thick. Most are donut-shaped and open in the center. Some have a ladder-like appearance with bands of tissue extending across the vagina. Others resemble honeycombs with multiple small openings. And in some women—most studies say one in one thousand—the membrane is so thick and the opening so small that fingers, tampons, and erections may not enter comfortably or at all (imperforate hymen). Gynecologists correct this by snipping hymenal tissue, enabling comfortable tampon insertion and PVI.

Imperforate hymens rarely cover the entire opening. If they did, girls could not menstruate. Over the past century, a few case reports have described girls who complained of persistent abdominal pain. They had completely imperforate hymens and could not discharge menstrual flow. Surgery resolved the issue.

Newborns' hymens tend to be prominent and thick. But as the years pass, most hymenal tissue thins and openings usually widen.

Like skin, hymens are flexible. In many girls, everyday activities—washing, exercise, masturbation—wear away some, most, or all of it. Little bits may remain (hymenal tags). In others, hymenal tissue remains largely intact despite strenuous athletics and vigorous masturbation.

What happens to any remaining hymenal tissue during first PVI? No generalizations are possible. Some women feel no pain and don't bleed at all. Others feel some discomfort and may bleed a little. And some suffer considerable pain and bleeding.

Because of hymen mythology, many young women *expect* first intercourse to hurt, setting up a self-fulfilling prophecy. The expectation causes anxiety, which may turn minor discomfort into pain, especially when so few young men know what they're doing.

Meanwhile, young women should not assume that pain during first PVI is hymenal. It may have other causes. Pain on intercourse is a common gynecological complaint with many possible causes. Women who suffer significant pain during first—or any—intercourse should consult a physician or gynecologist.

Some surgeons offer hymen restoration, either sewing tags together or stretching vaginal tissue. Few women opt for it. Most who do are sexual assault survivors who want to feel "whole" again or brides who fear their new husbands will know they're not virgins—even though it's impossible for men to tell.

Finally, what about those bloody sheets? Rough or poorly lubricated intercourse might abrade sensitive vaginal tissue sufficiently to cause bleeding. But in cultures that insist on bridal virginity, no blood on wedding-night sheets disgraced brides, dishonored their families, triggered lawsuits for marital fraud, and sometimes ended with brides' "honor" executions. Many women have taken no chances. Often with their mothers' urging, they've filed a fingernail to a point and on their wedding nights, pierced their inner thighs, which produced enough blood to stain the sheets, satisfy tradition—and perpetuate hymen mythology.

On the Way to Losing It, Negotiate How Far You're Willing to Go

Teen sex-education programs condemn "peer pressure," the way many teens, mostly boys, push others, mostly girls, to spread their legs when they'd rather not. These programs urge the sexually reluctant to "just say no."

Most adolescents expect boys to initiate erotic escalations and girls to either go along and risk slut-shaming or say no and risk prude-shaming. According to the National Health and

Social Life Survey, one-third of women recall not welcoming first PVI, but doing it to shed virginity, feel like adults, please boyfriends, defy parents, brag to friends—or during sexual assault. However, peer pressure plays a role not only in saying yes or no to initial PVI, but in negotiating *every step* up the erotic ladder.

Men often invoke a baseball metaphor to describe how far sex goes. Stepping up to the plate is deep kissing. First base is breast fondling. Second, hand jobs. Third, oral. And a home run, intercourse. The analogy is crude but useful. Absent coercion, most young people become sexual on a ladder of lovemaking that typically takes several years to culminate in PVI.

Progressive sexual play usually includes four milestones:

- Above the neck: kissing, then kissing with tongue play
- Above the waist: breast play with young women fully clothed, revealing bras, or topless
- Below the waist: hand jobs, oral sex
- PVI

No matter where you stand on the ladder, some suggestions:

Play solo. If you self-sex regularly, enjoy yourself. If not, as you start to play with others, consider more solo sex. Masturbation is our original sexuality and the foundation of enjoyable partner sex. It teaches us to respond to erotic stimulation and work up to orgasm. If you're uncomfortable making love with yourself, it's difficult to enjoy it with anyone else. As long as self-sexing is private and doesn't interfere with school, work, family obligations, or partner sex in a relationship, it's not only fine, but beneficial.

No coercion ever. No one should ever feel pressured to be sexual. You are *never* under any obligation to any partner to do anything that unnerves you. Think carefully about your individual comfort level so you're at peace with how far you're willing to go.

Review chapters 4–7. As you round the bases, the information should help you gain comfort with sexual skills.

Know your mind. Think about which step you're on and how you feel about taking the next one. The first few times at each step, you're likely to have mixed emotions—excited to get there, awkward about being there, and eager, apprehensive, or ambivalent about going further.

Some fourteen-year-olds are eager to try hand jobs, oral, or intercourse while some eighteen-year-olds would rather wait. There's no right and wrong, just what you decide for yourself. In the heat of passion, you may change your mind, but if you have limits, you'll probably be happier if you commit to them.

"Let's have great fun going this far." Once you're clear about your limits, speak up. *I enjoy doing A. I'm nervous about B—let's discuss it. And for now, I'm not into C.* If you're assertive, you gain valuable experience in sexual negotiation and limit setting. You also learn if your partner respects your boundaries. If you feel ignored, disrespected, or pushed beyond your limits, perhaps it's time to reconsider your relationship.

Another advantage of speaking up—it proves you're not a tease, which is unfortunately still a sexist stereotype today. *I never teased you. I told you exactly how far I was willing to go. Didn't you listen?*

Initiators, control your lust. Usually it's young men who push round the bases. An old saying goes: *Men have two heads and the little one does the thinking.* Many young men feel so eager for intercourse that they push too hard, and persuasion may become coercion.

Gentlemen, here are three reasons not to think with your little head:

• The girl is likely to tell her friends that you're an ass who should be avoided.
• Forced sex is *never* sizzling sex. It greatly increases risk of premature ejaculation, trouble coming, and erection problems.
• Sexual assault is a felony that might land your sorry butt in prison.

If you've been sexually pushy in the past, consider masturbating to orgasm a few hours before connecting with your girlfriend. Solo sex is calming. It may help you be a sensitive lover, not a jerk, or worse, a rapist.

"Okay?" At every step up the erotic escalator, initiators should ask, *Is it okay if I—?* Asking respects your partner. It acknowledges that sex involves mutual consent. Not conquest.

In addition, the discussions engendered by asking also slow the pace. Young women often complain that young men rush things. Slowing the pace provides the time most young women need to become erotically responsive.

Of course, it's no fun to feel highly aroused and have a partner say *stop.* In sex (and life), it's hard to hear *no.* But life involves disappointments and maturity involves accepting them graciously. If you stop when asked, you just might get a *yes* down the road. But if you don't stop, you're a creep and maybe a criminal.

"Take my hand in yours and show me." If porn is your model for caressing women's breasts and genitals, your girlfriend may recoil from touch that's too rough. Unless women specifically request otherwise, always touch their breasts and genitals tenderly. During erotic caressing, do everything at half speed. Keep lubricant handy and use it. Consider placing your hand in hers and saying, *Show me how you enjoy being touched.*

The same goes for cunnilingus. In porn, the men lick the women like machine guns. Always ask, *Is this okay? More gentle?*

Blue Balls/Lover's Nuts: No Big Deal

Blue balls and lover's nuts are colloquial terms for the ache young men feel between their legs following extended arousal without orgasm/ejaculation. Some men call it excruciating and appeal to partners for relief by hand, mouth, or PVI. Blue balls is real, but any aching is minor. Women are under no obligation to provide relief if they'd rather not.

When men become sexually aroused, extra blood flows into their genitals, causing erection and a feeling of congestion in the scrotum. Without orgasm/ejaculation, this extra blood may trigger aching. Any discomfort subsides on its own in around thirty minutes.

Girls, when boys plead for relief, you can choose to lend a hand or just say, *Do it yourself.*

When Young Women Push Young Men

Sometimes, girls initiate and boys would rather not. Some feel bored with how far they've gone and want the next step. Others become pushy after overindulging in alcohol. Whatever the reason, when girls push, boys may feel stressed. Sexual aggressiveness by girls contradicts cultural expectations. It's disconcerting to expect events to unfold one way and then have them proceed in another.

Boys should deal with pushy girls the same way girls should deal with aggressive boys: resist coercion. Be clear about your limits. Have fun within your comfort zone. Then stick to your guns. If you're prude-shamed, say something like, *Actually, I'm just not that into you.*

How to Lose It—Happily

Eventually, almost everyone rounds the bases and scores. Some first PVI is wonderful, but most people recall mixed feelings—happy to cross it off the list but not thrilled with the sex. Some didn't want to go all the way but were assaulted. Harvard researchers surveyed a representative sample of 13,310 US women, age eighteen to forty-four. Those saying their first time was forced—6.5 percent, millions of women.

Even when first PVI feels fine, many new lovers feel disappointed. Our culture hypes first PVI as a big deal. But for many, it's over in a drunken flash and bells don't ring. That's sad but normal.

Recall the first time you rode a bicycle. You probably wobbled and fell. But with practice, you mastered it. Sex is similar. It takes practice to enjoy. At every step, you may feel anxious and awkward. But eventually, you gain comfort with erotic play and the negotiations involved in mutual satisfaction.

Some suggestions . . .

Have you been sexually abused? If either of you has any history of unwanted or abusive sex, you can recover and enjoy fulfilling relationships and sizzling sex. However, involuntary sex complicates freely chosen lovemaking. As you contemplate your first time affirmatively consenting, if you haven't already, this would be a good time for therapy to recover from your sexual trauma.

Young women, check your hymens. Can you insert tampons comfortably? A lubricated finger? If not, PVI may feel uncomfortable, painful, or impossible. Consult a doctor or gynecologist. Minor hymen surgery may be necessary.

Admit your virginity. Many people, especially boys, wonder if this is wise. There's no right or wrong, just what you decide for yourself. But as loveplay moves below the waist, I encourage those who have not had PVI to say so. Coming clean usually enhances first intercourse.

Sexual relationships involve intimacy, revealing who you really are and hoping your partner accepts you. Such hopes may be rewarded or dashed. That's life. Young people can be kind or cruel, and fear of prude- or slut-shaming propels many to lie about their sexual experience.

Who's more likely to lie about virginity? Men. Almost everyone still expects young men to be more experienced and orchestrate the erotic dance. Dishonesty about virginity is likely to trigger anxiety. *Can I get away with faking experience? Will he/she know?* But honesty can also be stressful. *Am I pathetic? Will I be shamed?* Either approach may provoke stress that's bad for sex.

If you lie about your situation, you're likely to remain stressed throughout whatever happens—with the nasty stress hormone, cortisol, impairing erotic pleasure. But if you admit your virginity and your partner is reassuring, you can relax, which enhances responsiveness. Of course, immature partners may shame you. Either way, you're rolling dice.

Still, I encourage honesty. Your lover may not be experienced either, and may well admire your honesty or, if already familiar with PVI, feel fine about introducing you.

Finally, what if you're prude-shamed? *You haven't done it? What's wrong with you?* Here's a snappy comeback: *I could have. Several times. But I wanted it to feel special and it never did—until now.*

Limit alcohol. During first PVI, many, if not most, young people are intoxicated. Bad idea. Drunk sex is usually lousy sex.

The first drink is disinhibiting, which is why seducers offer alcohol so eagerly. But subsequent drinks impair judgment and interfere with erection and ejaculatory control in men, vulvar and clitoral sensitivity in women, and pleasure and orgasm in all genders. Alcohol also substantially boosts women's risk of sexual assault.

Don't do it drunk. If you want to get laid in an altered state, consider cannabis. Two-thirds of lovers consider it sex enhancing. And compared with booze, it's much less likely to trigger assaults.

Carry condoms. This applies to both young men and women. Use condoms your first time and every time. Keep them handy, but don't store them in wallets kept in pockets. Prolonged exposure to body heat may contribute to breakage.

Many young women underestimate young men's willingness to use condoms. That's what Australian researchers discovered in a survey of 819 young adults. Increasingly, young men are fine with condoms. If not, ladies, tell your guy, *Either you do, or I don't.*

Use lubricant. Even if first intercourse is totally consensual, anxiety may reduce young women's natural vaginal lubrication and cause discomfort or pain. In seconds, saliva or commercial lube makes PVI more comfortable.

Consider the setting. Discuss what you both consider romantic: candlelight, music, clean sheets, privacy—whatever. To maximize pleasure your first time or any time, arrange a romantic setting that shows consideration for the woman. She wants you to see her as special. She fears you see her only as *pussy.* Show her that you value her and are willing to expend effort on her comfort and pleasure. If you make her feel special, the sex is more likely to feel special, too.

Schedule it. For most first-time lovers, sex just happens. You drink too much and suddenly, you're in the throes—with possible regrets after. For a satisfying first time, plan it.

Now, many people young and old object to scheduled sex. They raise two objections: *What if I'm not in the mood?* And *Spontaneity is more romantic.*

Being in the mood is rarely an issue for horny teens and young adults. And who says scheduling isn't romantic? Making a date creates anticipation, which piques arousal. It also allows time to assemble condoms and lube, arrange music, change the linen, and place flowers on the nightstand. Except for the occasional quickie, sex coaches and therapists almost universally recommend scheduling nookie in advance.

Review the basics. Top athletes never stop working on the fundamentals. If sex is your sport, review chapters 1–10.

Don't imitate porn. See chapter 46.

Coach each other. Never assume you know what your partner wants. *Ask.* And don't assume that your lover knows what you enjoy. *Speak up.* Ideally you've been doing this since your first deep kiss. If not, start now.

Don't expect women to come during intercourse. PVI brings 95 percent of men to orgasm consistently, but only 25 percent of women of all ages—no matter how long it lasts, how large the erection, or how deeply in love the couple may be. The old in-out is great fun, but it usually doesn't supply what most women need for orgasm—direct, gentle, extended clitoral caressing.

Ask your partner how she'd like to climax—clitoral/vulva hand massage, cunnilingus, vibrator, or some combination. If hand massage, place hers on yours and encourage her to show you how she likes to be touched. If cunnilingus, check in about intensity. If she needs to bring herself off by hand or vibrator, that's not necessarily any reflection on who she is or your skill as a lover. Many women (and some men) have difficulty with orgasm, especially those who are young, inexperienced, and anxious.

Try these two positions. Many couples love the man-on-top (missionary) position. But for inexperienced lovers, it's often problematic. Young men may have trouble finding the vaginal opening. Men may hurt women by pushing in too forcefully. And in the missionary position, few women come.

A better position for young lovers is woman-on-top. He's on his back. She kneels over his hips. It's easy for one or both to apply lubricant to themselves or each other. One holds his erection as she slowly sits down on it. She controls the speed and depth of insertion, which keeps her comfortable. And while she's unlikely to climax from the intercourse alone, the woman-on-top position makes orgasm much more likely. Either can easily reach her clitoris and caress her or use a vibrator. Or he can place a fist where their pelvises meet and she can lean into it, which also provides direct clitoral stimulation.

Some men think woman-on-top is "not masculine." Nonsense. Using the suggestions just mentioned, she's more likely to enjoy sex and come. She's also more likely to consider you a good lover, which boosts your odds of getting lucky again. What's not masculine about that?

The other good position for inexperienced lovers is rear entry (doggie style). She stands bent at the waist or is on her hands or elbows and knees. He stands or kneels behind her. It's easy for him to insert. Ideally, he should place the head of his penis at the opening, remain still, and invite her to move back onto him. That way she controls the speed and depth of insertion. And either can easily provide direct clitoral caresses.

Never expect simultaneous orgasms. In Hollywood sex, the man is usually on top. He pumps, they both moan, and after a few strokes, it appears they both climax together. In real life, simultaneous orgasms are highly unlikely. Among the 25 percent of women who are consistently orgasmic during intercourse, few have them at the same moment as their men. Take turns helping each other work up to orgasm.

Keep your expectations low. Even with preparation and negotiation, it usually takes considerable practice to master lovemaking. Give it time.

If your penis doesn't cooperate . . . Try not to flip out. In all likelihood, your little buddy is fine, and the cause is alcohol, stress, fatigue, and/or inexperience.

Laugh. There's humor in two people trying to fit their genitals together. Try to laugh off difficulties. You're young. You have decades of sex ahead of you. So you fell off the bike. You'll master riding soon enough.

Afterward, cuddle. After you've both had orgasms, don't fall asleep or jump out of bed. Cuddling during afterglow increases sexual satisfaction, especially for women. That's what University of Toronto researchers concluded in a survey of 335 lovers (138 men, 197 women). Small increases in postcoital cuddling substantially boosted their sexual and relationship satisfaction.

"I love you." If you hear these three magic words, beware. They imply vastly different things to different people. To some, they mean it's time to plan the wedding. To others, they express appreciation for *this moment* with no future implications. Ask what your partner really means.

When do recent ex-virgins become "experienced"? There are two issues here—number of times and erotic skill. The two are surprisingly independent. It's quite possible to do it hundreds of times and still have lousy sex. It's also possible to make love just a few times and enjoy sizzling sex. It comes down to "having sex" versus "making love." Having sex happens to you. Making love is something the two of you *create together*. No matter how many times you've done it, you're experienced when you both consistently enjoy pleasure and help each other work up to orgasms.

Performance Anxiety Is Often *Transition* Anxiety

Anyone can feel nervous about sex. *Am I doing it right? Is my partner enjoying it?* Sexologists call this performance anxiety. But quite often, the issue involves transitioning from masturbation to partner sex.

Both are "sex," but they're quite different. In masturbation, the only person you have to please is yourself. That's comparatively easy. You get immediate feedback from self-touch and can quickly adjust however you wish.

In partner lovemaking, you must please another and help that person please you. It's an intricate dance that requires time, negotiation, coaching, and practice.

If you feel nervous, say so. Your partner might mock you. If so, perhaps that person is not for you. More likely, your partner also feels anxious. Coach each other, and all should be well . . . eventually.

Virgins' Wedding Nights: Probably Not Magical

Among the few percent of Americans who postpone PVI until marriage, some report magical first times. But over the years, I've received many queries from virgin newlyweds whose first rolls in the sheets left them disappointed, sometimes anguished.

This should come as no surprise. Mastering lovemaking requires practice. With no driver education, first-time drivers are likely to crash. The same goes for virgin first-time lovers with fairy tale expectations for their wedding nights.

Advice to virgin brides and grooms:

- Kiss, cuddle, and fool around on your wedding night, but consider postponing genital sex until the morning after. Right after the wedding, you're likely to feel exhausted and intoxicated, a combination that rarely produces sizzling sex.
- Understand that you have a lot to learn about your own sexuality and your new spouse's. Sizzling sex doesn't happen by magic. It takes negotiation, practice, patience, and a good sense of humor.
- If you haven't already, declare how often you masturbate. If infrequently, consider more. The more familiar you are with solo sex, the easier partner lovemaking becomes.
- Take turns reading part I of this book to each other. Discuss each chapter.
- Six months into your marriage, if you're still unhappy with your lovemaking, consider sex coaching or therapy.

The Secret Shame of Older Virgins

In *The 40-Year-Old Virgin*, Steve Carell plays Andy, a nerdy guy into his fourth decade who has never danced the horizontal tango. He admits it to friends, who decide to help. But their advice is worthless. On his own, Andy meets Trish (Catherine Keener), and eventually, well, it's Hollywood. . . .

The 40-Year-Old Virgin is a comedy, but for real older virgins, those who haven't experienced PVI by twenty-five, it's usually a tragedy filled with shame and isolation.

Older virginity was considered rare until the 1980s, when sex therapists began reporting a steady trickle of clients over twenty-five, three-quarters of them men, who had never made love with anyone other than themselves. Many had tried sex workers, but said it "didn't count," that they'd never had "real" relationships. By the 1990s, it was clear that a surprisingly large number of adults were involuntary virgins.

How many? University of California, San Francisco, researchers used data from the National Survey of Family Growth to track sexual abstinence among 7,589 American adults age twenty-five to forty-five. Among those not voluntarily celibate, 5 percent of the men and 2 percent of the women said they'd never had partner sex. One forty-year-old virgin man called it "my lifelong shame, my terrible handicap."

Sex therapists who counsel older virgins say most are shy, socially awkward, and uncomfortable with the whole idea of bumping bellies. One said: "I shut myself off. I can't really explain why, except that I was very shy. I was keenly interested in women, but they intimidated me. I had no idea how to get beyond friendships to anything romantic, no idea at all."

Fortunately, there's help—surrogate partner therapy. It began in 1966, when British sexologist Martin John Cole, PhD, introduced "sex surrogates," sexologically trained women, to facilitate sex therapy with men. He was attacked for running a brothel. A few years later, pioneering American sex researchers William Masters, MD, and Virginia Johnson also used surrogates at their St. Louis clinic and faced similar condemnation (but Masters was never arrested for pandering as depicted in the TV series *Masters of Sex*).

By the 1970s, the name changed from "sex surrogate" to "surrogate partner"—for good reason. Many surrogates never have genital sex with clients. Instead, they answer questions and introduce them to deep kissing, sensual touch, mutual nudity, and massage to help them become more comfortable with what happens in sexual relationships. Eventually, some surrogates include genital play.

To distinguish themselves from sex workers, most surrogate partners work closely with sex therapists and accept clients only by referral. Surrogate therapy costs more than regular sex therapy because both the therapist and surrogate must be paid.

Surrogates are available in many US locales. If not, prospective clients either travel to them or pay for surrogates' visits, which adds to the expense. One thirty-eight-year-old virgin lived on the East Coast. He found a psychotherapist near him to supervise his work with a surrogate and flew her out from Los Angeles—a total cost of $12,000, and for him well worth it. By the end of his therapy, he felt "finally, part of the adult world."

To find a surrogate partner, visit the International Professional Surrogates Association (IPSA, surrogatetherapy.org).

Losing It When Disabled

For those with disabilities, shedding virginity is especially daunting. The myth is that people with disabilities are neither sexual nor erotically attractive. Actually, everyone is sexual and everyone is sexually attractive to someone.

Depending on the disability, disabled young adult virgins must contend with possible lack of privacy, difficulty erotically touching another, energy and mobility problems, and possibly drug side effects that impair sexual functioning.

Disabled people who would like professional help losing their virginity might try surrogate partners. For more, see the film *The Sessions* with Helen Hunt and John Hawkes—he's quadriplegic and she's his surrogate. Visit the International Professional Surrogates Association (IPSA, surrogatetherapy.org).

CHAPTER 19:
Today's Young Adult Hookups Used to Be Called Dating

WHEN IT WAS launched in 2012, the dating/hookup app Tinder triggered breathless—often ominous—media reports of young adults consumed by casual, frenzied, quickie sex. The brouhaha lasted a few years, then subsided. But many mature adults and some young people remain concerned about hookup culture, fearing that Tinder and similar sites propel many young adults into bed with someone new almost nightly.

Actually, compared with previous generations, today's young adult sexuality hasn't changed much. The substantial research literature on hooking up shows that, since the 1920s, things have remained largely the same. Hooking up represents only a minor variation on what previous generations called dating.

Nothing New

In a sexual context, the term *hook up* dates from the late 1990s, though it didn't become prevalent until around 2006. Which raises a question. Did something change in young American sexuality during the first decade of the current century?

To investigate, University of Portland researchers analyzed data from the General Social Survey (GSS), the most comprehensive ongoing study of Americans' beliefs and behavior. The researchers compared GSS findings from two periods, shortly before "hooking up" entered the lexicon (1988–96) and as young adults embraced it (2004–12):

Total Number of Sex Partners among US Young Adults since Age 18		
	1988–96	2004–12
0	10%	15%
1	23%	23%
2	16%	13%
3–5	23%	24%
6–12	20%	17%
13–20	5%	5%
21+	4%	3%

Monto, A. M., and A. G. Carey. "A New Standard of Sexual Behavior? Are Claims Associated with the 'Hookup Culture' Supported by General Social Survey Data?" *Journal of Sex Research* 51 (2014): 605.

The only discernible difference—a larger proportion of today's young adults are *celibate*. Those reporting no lovers increased from 10 to 15 percent. Otherwise, the two sets of figures look remarkably similar. The term *hook up* may be newer, but bed-hopping among today's young adults appears quite similar to what today's parents and grandparents did in their youth.

Sexual Experimentation Peaks

In the chart above, one-quarter of young adults report six or more partners in their fairly brief lifetimes. They're highly sexual, a much larger proportion than in the general population.

Why the disparity? Largely because young adulthood is the time of greatest erotic experimentation. People can become sexually experimental at any age. Many try new moves after divorce. But young adulthood is the period of greatest erotic sampling. Largely liberated from parental constraints, young adults are free to follow their sexuality wherever it may lead.

In addition to young adults' widely varying number of partners, this stage of life also marks the time when people are most likely to explore the full range of their sexual interests: oral, anal, nonmonogamy, BDSM, and sex that's not exclusively heterosexual. This is a normal part of maturation, another step on the path to unique individual sexual identity.

How Sexual?

Some media reports have implied that hookups almost always lead to intercourse. This is not surprising. The term conjures hook-and-eye locks, with hooks slipping into eyes. It's only a small step to more intimate insertions.

But in surveys of hundreds of college students, researchers at Syracuse University and SUNY Binghamton discovered that most hookups are less sexual than media reports suggest:

Activities during Most Recent Hookup:
Kissing: 98%
Fondling the woman's breasts: 58%
Hands on genitals: 53%
Oral sex (provided and/or received): 36%
Intercourse: 34%

Garcia J. R., and C. Reiber. "Hook-Up Behavior: A Biopsychosocial Perspective." *Journal of Social, Evolutionary, and Cultural Psychology* 2 (2008): 192.

Only one-third of hookups included intercourse. A study of Northeastern University students showed similar results. Seventy-eight percent had hooked up, but only a third had rounded third and scored. One out of three might still appall social conservatives, but these findings show that the hook slips into the eye in only a minority of cases.

The Alcohol Connection

For college students, spring break is prime time for hooking up. Researchers at the University of Windsor, Ontario, surveyed students who hoped to have sex during spring break. Back on campus afterward, 61 percent of the men and 34 percent of the women said *mission accomplished*, usually within one day of meeting partners. This may sound hasty, but spring brings spring fever. Spring break is brief. Vacationing students are horny. And alcohol is everywhere.

A University of Illinois survey shows that 49 percent of college men and 38 percent of women reported having sex as a direct result of drinking. Canadian researchers at St. Mary's University in Halifax asked hundreds of college students about alcohol and hookups.

At My Last Hookup, I Was . . .
Sober: 27%
Mildly intoxicated: 27%
Very intoxicated: 35%
Passing-out drunk: 9%

Patrick, M. E., and J. L. Maggs. "Does Drinking Lead to Sex? Daily Alcohol-Sex Behaviors and Expectancies among College Students." *Psychology of Addictive Behavior* 23 (2009): 472.

The combination of alcohol and lust can be dangerous. When men and/or women drink, women face substantially increased risk of rape. Drunk lovers are less likely to use condoms. And drunk sex is usually lousy sex.

Intoxication and Sex through the Lifespan

Many, if not most, young people drink when they lose their virginity. Almost three-quarters of young people who hook up have sex intoxicated. And as adults mature, alcohol and sex often remain paired. University of Chicago researchers asked 3,432 Americans age eighteen to fifty-nine about alcohol during couple sex. In all age groups, half to three-quarters said they combined the two.

The first drink is disinhibiting. Prospective lovers are more likely to say *yes*. But intoxication raises risk of sex problems and sexual assault.

If you'd like to make love in an altered state but don't want to drink, consider cannabis. Several studies show that two-thirds of users call it sex enhancing. And compared with men who are drunk, those using cannabis are much less likely to suffer sex problems and be aggressive.

Do Hookups Exploit Women?

Critics uncomfortable with hookups often assert that they reflect male fantasies of porn-style, free-for-all sex, while ignoring young women's preference for lovemaking in the context of committed relationships. They charge that hookups hurt women, who afterward have regrets.

Of course, any coupling can produce regrets, but a Syracuse University study of 118 women undergraduates suggests that, far from feeling victimized, the large majority of young women feel enthusiastic about hooking up:

Why Did You Hook Up?
I wanted to have sex: 80%
It was an impulsive decision: 58%
I felt attracted to the guy: 56%
I was drunk: 51%
The guy really wanted it: 33%
I wanted to feel desirable: 29%
(Respondents could cite more than one reason.)

Fielder, R. L., and M. P. Carey. "Prevalence and Characteristics of Sexual Hookups among First-Semester Female College Students." *Journal of Sex and Marital Therapy* 36 (2010): 346.

Four of five young women affirmatively wanted to test the mattress. No doubt, some women feel used during hookups—some men, too. But the large majority of women participate because they want to.

After Hookups: Regret? Or Contentment?

Many mature adults disturbed by hookups assume that soon afterward, young people—particularly women—feel regret. Several studies have documented posthookup remorse.

However, these studies asked *only* about regret, ignoring other possible emotions. I've been happily coupled for close to fifty years. Looking back, I have some regrets. Who doesn't? Studies that assess only regret provide little insight into hookups' overall impact. Studies that have investigated the full range of possible reactions show that most young people feel fine about hooking up:

- University of Louisville researchers surveyed 187 students' reactions to hookups. Those who expressed mostly regret: 17 percent. Those expressing mostly enjoyment: 65 percent, almost four times as many.
- Researchers at SUNY Binghamton asked 311 students how they felt about their most recent hookup. More than half the women and four of five men said they felt happy—57 and 82 percent respectively.

These studies also show that serious hookup regret is most likely in just one circumstance—intercourse when very drunk. About one-third of hookups involve intercourse, and the participants are blotto in around half of them. This suggests that around 16 percent of young adults probably feel primarily regret, a figure in line with the Louisville study just mentioned. Meanwhile, around 84 percent feel okay or better.

As I came of age in the late 1960s, I had a fling or two I later regretted. That's life. That's also how young people learn to negotiate relationships. But even my worst romps left no lasting scars. I learned from them. The same appears to be true for today's hookup generation.

Do Hookups Derail Commitment?

Critics of casual sex consider hookups proof that young adults disdain long-term relationships. On the contrary, the Louisville researchers asked five hundred hookup-experienced young adults how they felt about commitment. Two-thirds of the women (65 percent) and almost half the men (45 percent) said they hoped their hookups would lead to lasting relationships. In addition, 51 percent of the women and 42 percent of the men said that during recent hookups, they'd discussed the possibility of greater commitment.

Friends with Benefits: How Friendly? How Sexual?

Many of today's young adults are products of divorce. They view marriage as fragile and risky, and they've a coined a new term for relationships somewhere between hookups and commitment, *friends with benefits* (FWB), emotionally attached buddies who also occasionally enjoy the horizontal bop. The term FWB may be fairly recent—the *Oxford English Dictionary* says it was coined in 1995—but FWB relationships are not. People of all ages have played that way forever.

How common are FWB relationships? Researchers at Michigan State and Wayne State Universities surveyed 125 young adults (65 women, 60 men). Sixty percent (40 men, 35 women) said they'd been FWBs and one-third claimed to be involved in such relationships when surveyed.

Can FWBs remain "just friends"? Almost two-thirds (62 percent) said yes. Among those experienced in FWB arrangements, 81 percent (34 men, 26 women) said it was quite possible to be happily FWB for quite a while.

FWB couples reported various sexual frequencies:

- Just once—19%
- Occasionally—52%
- Frequently—29%

They cited these advantages:

- Sex without commitment—74%
- A sex partner when needed—69%
- Sex with a friend, not a stranger—26%
- A relationship while remaining officially single—13%

They also recognized disadvantages:

- Developing romantic feelings—81%
- Risking the friendship—35%
- No commitment—16%
- Disliking the sex—12%

Bisson, M. A., and T. R. Levine. "Negotiating a Friends with Benefits Relationship." *Archives of Sexual Behavior* 38 (2009): 66.

Before they became sexual, FWB couples were friends for an average of fourteen months. Some remained long-term FWB (28 percent). But most such relationships changed after about six months. Many stopped having sex but remained friends (36 percent). Some became romantically coupled (10 percent). Or both the friendship and the sex ended (26 percent).

From Pregnant Puritans to Dating to Hookups

Every generation comes of age in a burst of sexual exuberance, and from time immemorial, many young adults have engaged in casual sex their elders found unsettling. Today's hookup culture is simply the latest iteration of this ancient truth.

Rebound and Revenge Sex: Beyond the Mythology

Somebody dumps somebody else. Soon after, conventional wisdom says both are likely to jump into bed with strangers. Dumpers have "rebound" sex to move on. Dumpees have "revenge" sex to soothe their distress. Actually, rebound and revenge sex are more the exception than the rule.

Two recent studies show that only one-third of young lovers engage in this type of sex, and when they do, it's not with strangers:

- University of Missouri researchers polled 170 college students who'd experienced recent breakups. Only a third said they'd ever had sex specifically to get over their breakup or to get back at the ex.
- ABC News surveyed 1,501 US adults of all ages. Among respondents eighteen to twenty-nine, only one-third said they'd had rebound sex and just 16 percent revenge sex.

This type of sex also supposedly involves strangers. But according to the Missouri survey, strangers were the *least likely* partners. Dumpers' and dumpees' first postbreakup partners were:

- Strangers met that day—5%
- Their most recent ex—20%
- A friend or acquaintance—21%
- A previous lover other than the most recent ex—54%

Barber, L. L., and M. L. Cooper. "Rebound Sex: Motives and Behaviors Following a Relationship Breakup." *Archives of Sexual Behavior* 43 (2013): 251.

Postbreakup sex is less about throwing caution to the wind than curling up with someone familiar.

Many people believe that sex with one's most recent ex hinders recovery from the breakup. Not so, according to Wayne State University researchers in Detroit. They analyzed diaries kept by young adults who'd recently broken up. Sex with the ex had no effect on the time it took them to say they'd recovered.

How long does rebound/revenge sex last? The more established the relationship, the longer the exes report distress. But interest peaks in the immediate aftermath and largely ends within six months.

The ABC sample included adults of all ages. With rising age, reports of rebound/revenge sex fall. As adults mature, they usually gain perspective on life's vicissitudes and cope with breakups in other ways.

Finally, some call rebound/revenge sex bad for the soul, an immature escape from "proper" grieving. Not according to researchers at the University of Illinois and Queens College in New York, who surveyed seventy-seven people (sixty women, seventeen men) age eighteen to thirty-nine who'd experienced recent breakups. Those who twisted the sheets soon afterward showed the greatest resilience and self-esteem.

In colonial New England, an estimated one-third of brides were pregnant at the altar. The Puritans frowned on premarital sex but tolerated it—if the couples married.

From the Civil War to the early twentieth century, proper courtship took place in young women's homes. Male suitors visited, and the couple spent chaste time together under the watchful eyes of the women's older relatives. But many courting couples also schemed ways to meet privately, for example, in the barns or stables adjacent to most of that era's homes, hence the expression *a roll in the hay.*

By the turn of the twentieth century, America was industrializing. Many young adults left home for cities where they had little older-adult supervision. It was the dawn of dating. The term was coined in 1896.

After World War I, risqué flapper fashions bared women's arms and legs, scandalizing matrons. Courtship increasingly involved telephone communication and automobiles, which removed courting couples from young women's homes. The Roaring Twenties also saw the founding of Planned Parenthood. Diaphragms and condoms separated intercourse from pro-creation as never before—and contributed to what moralists called rampant casual sex.

By World War II, dating was firmly established. Many young couples "necked," or more, at the movies. Young men reveled in "wine, women, and song." And many young women considered it their patriotic duty to send their boys off to war with a night to remember.

After the war, Alfred Kinsey's team surveyed eleven thousand adults, most eighteen to thirty-five, born from 1912 to 1929. Two-thirds of the men and half the women admitted premarital sex—and undoubtedly many of the naysayers also indulged but wouldn't admit it.

The post–World War II Baby Boom generation came of age just as the Pill finalized the separation of sex from pregnancy risk. "Wine, women, and song" morphed—but not much—into "sex, drugs, and rock 'n' roll," with parental critics decrying promiscuity.

Today, the Baby Boom generation's children are young adults who connect on Tinder and often do what comes naturally. But compared with their parents, they do it less and are more likely to use contraception, much less likely to have unplanned pregnancies, and considerably less likely to have abortions.

The Kids Are Alright

Instead of "dating," today it's "hookups" and "FWBs." Why has the vocabulary evolved? Largely because young adults delight in differentiating themselves from their parents.

In addition, another development has fueled casual sex among today's young adults. Compared with their parents and grandparents, they spend more time single. Census figures:

Average Age at Marriage		
Year	Men	Women
1950	23	21
1980	24	22
2016	29	27

Delaying marriage translates to hundreds of extra Friday and Saturday nights while single, plenty of time to explore casual liaisons.

Hooking up is nothing new. It's twenty-first-century dating, a normal, healthy part of maturation among young adults, most of whom act reasonably responsibly—unless drunk. Intercourse is the exception, not the rule. Hooking up rarely causes significant psychological distress. Most young women participants affirmatively desire their casual sex. And committed relationships are still on the agenda . . . in the future.

Older folks always worry about youthful erotic exuberance—often forgetting what they did as young adults. Hooking up is simply today's path to sexual adulthood. As that geezer band, the Who, once sang about the parents of today's young adults, "the kids are alright."

CHAPTER 20:
How to Prevent Sexual Assault and Harassment

SINCE 2000, THE media have spotlighted epidemic levels of college and military sexual assaults, everything from uninvited groping to gang rapes. And since 2017, when movie mogul Harvey Weinstein was revealed to have sexually harassed dozens of women, spurring the #MeToo movement, workplace sexual harassment has also become a major social issue. Sexual assault and harassment are horrible crimes, which are also usually preventable.

Most college and military sexual assaults result from a toxic combination of alcohol, poor understanding of risk, and friends who don't intervene in time. Based on these risk factors, several effective prevention programs have been developed that, in a few years, have consistently reduced rapes in the military and on college campuses by 50 percent.

The vast majority of workplace sexual harassment results from similar factors: alcohol, management denial, ineffective training, victim reluctance to report, and bystander silence. Many elements of the programs that have substantially reduced military and college rapes also help minimize sexual harassment.

Affirmative Consent: Great for Consensual Sex, but Useless for Rape Prevention

To prevent sexual assaults, college activists have advocated "affirmative consent," the idea that sexual initiators must obtain specific permission for every erotic escalation. Many campuses have incorporated affirmative consent into student handbooks and disciplinary actions. *Did she give you clear permission to finger her?*

Affirmative consent is a great boon to consensual sex—it builds trust, slows the pace, encourages mutual coaching and discussion of contraception and sexual infections, and helps prevent sex problems. But affirmative consent has nothing to do with preventing rape. Once the intoxicated spider captures the stumbling-drunk fly, it's too late for *Is this okay?*

Instead of emphasizing clear permission to proceed, successful rape-prevention programs focus on the moments shortly before assaults begin and the actions that either trigger or prevent them. By training young people to recognize assault triggers and react quickly, many colleges and the US Navy have reduced assaults substantially:

- In 1987, a first-year student at the University of New Hampshire was gang-raped in her dorm room—and the perpetrators stepped into the hall and invited others to join in. The incident sparked campus-wide soul searching and led to a survey showing that 37 percent of UNH's women students said they'd been sexually intimidated or assaulted

on campus. But in 2012, after campus-wide implementation of a prevention program based on assault triggers, rapes dropped by more than half.
- The University of Kentucky implemented a similar trigger-based rape-prevention program. Five years later, campus rapes had declined 50 percent.
- At the US Navy's boot camp in Illinois, a trigger-recognition program has reduced sexual assaults by 60 percent.
- At the Canadian universities of Calgary, Windsor, and Guelph, 893 first-year women students either read a brochure about sexual assault or took a twelve-hour rape-prevention course based on self-defense and recognition of assault triggers. One year later:

What happened	Brochure Group	Trained Women	Risk Reduction
Completed rape	10%	5%	50%
Attempted rape	9%	3%	67%

Trained women stopped two-thirds of attempted assaults and reduced completed rapes by half.
- Self-defense training was the *least* important element of the program. When women recognize assault triggers and take steps to stop escalations, rapes don't happen, so no need for self-defense.
- Finally, the Centers for Disease Control and Prevention evaluated 100 studies of sexual violence prevention programs. The verdict: prevention efforts substantially reduce rape.

One Woman in Five, One Man in Fifty

According to the CDC, at some point in life, 20 percent of women and 2 percent of men suffer some level of sexual assault.

Since 2000, record numbers of college women have reported sexual assaults and from 2010 to 2013, reports of military rape have increased 37 percent. These increases are unnerving, but they have less to do with any surge in rapes than with antiassault activism. Increasingly vocal advocates for women's safety have persuaded more victims to report assaults, documenting a serious problem that has remained veiled way too long.

For years, colleges and the military minimized women's rape risk, partly from ignorance of its prevalence, and partly because they feared that addressing it would threaten recruitment. Imagine parents hearing, *Your daughter faces a one-in-five chance of being hit by a campus bus.* Who would send their daughters to that college?

Who Gets Assaulted? Why?

As activism illuminated the epidemic of campus and military rapes, researchers identified the elements that govern risk:

- **Naivete.** Investigators with United Educators (UE), an insurance consortium of 1,200 colleges, found that 63 percent of college rape victims are first-year students. In the military, most victims are among the youngest recruits. Both groups, typically eighteen, have difficulty recognizing trouble and are often unable to extricate themselves from it—especially when drunk.

- **Alcohol.** In the vast majority of young adult sexual assaults, both perpetrators and victims are smashed. Almost two-thirds of military sexual assaults—62 percent—involve alcohol. A UE review of college rapes from 2005 to 2010 showed that 60 percent of accusers were so intoxicated they had *no clear memory* of the assault. In the military, the situation is similar. Even when victims and perpetrators aren't wasted, a University of Vermont study of 942 students showed that more than half of victims had been drinking before things got out of hand.
- **Power/prestige.** Throughout history, powerful men have considered subordinate women their sexual playthings. Most military sexual assaults involve perpetrators foisting themselves on victims of lower rank. In college, the issue is not rank but prestige, notably the cachet of being an athlete. Male athletes comprise only 10 percent of college student bodies, but according to UE, they commit 25 percent of campus rapes. Athletes are big men on campus and often believe the girls are theirs for the taking.
- **Bystanders.** Friends of perpetrators and victims often realize things are getting out of hand but take no action to stop it.

Sexual Assault Prevention 101

Details differ, but most successful prevention programs include reality checks, frank talk during orientation, alcohol abuse awareness, and bystander intervention.

Many young women believe they're most likely to be assaulted by strangers in deserted parking garages. In reality, they're most likely to be raped by dates and acquaintances at parties.

Successful rape-prevention programs begin on day one at college or in the military. All US Navy recruits train at one boot camp. On the bus there, before even reaching the gate, they watch a video featuring the camp commander. He declares in no uncertain terms that today's navy has zero tolerance for sexual assault.

During boot camp, officers of every rank reiterate this message loud and clear:

- *Do you think Ms. Sloppy Drunk can give real consent?*
- *If you cross the line, you're looking at prison.*
- *Not saying "no" is much different than saying "yes."*

Do Rape Victims Ask for It?

Accused rapists often say:

- *Her skirt was so short.*
- *She wasn't wearing a bra.*
- *She followed me into my room.*

In response, activists have insisted that focusing on women's behavior blames victims instead of perpetrators. At demonstrations, their banners say DON'T TELL ME HOW TO DRESS. TELL RAPISTS TO STOP.

Absolutely, rapists should stop. But women must remain aware and vigilant for their own protection, including using common sense and avoiding high-risk situations. Successful rape prevention programs don't counsel women how to dress. They emphasize sobriety, danger recognition, self-extrication, and bystander intervention.

Among colleges with rape-prevention programs, orientation programs are similarly blunt. In addition, many schools have instituted extraforceful orientations for incoming athletes, followed by ongoing reiteration by coaches. In recent years, several top collegiate athletes have been convicted of sexual assault, costing their schools likely championships. In order to keep top athletes playing, many coaches now read them the riot act about sexual assault. Some fraternities do the same with new members.

Many young adults drink too much, with binge drinking at parties quite common. Sexual assault is its collateral damage. When men drink, some become lusty and violent. And when women drink, many men believe they're more sexually available.

In the 1980s, when Mothers Against Drunk Driving first advocated designated drivers, pundits scoffed that partygoers would never voluntarily abstain to prevent drunk driving. Today, designated drivers are the rule—and drunk-driving deaths have plummeted. Assault-prevention programs advocate something similar. One person stays sufficiently sober to keep friends who drink out of trouble.

But one designated nondrinker is not enough. Rape prevention is everyone's responsibility. In an era threatened by terrorism, transportation authorities have promoted the mantra *If you see something, say something*. Rape-prevention programs tout a similar message: *Don't just stand there, do something*—anything to stop bad behavior before it becomes assaultive.

The navy emphasizes that bystander intervention need not be dramatic or heroic. It's not the cavalry riding to the rescue, but rather timely words to the not so wise: *Hey, asshole, that's not how you treat women*. The navy has also stepped up shore patrols to supervise sailors at ports of call.

The University of New Hampshire's Jane Stapleton says a little creativity goes a long way. If bystanders see trouble, she recommends the following: Turn on the lights. Turn off the music. Spill drinks on aggressors. Pull the girl away. Or tell the guy that someone in the next room wants to talk to him—anything to interrupt the interaction. One of Stapleton's favorite interventions came from a young woman who loudly told her drunk girlfriend—and the guy who was all over her: "Here's the tampon you wanted."

University of Kentucky researchers implemented a bystander-intervention training program at one college with 2,768 students, while taking no action at two others with 4,258 students. At the latter, sexual assaults continued unchanged, but at the school with bystander training, they dropped substantially.

New Focus on Young Men

Early rape-prevention programs focused on victims' trauma, hoping to foster empathy in young men. The new programs continue this, but also appeal to young men to keep their friends out of prison: *Do you want to see your friend's life ruined? If you were crossing the line, wouldn't you want someone to step in? If you see a friend going too far, it's your responsibility to intervene.*

Bystander intervention training exhorts young men to be proactive—and the message resonates:

- University of New Hampshire researchers enrolled a group of male students in the campus rape-prevention program. Months afterward, 12 percent of untrained men reported intervening in potential assaults, but in the trained group, 38 percent.
- At Georgia State University in Atlanta, 743 young men either completed a survey about sexual assault or attended a workshop on empathy for victims, sexual consent, alcohol's role in sexual violence, and bystanders' responsibility to intervene. Six months

later, men in the workshop were significantly more likely to have stopped friends from crossing the line.

Serial rapists account for 25 percent of college and military assaults. What about them? As prevention programs percolate through institutions, serial assailants are more likely to be identified sooner and stopped.

Of course, just as designated drivers haven't reduced drunk driving deaths to zero, sexual assault prevention programs don't stop all rapes. But in a year or two, programs based on assault triggers and bystander intervention typically reduce rapes by half.

Dating Violence Prevention in Middle and High Schools

Violence prevention programs have also proven effective in middle and high schools. Researchers asked 2,500 students at thirty New York City public middle schools about their experiences with sexual violence. Then they completed a six-session rape-prevention curriculum. Six months later, violence against girls had declined significantly.

Pediatricians at the University of Pittsburgh Medical Center asked 1,513 male athletes at sixteen area high schools if they'd ever committed sexual violence. Then half their coaches took no action while the other half implemented Coaching Boys into Men, a program involving repeated blunt talks about sexual violence prevention. A year later, those whose coaches spoke up were significantly less likely to have faced accusations of dating violence.

Sexual Harassment: New Focus on an Age-Old Violation

Since the beginning of cinema, movie people have snickered about the "casting couch." To win roles, many women have felt forced to put out for male producers and directors. Then in 2017 movie mogul Harvey Weinstein was unmasked as a serial sexual predator, a revelation that reverberated throughout American culture.

Workplace sexual harassment is rife. The federal Equal Employment Opportunity Commission (EEOC) says that, depending on the industry, 25–85 percent of women and 10 percent of men report offensive sexually loaded remarks, jokes, threats, groping, intimidation, and "sextortion," feeling required to provide sex to get hired, keep jobs, or advance.

The National Women's Law Center reports that harassment is particularly prevalent in:

- Traditionally male industries—construction, finance, banking—where some men view women as interlopers.
- Service industries that involve tipping. Workers often face unwelcome touching and demands for "special service."
- Low-wage industries—farm workers, hotel room cleaners—where union protections are rare and workers have little leverage.
- Jobs with gender disparities. When one gender substantially outnumbers the other, those in the minority may face harassment.

Sexual harassment represents the intersection of power and hostility. Those in charge, usually men, have power over subordinates, often women. But as increasing numbers of women rise to positions of power, some harass men. The EEOC reports that from 1990 to 2009, complaints by men doubled from 8 to 16 percent.

Compared with those not represented by unions, unionized workers usually face less harassment. Workers can file grievances with union representatives. But unionization is no guarantee against harassment. Union officials may be perpetrators.

Why Most Remain Silent

The EEOC estimates that 75 percent of sexually harassed employees never report it. Instead, they avoid harassers or ignore, downplay, or simply endure the abuse. Reporting is the *least* common response.

Employees don't report for many reasons. Some fear they won't be believed. Others suspect their complaints will be ignored. Some don't want to get harassers fired. And many fear retaliation.

Fears of reprisals are justified. One study showed that 75 percent of employees who protested workplace harassment faced retaliation: whispering campaigns, hostile confrontations, sneak attacks (computer sabotage, dead mice on desks), bad performance reviews, and demotion or firing.

Training and HR May Not Help

In 1986, the US Supreme Court ruled that sexual harassment violates employee civil rights. Since then, to avoid lawsuits, many companies have instituted sexual harassment training. But it's often perfunctory—a thirty-minute PowerPoint—developed more to shield employers from liability than stop harassment.

Meanwhile, human resources (HR) departments have an inherent conflict of interest. They're charged with both helping employees and protecting the company from liability. When the two conflict, HR departments may side with management against employees.

False Accusations?

Activists have long argued that false accusations of rape are rare. Accusers attract attention that's unwelcome. Even when treated sensitively by police and the criminal justice system—still not always the case—allegations subject accusers to invasive questioning, nasty cross-examination, and possible loss of income from time off work. Nonetheless, some rape accusations turn out to be false—around 5 percent, one in twenty:

- Dutch researchers reviewed all US police rape reports from 2006 to 2010. They judged 5 percent unfounded.
- Australian investigators analyzed seven studies of rape allegations in the US and Australia. The consensus—5 percent appeared false.
- University of Massachusetts and Northeastern University scientists reviewed ten years of rape accusations, a total of 136 at a New England university. Those later ruled false—6 percent.
- Arizona State University researchers reviewed all rape allegations reported to the Los Angeles Police Department in 2008. They judged 4.5 percent to be false.

True or false, allegations of sexual misconduct are horrible for those involved. The best way to prevent sexual violence is to stop it before anything happens. *If you see something, do something.*

But since 2010, the EEOC has recovered $700 million from employers who failed to prevent sexual harassment. Many corporate leaders have realized that harassment is bad for business.

Keys to Workplace Culture Change

Sexual assault became a political issue in the 1970s with the rise of the women's movement and the publication of such books as *Against Our Will: Men, Women, and Rape* by Susan Brownmiller (1975) and *Battered Wives* by Del Martin (1976). But it took twenty years of activism, lawsuits, and legislation for police departments to treat rape survivors sensitively and for the criminal justice system to punish rapists as the violent criminals they are. That struggle is far from over. Today, most Americans consider rape a heinous crime, but some still believe that "boys will be boys" and "women ask for it."

Sexual harassment is as old as patriarchal civilization, but it's become a political issue only recently. It will take time for workplace cultures to shift to the view that it, too, is a crime with perpetrators consistently identified and punished.

How can that period be shortened? The Surgeon General urged Americans to quit cigarettes in 1964, but in 2020, 14 percent still smoked. However, as rape-prevention programs have shown, when institutions revise their rules and officials at all levels embrace the new approach, culture change can occur surprisingly quickly.

Ongoing blunt talk at every level of the enterprise. Top executives, managers at every level, and HR departments must promote the same message relentlessly: sexual harassment is not tolerated. It's wrong—and bad for business. It doesn't matter who you are, your seniority, or how much rain you make, harassment will get you severely disciplined and quite possibly fired.

Every manager, not just HR, should have authority to receive complaints. Many employees feel more comfortable speaking to some superiors than others. When all managers can receive complaints, grievance filings increase.

Strength in numbers. Lone accusers typically feel isolated and suffer retaliation. But when several employees band together, their collective testimony carries more weight. If you experience harassment but don't feel comfortable reporting it, talk with coworkers. Discuss what you've endured. You're probably not the only one. Sexual harassers rarely stop at one victim. Group complaints are more likely to gain traction.

No compulsory arbitration. According to the Economic Policy Institute, more than half the nation's employment contracts require employees who file harassment complaints to submit to binding arbitration behind closed doors. It's secret, which discourages complaints and shields perpetrators.

In 2017, Microsoft became the first Fortune 500 corporation to stop requiring arbitration of sexual harassment allegations. Under Microsoft's new rule, employees who believe they've been sexually harassed are free to sue the company. Since then, other companies have abandoned compulsory arbitration of alleged sexual harassment, including Facebook and Google. In addition, several state legislatures and Congress are considering legislation to outlaw compulsory arbitration for sexual harassment.

No gag orders. Institutions want to protect their good names. When employees win sexual harassment actions, most employers insist on nondisclosure agreements. Harassed employees can't say a word without risking lawsuits and firing. This preserves the institutions' good names—but allows harassers to avoid public exposure.

All levels of government should outlaw gag orders. Complaints should be public. As of 2020, states taking this step include California, New Jersey, New York, Maryland, and Tennessee.

Bystander intervention. This is a cornerstone of successful rape-prevention efforts, and evidence is mounting that it's also key to ending sexual harassment.

- Bystanders can support victims. *I heard/saw that. Are you okay? If you complain, I'll vouch for you. Would you like me to accompany you to HR?* Bystanders can also refer victims to outside resources (below).
- Bystanders can help build strength in numbers. *Do you know anyone else who's had similar experiences?*
- Bystanders can challenge harassers. Confrontations can range from friendly questioning—*Are you aware of what you just said/did?*—to blunt recriminations—*I've seen you say/do that one too many times. I'm reporting you.*

Bystanders may not be present for the more sinister forms of harassment—grabbing, groping, assaults—but harassers often start with public obnoxiousness. Clamping down on it helps prevent escalations.

For culture to change, everyone must get involved. The EEOC says, "Workplace cultures don't change by themselves. The fight to stop workplace harassment depends on everyone."

If you see something, do something.

For Help Dealing with Sexual Harassment

- Equal Rights Advocates. equalrights.org/legal-help/know-your-rights/sexual -harassment-at-work/
- National Women's Law Center. nwlc.org/issue/sexual-harassment-in-the-workplace/
- AFL-CIO. aflcio.org/issues/sexual-harassment
- American Association of University Women. aauw.org/

CHAPTER 21:
If the Woman You Love Gets Raped

THE GOOD NEWS: since the 1990s, like other violent crimes in the US, the rape rate has decreased considerably. According to the US Department of Justice, from 1995 to 2010, the rate of reported female sexual assaults declined 58 percent. In 1995, women's lifetime risk was around 20 percent. Today, it's less than 10 percent.

The bad news: around four hundred thousand US women are sexually assaulted annually. This figure comes from the nation's most authoritative crime statistics, the Justice Department's National Crime Victimization Survey, compiled from interviews with a representative 160,000 Americans about their crime experiences during the previous year, whether or not they called the police. Around 90 percent of rape victims were women. And 20 percent of assaults involved more than one perpetrator.

> ## Men Also Get Raped
>
> The overwhelming majority of rape victims are women, but this horrible violation also happens to some men. For poignant insights into male victimization, read *Deliverance* by James Dickey, *The Prince of Tides* by Pat Conroy, or *Fortune and Men's Eyes* by John Herbert, or see the movies.

Less Sexual Than Assaultive

Sexual assault has more to do with assault and power than sex and attraction. Any man who has ever been mugged can appreciate some of what women endure during and after sexual assault, in the sense that the typical mugging survivor fears being killed during the attack, followed by a haunting sense that personal safety is a cruel illusion.

Now instead of simply intimidating you with a weapon and taking your valuables, imagine that one or more muggers ripped your clothes off and forced one or more penises into your mouth and/or anus. Would you consider that a "sex" crime? It involves the genitals, so it's sexual, but like women, men who experience sexual assault focus much less on the sexual aspect than on the assault.

How Men Can Help Women Recover

If the woman you love experiences sexual assault, you can either help or hinder her recovery. How to help:

- **Support her survival.** Some rapists kill their victims and many threaten death. Anything the woman did to survive was the right thing to do. Never say, *You should have . . .* Survivors are certain to obsess for a long time about their reactions and if they might have responded differently. Men should consistently provide reassurance: *You survived a life-threatening situation. Everything you did was the right thing to do.*

- **She's in charge.** The survivor should make every decision in response to the assault. She was the one victimized. Her dignity was trampled. Healing involves regaining feelings of personal sovereignty. Whatever she decides, support her decisions—even if you disagree with them. Rapists are most likely to be convicted if survivors call the police immediately and don't bathe or clean up until any evidence—semen, hair—has been collected. But survivors may want to bathe and not call the police. Feel free to gently question their decisions and point out the implications. But once survivors have made their decisions, support them.
- **Avoid accusations.** Women don't "invite" rape by dressing provocatively, hiking alone, giving directions to strangers, or anything else.
- **Don't take revenge.** If the survivor can identify her attacker(s), don't grab a weapon and take off after him/them. She's just dealt with one or more men who were completely out of control. Don't become another. Stay with her. Be there for her.
- **Encourage her to get help.** Find the nearest rape crisis center. Offer to take her there. Find a therapist who deals with sexual trauma. Offer to help pay for counseling. Some survivors crave professional help. Others don't want it. Whatever she decides, support her decision.
- **Get help yourself.** A lover's sexual assault may raise difficult issues for men: the urge to seek revenge, self-criticism over failing to prevent the assault, and perhaps memories of times when you might have crossed the line. This might be a good time to consult a therapist.
- **Reassure her of your love.** Tell her you still love her and don't consider her "damaged."
- **You may become her target.** You're not the rapist, but trauma survivors often berate those closest to them. Brace yourself. If she assails you, don't take the bait. Gently say that you're not *him*, that you love and respect her.
- **Don't press for sex.** Most survivors need to take a break from partner genital sex. Respect that. Tell her you care about *her* more than you care about sex with her. Say that often. Let her decide when to resume the sexual part of your relationship.
- **Offer nonsexual sensuality.** She might not want genital sex, but she may enjoy baths, cuddling, and massages.
- **Continue to listen.** As time passes, it's natural to say, *It's over. Don't dwell on it.* But many survivors need to process their reactions for what may seem "too long." Give her all the time she needs.
- **Arrange fun together.** Offer to organize activities she enjoys. She may demur. Keep offering. You both may feel you're just going through the motions, but over time, fun together aids recovery.
- **Consider couple counseling.** After several months, if survivors can't move beyond the assault and your relationship suffers, suggest couple counseling.

Supporting Those Being Stalked

Stalking is a form of harassment that causes reasonable people—overwhelmingly women—to fear harm. Stalking includes unwanted phone calls, messages, texts, or emails; approaching or confronting victims in places when they neither expect nor want contact; and spying on victims with cameras or listening devices. Stalking is a crime in all fifty states. Compared with sexual assault and child sex abuse, stalking gets little media attention, but it's fairly prevalent and always unnerving. According to the National Center for Victims of Crime:

- At some point in life, 15 percent of women and 6 percent of men get stalked.
- Most stalkers are current or former lovers, friends, or acquaintances.
- Around 15 percent of victims are teens. Half are in their twenties.
- About half of victims experience at least one unwanted contact a week.
- Among women killed by current or former lovers, 76 percent were stalked beforehand.
- Before being killed by stalkers, half of women reported the stalking to police.

Few women mention they're being stalked or have been, so few men have any idea. Tip-offs include suddenly switching jobs, changing contact information, or moving for no apparent reason, and being unusually apprehensive.

If you suspect a woman you know is being stalked:

- **Ask her.** Don't demand to know. Telling you is her decision. Assure her that you care about her, abhor stalking, and want to help.
- **Ask if she feels threatened.** If so, encourage her to contact police. Many women refuse, saying police don't do anything. That may sometimes be true, but it's changing. If she won't call the cops, contact them yourself and ask how they deal with stalking. Many police departments have become more responsive, confronting stalkers and insisting they stop immediately or risk jail. If the police appear sensitive, gently share your findings with the woman and encourage her to report. Then abide by her decision.
- **Never stalk an ex.** If a woman dumps you, you have every right to feel sad, confused, betrayed, and angry. But relationships require mutual consent. She has every right to break up with you—for any reason. Grieve your loss. Vent to your friends. But leave her alone. Stalking won't bring her back. It's more likely to convince her she was right to end things. And stalking might land you in jail.

CHAPTER 22:
"You're Insatiable!"
"You Never Want To!"
How Sex Therapists Recommend
Overcoming Desire Differences

A N OLD JOKE asks: What's foreplay to men married ten years? *An hour of pleading.* In most long-term relationships—but by no means all—the men feel hornier than the women.

When couples first fall in love, they can't keep their hands off each other. But the hot-and-heavy period rarely lasts more than a year. Then sexual heat cools for one partner or both, and frequency declines as relationships evolve from passionate to compassionate.

When both lovers agree on less sex, there's no conflict. But typically, one craves sex more than the other. Canadian researchers interviewed 117 long-term couples. Their top sexual complaint was conflict about sexual frequency, reported by 36 percent of the women and 39 percent of the men. Desire differences often cause rancor and drive people crazy. They're one of the leading reasons couples consult sex therapists.

How Often Do Americans Do It?

Everyone is sexually unique. Put two singular individuals together, and the couple is sexually like no other. Consequently, there's no "right" sexual frequency couples "should" enjoy. And we must be careful generalizing about "average" or "typical" sexual frequency. But researchers keep peeking between the sheets. Everyone wants to know how often everyone else does it.

I reviewed the half dozen most widely cited studies. In every age group, no matter how long lovers have been together, frequency varies substantially, but on average, couples under forty-five typically do it about once a week, older couples two or three times a month.

Demographics impact frequency. A team led by Brigham Young researchers analyzed interviews with 6,785 married Americans about what contributes to sexual frequency. First, what *doesn't*:

- **Race.** Race has no impact.
- **Region.** Geography has nothing to do with frequency.
- **Work.** Couples with one stay-at-home spouse generally have the same frequency as two-income couples.

What *does*:

- **Stage of relationship.** The hot-and-heavy period typically lasts six months to a year, after which frequency almost always declines. This happens independent of all other factors including age. Couples who fall in love in middle age or older typically experience a burst of passion, but it's usually brief.
- **Age.** Frequency almost always declines with age, but the decrease is rarely steady. It's usually happens in steps—plateaus and drops. After initial heat, most young adult couples negotiate or fall into a frequency and maintain it until around forty-five. Then frequency usually drops and slowly continues to decline, with some older couples retiring from sex altogether while others continue making love regularly—some frequently—into very old age.
- **Happiness.** Frequency generally tracks relationship satisfaction. Compared with unhappy couples, happy partners usually—but not always—have more sex. However, sexual frequency among self-described happy couples ranges from never to several times a week.
- **Affairs.** Compared with monogamous spouses, those who dally generally have more sex, just not entirely with their primary partners.
- **Health.** Sex is one way the body celebrates vitality. Both acute and chronic illnesses reduce frequency. Still, among robustly healthy individuals, frequency varies tremendously. The same is true for those with chronic medical conditions.
- **Education.** The curve is an inverted U with the right arm truncated. Those with less than a high school education typically have the least sex. Frequency increases with high school diplomas and bachelor's degrees. But advanced degrees often mean somewhat less whoopee.
- **Religion.** Faith has little to do with frequency, but those who consider nonprocreative sex sinful do it less.
- **Long-term cohabitation.** Compared with married spouses, committed unmarried couples generally have somewhat more sex. If they marry, they usually continue to have a bit more.
- **Pregnancy.** Expecting has no consistent impact on frequency. Some pregnant women want more sex, others less, and some experience no change. However, frequency typically declines during the third trimester. A huge belly can get in the way. And after babies arrive, most couples don't return to prepregnancy frequency until new arrivals sleep through the night.
- **Young children.** The myth is that parents of young kids don't have the time or energy for sex. That's true for some, but parents who prioritize lovemaking may do it as often as they did before parenthood.
- **Divorce.** Those in miserable, sexless marriages often hope for more romps soon after divorce. Unlikely. Divorce is traumatic. The adjustment takes time and usually reduces libido and frequency for around a year afterward.
- **Remarriage.** After divorce or widowhood, some people who remarry have more sex in subsequent marriages. Others have the same frequency or less.
- **Single parenthood.** Some single parents don't have much sex. Others maintain their preparenthood frequencies. And some make love more.
- **Shared housework.** As women joined the labor force and more men participated in housework, some social scientists predicted the increase in domestic teamwork would boost frequency. Actually, with shared housework, sex typically *declines* a bit.

- **A history of child sex abuse or other sexual trauma, especially when it's unacknowledged.** In both women and men, a history of sexual trauma may diminish desire years later.
- **Individual differences.** The Brigham Young team analyzed what proportion of frequency differences the factors just discussed accounted for—only 20 percent. All of the above predicted just one-fifth of couples' sexual frequency differences.

Which means that individual differences account for 80 percent of the variance. Our sexual desire, frequency, and repertoire are as unique as our taste in food. Some people love liver, others can't stand it. Similarly, some folks want sex more or less than others. That's just who they are.

Of course, it's difficult to resist headlines about research purporting to reveal Americans' sexual frequency. But there is no "normal" amount. What matters is what lovers negotiate. Unfortunately, for many couples, that triggers conflict.

Reported Frequency and Repertoire: Why Do Men and Women Differ?

Dozens of studies have shown that compared with women, men consistently report more partner sex. How is that possible? Every time a man has heterosex, a woman also has it, so what explains the well-documented gender difference? Self-image and sex work.

Most men like to think of themselves as studs. Consequently, at every age, they overestimate the number of women they've bedded. Meanwhile, most women view too-frequent sex (whatever that is) as slutty, a label they'd rather avoid, so they underestimate their frequency.

In addition, some 15–20 percent of male Americans patronize sex workers. Women sex workers number fewer than 1 percent of the adult female population. Many men's estimates include sex worker encounters, but sex workers generally elude researchers, so their great frequency doesn't get tabulated. This raises men's average and reduces women's.

Men also say they give and receive more oral sex than women say they provide and receive. The same two reasons apply: men overestimate; women underestimate. And with sex workers, men receive a great deal of fellatio and provide some cunnilingus, but sex surveys rarely include sex workers' experiences.

Why the Hot-and-Heavy Period Ends

Over the decades, I've received a steady stream of pained inquiries about desire differences. Stories differ, but the problem usually develops after six months to two years, as one partner's initial enthusiasm wanes. Accusations of bait and switch are common. *You fucked me to the altar, but now I don't get any. You misled me.* To which the other usually replies, *This is what happens in long-term relationships. How was I supposed to know you're so different?*

The hot-and-heavy period ends for many reasons:

- **Routines.** New love releases dopamine, the neurotransmitter of erotic heat and frequency. But over time, as sex and life together becomes routine, dopamine levels return to normal and desire and frequency decline.

- **Familiarity.** Initially, couples have fantasy pictures of each other—the "perfect stranger." But over time, fantasies fade, leaving you with who your honey really is, warts and all. You and your mate may enjoy a long, happy relationship. But fantasies ignite libido. Reality usually cools it.
- **Responsibilities.** When couples first connect, they give each other undivided attention. Then daily life intrudes: jobs, family, friends, bills, chores. Daily hassles often distract from sexual desire and frequency.
- **Complacency.** As time passes, most couples take their relationships increasingly for granted. There's less mutual courting. Complacency depresses frequency.
- **Relationship problems.** If resentments and anger develop, sexual quality declines and frequency suffers. Relationship harmony doesn't exempt couples from desire differences, but in fraught relationships, one or both spouses often withdraw from sex.

Whatever the reason(s), after a while in almost all long-term relationships, sexual urgency subsides, frequency declines—and toxic desire differences may develop.

The High Cost of Desire Differences

When desire differences fester, good will erodes and a grim chill descends. Sexual enjoyment declines, and irritability, bickering, and recriminations increase.

The one who wants more sex typically feels rejected, unloved, angry, unattractive, and deceived. The one who wants less typically feels besieged and unloved and resents feeling like a sex object. Chronic, festering desire differences often make both partners miserable.

A major casualty of desire differences is nonsexual affection: playful hugs, cuddling while watching TV, and morning and nighttime kisses. The higher-libido partner typically initiates such affection and interprets any positive response as a shot at getting lucky. The lower-libido spouse shrinks from nonsexual affection for fear of being misinterpreted. One complains, *You're as cold as ice.* The other retorts, *Can't you experience affection without immediately assuming it's sexual?*

As resentments deepen, what began as one problem becomes two: the desire difference and the chronic resentments it engenders.

Who Wants Sex More—Men? Or Women?

Men. Duh! The conventional wisdom says men are insatiable, women equivocal. Actually, the issue is more complicated. Since the 1980s, I've informally surveyed dozens of sex therapists about couples they counsel for desire differences. Their consistent estimate: men have more libido in half to two-thirds of cases. Women want sex more in one-third to half. An analysis of Google searches corroborates my findings. Women frequently search "Why doesn't my boyfriend/husband want to have sex with me?"

When the man wants more, the couple may experience distress, but their problem feels culturally expected, therefore, "normal." But when the woman wants more, the stress of the desire difference gets compounded by viewing their situation as "abnormal," therefore, more fraught.

Just as it's impossible to predict sexual frequency, there's no predicting who's hornier. Most of the time, the man but fairly often, the woman.

Who Controls Your Sex?

In counseling for desire differences, sex therapists often ask, *In your relationship, who controls the sex?*

Invariably, each partner points at the other—and both are astonished to discover that their other half thinks *they* wield the power, when each feels utterly powerless. Lower-libido partners have the power to shut things down by saying *no*, which leaves those who want more sex feeling powerless, hurt, and unloved. Meanwhile, higher-libido mates often browbeat their other halves for sex, leaving the latter feeling powerless, beleaguered, and unloved. Powerlessness leaves both people feeling frustrated, depressed, and angry.

What Do You Really Want?

Sex therapists typically ask higher-libido partners, *What do you really want? Sex? Or something else?* Inevitably, they reply: *Sex.*

Therapists also ask lower-desire partners, *How often do you want sex? Is there anything else you want?* They typically reply: *I have no idea how much sex I want. I never get the chance to experience my own libido. I'm either fending off advances or giving in.*

Desire differences often obscure the fact that both lovers have nonsexual desires, typically for more nonsexual affection and fun together. But they get sacrificed on the altar of the desire difference. Goodwill erodes, and that stings.

Ironically, the realization that desire differences often mask nonsexual issues may create room to negotiate. The hornier spouse might decide, *I'm willing to make do with less if you pay more attention to me out of bed.* The other might concede, *I could live with more sex if you make me feel special out of bed.*

It's not easy to negotiate chronic desire differences. But when couples understand that they usually want more than just more or less sex, the door to productive negotiations often cracks open.

How to Negotiate Sexual Frequency

No magic formula can deliver couples from desire differences. But these suggestions may help:

- **Count your blessings.** You want sex twice a week. Your lover would be happy with once a month. That's a drag, but at least the low-desire partner wants *some* sex. Many people don't want any. Be thankful low libido isn't *no* libido.
- **Be flexible.** Some people prefer sex late at night, others mornings or afternoons. Some like to play under warm quilts, others atop the bedspread. Some like locking legs in silence, others prefer music, conversation, or talking dirty. Some love sex toys, others don't. And some enjoy a bit of kink—blindfolds, spanking, or more—while others recoil from anything unconventional. Over time, such disagreements can aggravate desire differences. If you're the lover who wants more sex, accommodating your partner's preferences just might get you more of what you want.
- **Talk to a friend on the other side.** All the long-term couples you know have probably wrestled with desire differences. Ask around. Try to find a friend, ideally of your gender, on the opposite side of the difference. That person's views might provide perspective.
- **Experience your power.** You feel your partner controls your sex life. Actually, you have more clout than you think. It doesn't matter who wants sex more or less. You have the power to make your spouse think you control it, to make your mate miserable. And you have the power to destroy goodwill by obsessing about your complaints.

  Consider a walled city under siege. The besieging forces have not broken through, but their demand for surrender places tremendous pressure on every aspect of city life. That's not victory, but it is power. Meanwhile, the defenders haven't repelled the attackers, but their resistance keeps the besieging army pinned down. That's not victory either, but it is power. Understanding your power often reduces feelings of victimization.

- **You can't change your lover's libido.** In couples plagued by desire differences, each hopes the other will "come around" to their level of libido. Desire can change. But any change must come from within, not from cajoling. In fact, pressure to "see the light" is likely to cement intransigence.
- **Work on other issues, too.** Desire differences reflect a loss of teamwork. Make every effort to collaborate productively on other issues. If one partner feels stuck about school, work, family, or money, work together to resolve those issues.

Three Choices

Toxic desire differences create three stark choices: You can (1) break up, (2) live in misery—with the lustier partner possibly having affairs—or (3) negotiate a mutually workable compromise. Which will it be? If you don't want to separate or feel miserable forever, you have only one choice—finding a frequency you both can live with.

Resolving desire differences employs the same skills involved in negotiating any conflict:

- **Begin sentences with "I want" or "I need," not "You should."** State your own desires, not what you want the other to do. Not: *You should want sex more. You should meet my needs.* Rather: *I want sex at least once a week. I absolutely need it at least twice a month.*
- **Be succinct.** Once you've stated your position, don't belabor things. Your partner knows how you feel.
- **Listen respectfully.** Don't interrupt. Don't roll your eyes. You've heard it all before, but keep listening. You have two ears and one mouth. Use them proportionately.
- **Separate your love for the person from your disagreement over frequency.** If divorce is off the table, there must be good reasons why you're staying. List them. Remind yourself of the things you love about your partner.
- **Avoid contempt.** Relationship therapists say it takes ten endearments to neutralize the sting of one nasty zinger. Don't descend into name-calling. Avoid sarcasm. Bend over backward to be kind and gracious.
- **Try to maintain a sense of humor.** If you can't laugh about your desire difference, laugh about something else. Watch a comedy. See a comedian. Share jokes. Anything to inject levity into the acrimony.
- **Remember, you're teammates.** If you're not going to separate but can't stand the status quo, you have no alternative but to work together. With any luck, you'll be able to thrash out a compromise you can both live with.

Note: compromise does not produce happiness. It merely reduces mutual unhappiness to acceptable levels. If one person wants sex twice a week, while the other would feel fine with once a month, a reasonable compromise might be once every ten days. Neither of you gets what you truly want. But your flexibility shows that you value your relationship over winning.

No negotiated frequency is set in stone. You might agree to a trial frequency for a few months, then reevaluate.

Compromise should include flexibility. Weekly lovemaking doesn't mean sex absolutely once every seven days. People get sick. Obligations arise. Adjustments become necessary.

Of course, it's no fun to compromise, but the sooner you negotiate a mutually workable frequency, the better off you and your relationship are likely to feel.

Schedule It

One maddening aspect of desire differences is seemingly constant bickering about sex. One begs, pleads, and grovels: *Tonight? Tonight? Tonight?* The other says *No*, or *I'm not in the mood*, or *I have a headache*. Or the worst retort, *Maybe*.

Maybe drives the more libidinous partner crazy. *So, what'll it be? Yes? Or no?* That person becomes even more miserable and plaintive, which makes the lower-desire partner feel even more beleaguered and defensive.

The battle usually ceases when you open your calendars and schedule sex dates per your negotiated frequency. Many people object to scheduling, insisting the best sex is spontaneous. But after the hot-and-heavy period, spontaneous sex fades. In established relationships, sex therapists are virtually unanimous in the opinion that scheduled sex offers couples the best chance for long-term erotic happiness.

Scheduling means you both know exactly when you'll make love. That's usually a tremendous relief. Those who want more sex can look forward to it. Those who want less know sex will happen *only* when it's scheduled. They're freed from repelling constant advances. Conversations become less strained, resentments less stinging. Sexual uncertainty and accompanying rancor get replaced by certainty and, over time, usually by grudging acceptance of scheduled lovemaking.

"What If I'm Not in the Mood?"

When higher-libido lovers suggest scheduling, this is lower-libido lovers' immediate retort. A pervasive myth holds that sex should "just happen" when lovers are "in the mood." But by the time couples have been together long enough for desire differences to fester, sex rarely "just happens." One partner always seems to be in the mood, the other seldom if ever.

In the classic formulation, libido precedes sex. You want it, and go after it. That's true for most men and some women. But studies by University of British Columbia psychiatrist Rosemary Basson, MD, show that before sex, many women say they experience *no particular desire for it*. Then, assuming they enjoy the loveplay, they heat up. For these women, sexual desire is not the *cause* of sex, but its *result*. Basson's research has focused only on women. But it's not much of a leap to extend her findings to low-desire men.

If these women (and presumably men) don't experience a drive for sex, why do they do it? For one or more of the many reasons listed in chapter 1.

Women's top five:
1. I felt attracted to the person.
2. I wanted to experience the physical pleasure.
3. It feels good.
4. I wanted to show my affection for my partner.
5. I wanted to express my love for my partner.

And men's:
1. I was attracted to the person.
2. It feels good.
3. I wanted to experience the physical pleasure.
4. It's fun.
5. I wanted to show my affection for the person.

Note that in addition to experiencing the physical pleasure of sex, both men and women often say they have sex for reasons that are not strictly sexual—wanting to express love and affection.

What about new relationships when lovers can't keep their hands off each other? Basson's model still holds. People who feel a classic sex drive revel in it as they fall in love and enjoy lots of hot sex. Meanwhile, those more interested in emotional closeness know that sex opens a door to it, so early in relationships when they feel especially hungry for closeness, they, too, are up for frequent sex. But as the relationship develops and lovers settle into life together, the hunger for emotional closeness subsides and people who primarily experience those needs experience less libido.

Those who want more sex shouldn't pressure lovers by saying, *If desire doesn't precede sex for you, then just have sex with me whenever I want and you'll get in the mood as we make love.* This misconstrues Basson's findings.

Imagine your partner loves socializing with certain friends. You like them, too, but not as much. How would you feel if your partner said: *It doesn't matter that you like them less. Just play along and by the end of the visit, you'll enjoy it.* That may be true twice a month—but not twice a week. The key is to negotiate a compromise frequency you can both live with long term. Sex should never feel coerced.

But while resolving desire differences, it's equally important for those with less interest to let go of the idea that before proceeding, they must feel "in the mood." Scheduling allows you time to psych up for lovemaking, to work up anticipatory excitement so you enjoy it.

Scheduling frees couples from constant bickering. It enhances relationships. And after a few months, chances are you'll feel good about scheduling and better about your lovemaking.

Embrace Your Schedule in Good Faith

Once you've negotiated a compromise frequency, accept it. You haven't gotten what you truly want, but you've both demonstrated sufficient flexibility to negotiate a frequency you can live with—at least for the time being. Try to view the glass as half full. Avoid snide remarks about the huge sacrifice you've made. Your lover already knows—and has made a similar sacrifice. Do your best to put bickering behind you.

Restore Nonsexual Affection

Scheduling produces an immediate dividend—the return of nonsexual affection. Being touched, held, and cuddled are among life's most satisfying pleasures. Affectionate touch is the physical expression of the emotional connection you and your partner share. It's a tremendous boon to relationships. Once you schedule sex, affectionate touch loses its sexual charge. Both of you can initiate hugging and cuddling secure in the knowledge that all you're doing is sharing affection. That's usually a relief—and it allows affectionate touch to return to your relationship.

Note to the more libidinous partner: don't misinterpret spontaneous affection as a sexual invitation. Stick to your schedule.

Work to Restore Good Will

When lovers experience chronic conflict, they typically think the other person should be nicer. But you don't control your partner. You control only yourself. If you want to restore relationship harmony, make every effort to be nicer *yourself*. Perform at least one act of loving kindness a day, preferably several.

Savor Your Solution

When couples negotiate a frequency and schedule it, at first, both usually feel wary. That's to be expected. Goodwill has eroded. Trust has been damaged. And both people may focus more on what they've given up than gained.

But over time, assuming you both honor your agreement, tensions usually subside. You still have a desire difference, but its pain fades, and your relationship—and lovemaking—improve. Over time, you both realize you've accomplished something important. You've negotiated an agreement you can both live with. Congratulations.

If Self-Help Doesn't Resolve Things

Self-help may not be able to repair the damage if:

- One or both insist the problem is all the other's fault. *You're impossible!*
- One or both claim all the distress. *You're driving me crazy.*
- One or both insist the other is deranged. *What's wrong with you?*
- One or both claim the other is intransigent. *You'll never change.*

If these accusations sound familiar, consider sex therapy. Desire differences are one of the leading reasons couples consult sex therapists, so most therapists have substantial experience helping couples overcome them.

CHAPTER 23:
Sizzling Sex During Pregnancy, Nursing, and Parenting

SEX IS USUALLY necessary for procreation, but once the pregnancy test turns positive, many think expectant and child-rearing parents should sacrifice lovemaking to raising the kids. You can if you like. But many parents value sex, derive emotional sustenance from lovemaking, and enjoy it regularly. Of course, pregnancy and parenthood require sexual adjustments, but with a little planning and creativity, sizzling sex is quite possible—and it improves parenting.

Pregnancy and Libido: Completely Unpredictable
Here's the conventional wisdom about desire during pregnancy: women's libidos collapse during the first trimester, often rebound during the second, and fall again during the third. This pattern makes some biological sense. Women's libidos may initially fall because of fatigue, morning sickness, and the emotional shift into living for two. During the second trimester, morning sickness usually—but not always—subsides, and libido often rebounds. But it falls again during the third from fatigue, the awkwardness of a huge belly and swollen breasts, and other discomforts, for example, hemorrhoids.

But the conventional wisdom obscures a greater truth: individual sexual uniqueness extends to sexuality during pregnancy. Expectant mothers'—and fathers'—libidos vary tremendously and cannot be generalized or predicted.

For their book, *Sexy Mama: Keeping Your Sex Life Alive While Raising Kids,* Cathy Winks and Anne Semans surveyed more than seven hundred women about their sexuality during and after pregnancy. They reported an enormous range of experiences, from reveling in an erotic awakening to feeling totally turned off and everything in between.

Many men in pregnant couples also experience libido changes. Most expect to feel turned on by their wives' changing bodies. *It's like sex with different women—all my wife.* Actually, many feel turned off. Swedish researchers studied 112 expecting couples. Some of the men couldn't get enough sex with their pregnant wives, but many previously horny goats completely lost interest, especially during the third trimester.

Does Sex Harm the Fetus or Trigger Premature Labor?
During pregnancy, genital blood flow increases, and some of Winks's and Semans's respondents said their orgasms became more intense and pleasurable, the best of their lives. Some who'd never experienced orgasms had them. And many said that while pregnant, it was easier to come. But others noticed no sexual changes. Some said their genitals became uncomfortably sensitive, that clitoral caresses felt disconcerting or painful. And some tried to avoid sex and especially orgasm for fear it might harm the fetus.

Many couples fear sex might hurt the baby. Highly unlikely. Fetuses develop in a sturdy sack filled with amniotic fluid, mostly water, an excellent shock absorber. A savage beating might rupture the sack and trigger miscarriage, but the amniotic sack is sufficiently resilient to stand up to even bed-shaking sex and volcanic orgasms. In addition, pregnancy-related hormonal changes cause cervical mucus to form a plug that seals the uterus, largely eliminating risk of harm from vaginal insertions.

In medically uncomplicated pregnancies, intercourse and women's orgasms are unlikely to trigger premature labor, even during the third trimester. In fact, orgasms close to term may help *prevent* prematurity:

- Scientists with the National Institute of Environmental Health tracked the lovemaking of 596 pregnant North Carolina women. Third-trimester intercourse and orgasms were associated with 66 percent *less risk* of prematurity.
- Ohio State University researchers asked ninety-three pregnant women at term if they'd had orgasms during the previous week. Compared with abstainers, those who'd climaxed shortly before delivering went into labor no sooner. In fact, they delivered slightly *later*.
- Researchers in Malaysia asked third-trimester women to track their orgasms. Climaxing did not trigger labor.
- University of Chicago obstetricians analyzed preterm deliveries. The women's orgasms didn't matter. The only sexual risk factor was man-on-top intercourse near term.

If intercourse and orgasm don't trigger premature labor, what does?

- Lack of prenatal medical care
- Use of alcohol, tobacco, and/or cocaine
- Infections: UTI, bacterial vaginosis, trichomoniasis, gonorrhea, and chlamydia
- Age over thirty-five
- Previous preterm delivery
- Obesity or anorexia
- Severe emotional stress—violence, money woes, or serious illness or a death in the family
- Skipping meals
- Possibly: antidepressant medication, previous induced abortion, strenuous work, working the night shift, very spicy foods, or jobs requiring standing more than two hours a day

Not sex.

However, a few complications of pregnancy warrant abstinence: placenta previa, multiple fetuses, vaginal bleeding, serious uterine irritability, or high-risk pregnancy. Consult your prenatal care professional.

If a medical provider advises suspending intercourse, it's still quite possible to make love—mutual whole-body massage, hand jobs, oral, toys, and perhaps some kink. If you're advised against orgasm, kissing, cuddling, and massage are still available.

Does Cannabis Harm the Fetus?

Cigarettes and alcohol abuse, but not an occasional drink, damage unborn children. What about marijuana? Researchers at Washington University in St. Louis analyzed thirty-one studies. Their conclusion: "Maternal marijuana use during pregnancy is not a risk factor for adverse outcomes."

Doing It While Pregnant

During the first trimester and into the second, play any way you both enjoy.

But after around twenty weeks, as breast and belly swell, the man-on-top (missionary) intercourse position may become uncomfortable—and trigger premature labor. Better positions include rear entry (doggie), woman-on-top, or spooning, her back to his chest. If you love the missionary position, wedge a fat pillow under one of the woman's hips. This reduces pressure on the placenta.

Many pregnant women develop hemorrhoids. If so, sex, especially anal play, may become painful or impossible. A lubricant might help, but if anything feels uncomfortable, avoid it.

Finally, every pregnant couple is sexually unique, so this advice goes only so far. Discuss how and how much you'd like to play. Continue the conversation as the pregnancy progresses.

University of Wisconsin researchers followed the sexuality of 570 pregnant couples. Through the fifth month, 85 percent continued to make love. But as due dates approached, the proportion declined sharply.

When Can New Parents Resume Lovemaking?

Some baby books advise waiting three weeks after uncomplicated deliveries without episiotomy, six weeks with episiotomy, and two to four months after C-sections. Actually, it's impossible to generalize. Couples should decide for themselves. Considerations include:

- **Priorities.** Many new mothers told Winks and Semans sex was no longer a priority. They wanted some but had neither the time nor energy.
- **The baby's sleep schedule.** Until the baby sleeps through the night, most new parents feel so exhausted that when they see a bed (or sofa or chair), they crave sleep, not sex. Most infants don't sleep through the night until around twelve weeks. Don't expect much libido or nookie until then.
- **Nursing.** Breasts engorged with milk can feel uncomfortable. Some women don't produce sufficient milk. Some infants have trouble latching on, and nipple problems may cause pain. Few nursing mothers feel very sexual during the first few months of breastfeeding, and some don't regain interest until they wean. Milk-filled breasts excite some men but repel others.
- **Hormonal changes.** After delivery, new mothers' blood levels of estrogen drop, offset by higher levels of two other hormones, prolactin and oxytocin. They facilitate mother-infant bonding, but usually reduce libido.
- **Anxiety.** New parenthood causes stress, which may sabotage libido.
- **Depression.** Another libido killer. Ordinary new-parent anxieties may be complicated by postpartum depression (PPD), which affects 10–15 percent of new mothers. Symptoms vary from unexplained weeping to harming themselves and their infants. A history of previous mental health problems increases risk.

- **Vaginal pain.** Some women suffer persistent delivery-related vaginal pain, which may take a while to subside.

Be patient. Many women and some men need many months to regain their prepregnancy libidos.

If you take a break from genital play, try to maintain a sensual connection. Kiss, hug, cuddle, trade massages. Locking hips may be on hold, but most new parents find nonsexual affection welcome and reassuring.

The Wisconsin researchers just mentioned continued tracking their 570 couples after delivery. At one month postpartum, only 16 percent made love, by four months, 88 percent, and at twelve months, 91 percent.

If Your Sexual Hiatus Lasts "Too Long"

Too long is a matter of opinion. For some couples, it's four months, for others six, for some, weaning, and for a few, when they start to go crazy. If you feel sex-starved and your spouse has no libido, consider sex therapy.

Sex Suggestions for Parents

If you want to maintain a sexual relationship, prioritize it. With children, impulsiveness and spontaneity go out the window. Everything must be scheduled, including sex. If either new parent feels reluctant to make sex dates for fear of not being in the mood, review chapter 22 or consult a sex therapist.

Once you've made peace with scheduled sex:

- **Discuss any new limits.** Over time, lovers' taste in erotic repertoire evolves. New parenthood may call for new moves. Coach each other.
- **Enjoy nap times.** Most infants nap during mornings and afternoons, and toddlers in the afternoons. Most naps last at least an hour—that's enough time for parents to play. In addition, new-parent fatigue may preclude sex at night. You may have more erotic energy while your baby naps. Some people can't imagine making love with a baby napping in the room. That's rarely an issue. Babies sleep like babies.
- **Get a babysitter.** With babysitting, you can visit commercial hot tubs, or check into a hotel, or, if friends are out of town, use their homes.
- **Arrange sleepovers.** Kids love sleepovers. If relatives live nearby, they might host. Otherwise, cultivate other new parents and take turns hosting. With little ones away, parents can play.
- **Don't discuss the kids.** Some new parents obsess about their children and talk about little else. But parents also need to maintain their couple relationships. During sex dates, do your best to focus on each other.

Regular Lovemaking Improves Parenting

"Growing up," *Sexy Mamas* coauthor Cathy Winks explains, "women are told to be hot babes. But once they become moms, many believe they're no longer sexy—or sexual. They think they're supposed to sacrifice pleasure for the sake of the children. So many women (and some men) struggle with being sexual parents."

"We were surprised," coauthor Anne Semans adds, "by the number of new moms who bought into the idea that sex is self-indulgent, and consciously backed away from it."

Actually, Semans explains, active lovers make better parents: "The qualities required for satisfying lovemaking—listening, generosity, patience, nurturing, imagination, partnership, loving touch—all translate well into parenting. Many of our respondents said parenthood had deepened their relationships and lovemaking. That was heartwarming, and we heard it often."

Sex and Single Parents

If coupled parents have little time or energy for sex, then single parents should have even less. Solo parents must devote a huge proportion of their time, energy, and income to child-rearing. Hence the myth they dispense with dating and sex. But a Dartmouth study shows that single parents typically have sex just as often as childless singles—sometimes more.

The researchers mined data from Match.com's "Single in America" survey that polled 5,481 single adults, including 2,121 parents. Compared with childless singles and coupled parents, the single parents worked fewer hours and made less money. But they thought about sex as often as childless singles, dated as often, and were equally sexually active.

How do single parents manage this? One possibility is that they crave remarriage and focus on finding new co-parents. The study provides some support. As single parents' number of young children increased, so did their dating.

But single parents' main reason for dating and sex was *pleasure*. Most said they parent best when they feel happy and don't resent their children for denying them a social life.

On my blog, one single mom commented: "I'm raising my daughter entirely myself, and I have more sex now than I did when I was with her father, more than when I was single with no kid. I want a long-term partner, but I date and have sex mainly to soothe my stress with pleasure. The fun I have dating extends to the rest of my life. It makes me happy—and I'm a better parent."

CHAPTER 24:
Over Time, Does Sexual Quality Decline?

A N OLD JOKE asks: What's the fastest way to destroy couples' enjoyment of sex? *Get married.*

Actually, after the wedding, the overwhelming majority of spouses continue to make love and most say they enjoy it. But the joke reflects the conventional wisdom that, like an old sweater, as time passes, the quality of sex unravels.

Does it? A sociologist at Wagner College, Staten Island, analyzed 1,550 married couples' interviews for the National Health and Social Life Survey. He discovered that relationship duration has only a "small" negative effect on sexual quality—much less than the joke suggests. Meanwhile, with a little effort, longtime couples can enjoy sexual *enhancement*.

Why Quality Erodes
The Wagner researcher identified four factors that predict sexual deterioration. In order of importance:

- **Gender.** Plenty of married men nurse sexual grudges, but usually, quality decline reflects women's chronic dissatisfaction.
- **Routine.** Novelty usually fades and with it sexual excitement.
- **Children at home.** Compared with childless couples, those raising children, especially preschoolers, are more likely to report erotic cooling.
- **Cohabitation.** A marriage license is more than just a piece of paper. Compared with married spouses, over time, unmarried couples usually report greater deterioration of sexual quality, even if they do it frequently.

The Wagner researcher did not explore what couples do in bed, but two teams of psychologists did—one Canadian, the other from several US universities. They asked 1,176 married couples, age twenty-two to seventy, how they played and how their sexual moves affected the quality of their lovemaking. In descending order:

- **Genital preoccupation.** Compared with lots of kissing, cuddling, and mutual whole-body massage, those who quickly plunged into intercourse generally reported reduced quality and satisfaction.
- **Women not having orgasms.** Women who don't come resent it.
- **Coaching.** Some lovers coach one another. Others do not. Silent couples report greater sexual deterioration.

- **Ruts.** The same old moves get boring.
- **No oral.** Without fellatio and cunnilingus, most people feel disappointed.
- **Infidelity.** For the vast majority of folks, spousal unfaithfulness destroys both trust and sexual quality.
- **Poor health.** From aches and pains to serious conditions, health problems may ruin sex.

How to Maintain Sizzling Sex

Now that we understand what reduces sexual quality, it's not difficult to enhance it:

- **Schedule it.** This helps resolve desire differences, encourages anticipatory excitement, and allows time to plan novelty.
- **Work to stay healthy.** Age is just a number, no matter if it's your age, your relationship's duration, or both. Of course, as candles pack the cake, vitality ebbs and chronic conditions may reduce sexual quality. But no one is ever too old or infirm to get healthier, and as health improves, so does erotic enjoyment.
- **Kiss and cuddle more.** Genital preoccupation is a major sex killer. Forget "foreplay." Cultivate loveplay, leisurely, playful, mutual whole-body massage that eventually—after twenty minutes or so—extends to the genitals.
- **Do something different—anything.** Introduce novelty. It boosts brain levels of dopamine, the neurotransmitter of lust. What's new need not vastly differ from routine play as long as it feels fresh. Trade foot massages. Bathe or shower together beforehand. Add music, scented candles, lubricant, sex toys. Make love in a new place in a new way.
- **Coach each other.** Everyone is sexually unique. No one can read anyone's erotic mind. To communicate likes and dislikes, lovers *must* say so directly and specifically. It doesn't matter when you coach—before, during, or after sex. Declare your preferences and gently remind your partner until, within declared limits, you get as close as possible to what you want.
- **Share more oral sex.** In porn, fellatio is ubiquitous, endless, and often culminates in ejaculation. Meanwhile, cunnilingus is sporadic, perfunctory, and almost never produces orgasm. No surprise there. Porn depicts men's erotic fantasies, which are more concerned with receiving pleasure than providing it.

For most women, cunnilingus is crucial to orgasm. Little or none means that many women don't come, which fuels dissatisfaction with marital sex. Gentlemen, if this is news to you, review chapter 8 and ask your partner to coach you how and for how long she enjoys being caressed, kissed, and licked down there.

- **Get away from the children.** Sleepovers are fun for kids and godsends for parents interested in finding time to make love.
- **Tie the knot.** Why would long-term cohabitation compromise sexual quality? Compared with men, women tend to place more value on that commitment. If they remain unmarried, women's sexual satisfaction often suffers.
- **If you've agreed to monogamy, honor your agreement.** Cheating annihilates sexual quality. Some couples negotiate occasional nonmonogamy: visits to sex or swing clubs, or some form of open relationship or polyamory. That's not cheating. But secret infidelity destroys sexual quality.

Straight versus Lesbian/Gay Relationships: Any Differences in Quality and Satisfaction?

Many people assume that men and women are so different that neither can comprehend the other's sexual sensibilities. If that's true, then same-gender couples should enjoy greater long-term sexual satisfaction. Canadian psychologists surveyed 423 coupled individuals, 253 heterosexuals, 170 gay/lesbians. They found "far more similarities than differences." Sexual quality over time has less to do with gender disconnects than with mutual erotic coaching.

Play a Game, Read a Book

Sexual quality decays primarily because lovers get lazy. Fortunately, it doesn't take much to keep things fresh. A substantial cottage industry offers all sorts of items that promise to keep sex sizzling. Two of my favorites:

"An Enchanting Evening." Barbara and Michael Jonas of Scottsdale, Arizona, had a spat before he left on a business trip. Barbara wanted his homecoming to be happier—but how? She typed questions on index cards and created a rudimentary game board. Then she tacked a note to their door and held her breath.

On his way home, Michael wanted to tell Barbara how much he loved her but wasn't good at expressing his feelings. He saw Barbara's note: "Change into something comfortable and meet me in the living room."

In the living room, he found the lights low and Barbara dressed alluringly. She handed him a glass of wine, a pencil, and index cards, and asked him to write a wish for later that evening. Barbara also penned a wish. "First one around the board wins the wish."

They rolled dice, moved game pieces, and drew index cards. Some asked questions designed to celebrate their relationship: *What attracted you to your spouse?* Others contained playful directions: *Kiss your spouse where it's unexpected.*

The Jonases don't recall who won that first game, but their memories of that evening remain vivid. "Barbara's game was very powerful," Michael recalls. "It helped me say the loving things I'd always felt but couldn't express."

"We had a wonderful reunion," Barbara recalls. The game led to another form of play they both enjoyed.

Afterward, Barbara shelved her game, but Michael kept thinking about it. He suggested generalizing it—changing "spouse" to "partner" and "marriage" to "relationship." They called it "An Enchanting Evening" and eventually quit their jobs and launched a business, Time for Two, to market their game and others they subsequently developed.

The game reminds couples why they fell in love. It promotes intimate conversation and creative erotic play. Bias-free, it can be enjoyed by young and old, straight and gay, from initial infatuation to fiftieth anniversaries. The "talk" cards foster loving support. The "touch" cards are deliciously ambiguous. One says, *Gently fondle something your partner has two of.* That might be ears or breasts. There's no pressure. Couples can play at any comfort level.

The game has become a popular wedding gift, and many couples counselors and sex therapists assign it as homework. The Jonases still play it. "For love and intimacy to flourish," Barbara says, "they must be nurtured."

"An Enchanting Evening" and the Jonases' other games are available at TimeForTwo.com.

The Book of Love, Laughter, and Romance. As sales of "An Enchanting Evening" took off, the Jonases included a postcard in each box asking how their customers kept their relationships fresh and erotic. Thousands replied. The Jonases collected their responses into *The Book of Love, Laughter, and Romance*, which contains hundreds of delightful suggestions for keeping long-term love fresh and exciting. It's also available on their site.

CHAPTER 25:
My One and Only?
Infidelity and Sex Work

MOST COUPLES DEMAND monogamy. For many, any breach of sexual exclusivity spells disaster. *He cheated. It's over.* Even when infidelity doesn't precipitate breakups, it may cause severe relationship damage.

If you require monogamy, you have every right to do so—but you may be disappointed. Sexually, we're all unique and that extends to how we feel about limiting ourselves to one lover.

Are Humans Naturally Monogamous?

Many insist that monogamy is "natural." Actually, only around 9 percent of mammal species mate for life, and among humans, the high prevalence of infidelity makes it difficult to argue that sexual exclusivity is innate:

- In the Bible, polygamy was common—several wives or one official wife plus concubines. In Genesis, patriarch Jacob has two wives, Leah and Rachel, and two concubines, Bilhah and Zilpah. He fathers children with all four.
- Infidelity is the only sin proscribed in *two* of the Ten Commandments: *Thou shalt not commit adultery* and *Thou shalt not covet they neighbor's wife.* Don't do it. And don't even think about it. If the ancients were monogamous, these commandments would not have been necessary.
- Mormons were publicly polygamous until 1890. Some still are.
- Members of the Lusi tribe of Papua, New Guinea, believe that healthy fetal development requires pregnant women to have intercourse with many men.
- A few cultures have institutionalized polyamory. In 1985, anthropologist Thomas Gregor counted eighty-eight ongoing sexual relationships among one Amazon village's thirty-seven adults.
- Every US metropolitan area and many rural areas boast sex and swing clubs—search "sex/swing clubs" and any locale. The former are typically open to all adults, the latter to couples and single women.

Advocates of strict monogamy often claim that nonmonogamy just doesn't work. For most, that may be true, but I know several happy long-term couples who have practiced occasional nonmonogamy for decades:

- One, married twenty years, is basically monogamous, but each month the woman spends a long weekend with her secondary man who lives fifty miles away.

- Another, together fifteen years, is generally monogamous, but for the woman's birthday, the man annually arranges for threesomes with other men.
- A third, together twenty-five years, maintain monogamy at home but grant each other "hall passes," permission to play, when either travels for business.
- Another, married thirty years, meets secondary lovers periodically. The woman explains, "I'm in love only with my husband, and he's in love only with me. But we both enjoy playing on the side. It's fun and keeps our marital sex fresh and exciting. Occasionally, around town, we run into one of our secondaries. We make introductions and chat a bit. Everyone smiles. It's fine."

If monogamy is natural, why do so many novels, plays, movies, songs, and TV shows revolve around its violation? Some observations:

- "Confusing monogamy with morality has done more damage than any other human error." —Playwright George Bernard Shaw (1856–1950)
- "A knight off to the Crusades fitted his wife with a chastity belt and, in case he died, entrusted the key to his best friend. He'd ridden only a few miles when his friend, riding hard, caught up with him. 'You gave me the wrong key!'" —Author Anais Nin (1903–77)
- "We drove back to the hotel and said goodbye. How hypocritical to leave the man you want to fuck to be with a man you don't want, and then, in great excitement, fuck the one you don't want while pretending he's the one you do. That's monogamy." —Author Erica Jong (1942–), in *Fear of Flying* (1973)
- "I told my wife I was seeing a psychiatrist. She told me she was seeing a psychiatrist, two plumbers, and a bartender." —Comedian Rodney Dangerfield (1921–2004).

Author Dan Savage observes that until the twentieth century, most cultures assumed men were naturally nonmonogamous. Monogamy was only for women, enforced by men to control women's sexuality and guarantee paternity. That's still the case in many societies.

In the West, women have increasingly become men's political and economic equals. But they have not gained the sexual freedom men have historically enjoyed. Instead, men have had their sexual freedom curtailed by increasing expectations of lifelong monogamy. For many, it's a struggle; for some, impossible.

Savage notes that we humans are decidedly imperfect, yet when it comes to sexual exclusivity, many demand perfection: "Monogamy is like sobriety. You can be sober for years, then fall off the wagon and sober up again. If couples have been married thirty years and each steps out a few times, they're not reprehensible. They're actually *very good* at monogamy." Savage coined the term *monogamish* to describe ostensibly monogamous couples who accept occasional lapses.

Infidelity: How Prevalent?
Infidelity is difficult to research. Few admit it. I recall a survey showing that only a tiny percentage of married folks had ever been unfaithful. The researchers interviewed subjects *in the presence of their spouses*. Duh!

Admissions of nonmonogamy depend on how researchers ask about it. University of Colorado scientists asked 4,800 married women about infidelity during the previous year using face-to-face interviews and an anonymous questionnaire. In the interviews, only 1 percent admitted straying, but in the nameless questionnaire, 6 percent.

Meanwhile, controversy clouds the definition of *infidelity*. Most say it's sex with anyone other than your mate. But what about spouses who are separated but not divorced? Or mates separated for extended periods by work or military deployment? Is infidelity any sex outside of marriage? Or just secret sex? Or only sex with emotional involvement? And does cheating require intercourse? What if you simply kiss passionately? Or trade hand jobs? Or oral sex?

A huge research literature has explored infidelity. I reviewed fifty studies. Some highlights:

- One mate at a time is the current norm, but historically, 84 percent of known human societies have permitted men more than one ongoing sexual relationship.
- Since Kinsey's studies in the late 1940s, credible estimates of heterosexual Americans' lifetime infidelity have varied wildly—for men, from 12 to 72 percent, for women, from 7 to 54 percent.
- Three-quarters of Americans call extramarital sex "always wrong," yet a majority of unfaithful Americans call theirs justified.
- Infidelity is associated with alcohol, previous cheating, spousal boredom, relationship dissatisfaction and duration (likelihood rises over time), expectations of imminent breakups, and low-frequency, poor-quality lovemaking. Among men, a pregnant wife and having an infant also increase risk of affairs. However, among spouses who have been unfaithful, 56 percent of men and 34 percent of women call their marriages "happy."
- Strict monogamy is associated with regular religious observance. Infidelity is linked with loneliness, extroversion, anxiety, depression, moodiness, narcissism, openness to new experiences, a history of child sexual abuse, and knowledge that one or both of one's parents had been unfaithful.
- With regard to education, the curve is U-shaped. Those without high school diplomas or with graduate degrees have the greatest likelihood of infidelity.
- Working outside the home doesn't matter much. Half of both male and female cheaters meet their paramours through work, half in other ways.

Researchers at Rutgers and SUNY Stony Brook reviewed 148 studies worldwide and concluded, "Despite near-universal disapproval, infidelity is a global phenomenon that occurs with remarkable regularity."

Infidelity has been so prevalent for so long that some researchers have suggested the inclination may be genetically hardwired and provide an evolutionary survival advantage. Our thirst for novelty appears to be genetically inherited. That would include not just new sexual moves, but also quite possibly new partners.

The evolutionary mission of life is to reproduce. The best way for men to do this is to mate with as many women as possible. As early primates evolved into apes and humans, males who mated with the most females were more likely to father offspring who may well have gained genes that tilted them toward philandering.

Meanwhile, the best way for women to send their genes into the future is to raise children to sexual maturity, a challenge made easier with a man. Hence assertions that compared with men, women are "naturally" more monogamous. Women's need for parenting help may explain why their rate of infidelity appears lower than men's. Nonetheless, many women stray, by some estimates up to half. Why?

Several researchers speculate that women and their offspring gain a survival advantage by having "backup" mates who can provide resources if their primary man dies or leaves. In addition, women may use infidelity as a way to "trade up" to mates who can offer more and better support. The children of unfaithful women may well have been more likely to reproduce—and carry genes that pushed their offspring toward continued infidelity.

The Rutgers-Stony Brook researchers concluded, "Throughout prehistory, infidelity had payoffs for both men and women, thus perpetuating its genetic underpinnings and a taste for infidelity in both genders today."

Our species' Latin binomial is *Homo sapiens*. The second term means *wise*, implying that we have transcended base animal instincts. But civilization is only ten thousand years old, in evolutionary terms, practically brand new. More than we'd like to admit, we're still beasts driven by animal instincts. Two popular sexual metaphors illustrate this: Men are *wolves*, women *foxes*.

Despite a mountain of research, we're still not sure of the true prevalence of infidelity or why it occurs, nor can we reliably predict it. All we know is that infidelity occurs so frequently that when we hear about its icy finger touching couples we know, we're saddened—but not necessarily surprised.

Why Do So Many Men Pay for Sex?

Most men may pay for sex either directly or indirectly. Dating and infidelity involve indirect payment. The sex itself is free, but men usually pay for drinks, dinners, gifts, and maybe hotel rooms. Commercial sex dispenses with the wining and dining. Customers ("johns"), almost always men, pay sex workers directly for their services.

Why do men pay for sex? The biological reason is testosterone. Compared with most women, most men think about sex more, want it more, and masturbate more. And when lust, opportunity, and financial ability intersect, many pay for it.

Sex work may or may not be "the oldest profession," but there's no doubting its antiquity. In Genesis, patriarch Judah cavorts with a woman he believes is a harlot. Actually, she's his daughter-in-law, Tamar, in disguise. And in the book of Joshua, the Israelites conquer Jericho with help from one of the city's sex workers.

In patriarchal cultures, men have controlled the sexuality of all women—except sex workers. "Working women" gained sexual self-determination but faced social marginalization and condemnation.

Western literature is replete with stories of "whores with hearts of gold" who win a measure of social acceptance by providing more than just fleshy openings. In Dostoevsky's *Crime and Punishment*, a prostitute persuades Raskolnikov to confess his murder. Tarts with hearts are also a fixture of Hollywood—Jamie Lee Curtis in *Trading Places* (1983) and Julia Roberts in *Pretty Woman* (1990).

Few men admit paying for sex. It's stigmatized, and the myth is that only single losers with no social skills stoop so low, that "real men" can get lucky without cash payment. Despite the stigma, many men have participated in studies of commercial sex. The consensus of findings:

- Only around half are single. The rest are cohabiting or married.
- Johns are not necessarily losers with poor social skills. They come from all walks of life. Few get arrested (around 5 percent), but those who have include former New York governor Eliot Spitzer (in 2008), actor Hugh Grant (1995), televangelist Jimmy Lee Swaggart (1988), and Arkansas congressman Wilbur Mills (1974). Sex work researchers at the University of Gothenburg, Sweden, concluded, "No social characteristics distinguish johns from other men."

- Researchers at the Free University of Berlin, Germany, surveyed six hundred men who paid for sex. They were psychologically indistinguishable from other men, except they had more inclination toward risk-taking.
- Likelihood of visiting sex workers varies by country based on cultural tradition. From various surveys, here are estimates of the proportion of male adults in fourteen countries who have paid for sex at least once:

  Cambodia: 59–80 percent
  Thailand: 75 percent
  Italy: 17–45 percent
  Spain: 27–39 percent
  Japan: 37 percent
  Netherlands: 14–22 percent
  United States: 15–20 percent
  China: 6–20 percent
  Switzerland: 19 percent
  France and Australia: 16 percent
  Sweden: 8–14 percent
  Finland: 13 percent
  Norway: 10–13 percent
  United Kingdom: 7–9 percent

If 15 percent of adult American men have paid for sex, that's around fifteen million men.

- Most clients crave sex without responsibility. They pay, get what they purchased, and leave—no muss, no fuss.
- At a sex research conference I attended, J. M., a fifteen-year veteran Seattle sex worker in her forties, presented her survey of 225 clients, the only such study I know of. She characterized her single clients as attractive and charming—but sexually insecure. Most dated and had sex without paying for it (directly). So why visit her? They said:
  - "To learn more about pleasing women."
  - "I have regular sex, but I'm anxious. My dating relationships haven't progressed to the kind of comfortable sexual give and take I'd like."
  - "I get nervous on dates. The stakes are higher when you want an emotional connection. Here I can relax and just do it."
  - J. M.'s married clients made love at home, but not often enough to suit them.
  - Many complained that their wives weren't interested in sex or nonsexual affection.
  - Married johns often visit sex workers to obtain moves they don't get at home: fellatio, BDSM, and anal play—anally fingering the woman, anal intercourse, being fingered, or the sex worker using a strap-on dildo on them.
  - "At home I don't get much kissing and touching. I asked my wife to go into therapy. She refused. So this is my therapy."
  - "My wife and I are good friends but there's not enough affection or sex. So after much thought, I decided to make up for what I don't get at home without hurting anybody."
  - Many married clients told her, "I come here to save my marriage." Few expressed any guilt—just 8 percent.

Adult Sex Work: Legalize It

In 2015, the Nobel Prize–winning human rights organization Amnesty International provoked international controversy by advocating the immediate worldwide decriminalization of adult sex work.

"Sex workers," Amnesty said, "are among the world's most marginalized populations. They are at high risk for violence, arrest, detention, extortion, harassment, and exclusion from housing, health care, and occupational safety benefits available to other workers."

Amnesty argues that decriminalization empowers sex workers. "Gender inequality and discrimination promote women's entry into sex work. Criminalizing women for their lack of life choices is not the answer."

In 1999, New South Wales, Australia, legalized prostitution and brothels. Critics predicted a huge increase in the number of sex workers. The number increased slightly, but regular police checks largely eliminated trafficked women in brothels. Meanwhile, before legalization, sex workers had very high rates of emotional stress. Once prostitution was legalized, sex worker stress declined to same level as other women in the labor force.

In 2003, New Zealand legalized brothels and experienced the same results.

Opponents of legalization claim it increases pimping and trafficking. Researchers disagree. Barbara Brents, PhD, a professor of sociology at the University of Nevada, has studied that state's legal sex industry for twenty years. "In legal brothels, employees say they feel safe. They are bound by their work contracts, but otherwise are free to come and go. Most importantly, in legal brothels we have found no evidence of trafficking."

Legal sex workers also pay taxes and reduce criminal justice system costs for antiprostitution enforcement efforts that are largely futile. In 2013, the Canadian Supreme Court cited Brents's research in its decision to decriminalize adult sex work.

Even critics of legalization acknowledge that age-old suppression efforts have had no impact—other than driving sex work underground, where sex workers find themselves largely at the mercy of pimps, traffickers, and violent clients.

Joining Amnesty, two prominent antitrafficking groups support decriminalization—Anti-Slavery International and the Global Alliance Against Trafficking in Women. They all support strong penalties for human trafficking and sexual exploitation.

Amnesty argues that keeping prostitution illegal imprisons sex workers in the underground economy, where they have no rights. The criminal justice system stigmatizes them as "criminals," discouraging them from turning in pimps, violent clients, or police who rape them. It's also daunting for sex workers to transition into legitimate jobs and above ground lives.

Laws prohibiting so-called vices don't work. Prohibition didn't stop drinking. It simply drove alcohol underground and enriched organized crime. Laws against marijuana have never suppressed its use. As of 2020, most states have legalized medical marijuana or decriminalized its use, and ten states and the District of Columbia have legalized recreational use—with no major increases in crime, truancy, auto accidents, or other ills. Sex work cannot be suppressed, so why fight it?

Decriminalization doesn't solve all problems related to sex work. Psychopaths can still prey on sex workers and women can still be trafficked. But decriminalization improves sex workers' lives, encourages them to report and testify against pimps and traffickers, and facilitates transition to other occupations. Adult sex work and brothels should be legalized.

Some men fantasize they can develop actual relationships with sex workers. There's even a sex work specialty, the "girlfriend experience" (GFE), where, for an extra fee, the women pretend to be clients' gal pals and engage in conversation and kissing as well as genital play.

Meanwhile, a small proportion of clients have violent streaks and assault sex workers. Women at highest risk are those who walk the streets. Assaults are much less common, though possible, in brothels or private homes.

In some surveys, clients say they've never considered the possibility their providers might have been trafficked into sex work. In others, clients admit suspecting trafficking, especially when sex workers have foreign accents.

Why pay for sex instead of self-sexing? We're a social species, and sometimes, men want another's touch, even if it's not loving, even if they have to pay for it.

CHAPTER 26:
Chronic Illness and Disabilities: Sizzling Sex Is Always Possible

ILLNESS AND DISABILITY complicate sex, but *never* preclude it. Touch is the only sense we can't live without. Virtually everybody—every body—enjoys sensual touch. When there's a will, there's always a way. Even those with severe disabilities can enjoy erotic pleasure.

Sex and Acute Illness and Injury

Colds, flu, sprains, back pain—acute health problems interfere with sex.

Don't expect your libido—or anything else—to stand up if you can't. The body expends considerable energy fighting even minor illnesses, for example, colds, leaving less energy for sex. But as illnesses and injuries resolve, sexual desire and function almost always return. Be patient.

How patient? Ask your doctor to estimate your recovery time. It may take longer. If sex continues to be problematic after twice your doctor's estimate, consider sex coaching or therapy.

Patience can be especially challenging for couples with serious desire differences. If the illness affects the lower-libido partner, the other may level accusations of malingering. There's no easy answer. Try to remember that even medically minor health problems may cause libido loss that lasts longer than you think it should.

Sizzling Sex with Chronic Conditions

You've just been diagnosed with diabetes, high blood pressure, or another chronic condition. When your doctor says, *Any questions?* you don't usually ask, *What about sex?* Every chronic condition is different. But coping sexually is pretty much the same:

- **Expand your definition.** If you define "sex" as just vaginal intercourse and can't accomplish that, you might conclude you're erotically washed up. But if your definition is more flexible, then bidding farewell to intercourse is like passing up one dish at a buffet. Even those with health issues can usually kiss, cuddle, and enjoy massage and oral sex. Even with disabilities, you still have abilities.
- **Find information and support.** Ask your doctor(s) about the sexual implications of your condition and the possible sexual effects of all your medications. Then search the internet: *sexual effects of*—your condition and medications. That should produce a useful overview. Join the organization(s) devoted to your condition. All chronic condition and disabilities have national advocacy groups. Ask the organization about sexual coping and for referrals to experts on your condition's sexual implications. Finally, most

organizations sponsor support groups. Ask members how they cope sexually. You're likely to get an earful.

- **Stay as healthy as possible.** *But I'm* not *healthy. I have this damn condition.* Yes, you do. But you'll feel better, manage your condition more easily, and retain more sexual interest and ability if your lifestyle is as healthy as your circumstances allow. Many medications for chronic conditions may cause sexual side effects: antidepressants and pain and mood-altering drugs among others. A healthy-as-possible lifestyle might allow you to reduce your dose or eliminate some drugs.
- **Try lubricants and sex toys.** Many chronic conditions and disabilities reduce genital sensitivity. Lubricants often help. Vibrators, too, including vibrating penis sleeves, and depending on your situation, maybe other toys.
- **Consider sex coaching or therapy.** Coaches and therapists can suggest erotic adjustments.

Want Fewer Colds? Make Love Weekly

Don't kiss me. I have a cold. Who hasn't heard this? Close contact spreads colds, so sex with cold sufferers should spread them. But a study at Wilkes-Barre University in Pennsylvania shows that weekly lovemaking *reduces* cold risk.

The investigators asked 111 college students to estimate their partner sex frequency: none, less than weekly, once or twice a week, or three or more times. Then the students provided saliva, which contains the body's first line of defense against cold viruses, immunoglobulin A (IgA). As IgA rises, risk of catching colds falls. The once-or-twice-a-week group had the most IgA, suggesting that weekly lovemaking reduces risk of colds.

Why would weekly sex help prevent colds? It's relaxing and emotionally supportive, which provide immunological benefits that evidently outweigh the risk of proximity.

Many studies show that deep relaxation stimulates the immune system. Psychologists at Washington State University took blood samples from sixty-five people and counted their infection-fighting white blood cells. Then all participants watched a documentary about the immune system. One-third did nothing else. Another third learned to meditate and practiced twice a day. The final third twice daily visualized their immune systems growing stronger. A week later, the researchers obtained fresh blood samples. Controls experienced no white cell boost. But both the meditation and visualization groups did.

Lovemaking also provides powerful emotional support. University of Pittsburgh researchers asked 276 healthy volunteers about their social ties, and then squirted live cold virus up their noses. Those with the most social support were least likely to catch the cold.

Perhaps that old saying should be revised. *I feel a cold coming on. Let's do it!*

Osteoarthritis? Sex Often Helps

Make love regularly. That's a good prescription for the thirty-five million mostly older Americans with osteoarthritis (OA), the most common type of joint disease. In OA, after years of wear and tear, the shock-absorbing cartilage surrounding the joints breaks down, causing stiffness, pain, reduced range of motion, and possibly swelling. Symptoms are worst in the morning, then with movement often improve during the day.

To manage OA, doctors advise low-impact exercise that gently moves affected joints through their full range of motion: stretching, walking, gardening, yoga, water exercise—and sex. Lovemaking involves gentle range-of-motion exercise that reduces pain and inflammation. Sex also releases endorphins, the body's own pain relievers.

To incorporate sex into OA management:

- **Schedule it.** Chronic conditions require planning and adjustments. Scheduling sex allows preparation, so you can make love when symptoms are least bothersome.
- **Bathe or shower beforehand.** Warmth soothes the joints, and it's relaxing, which helps prepare the mind and body for lovemaking.
- **Take your medicine.** Consider taking pain medication before you undress: aspirin, ibuprofen (Advil, Motrin), acetaminophen (Tylenol), or naproxen (Aleve). High-CBD cannabis, a natural pain reliever, may also help.
- **Massage each other all over.** Whole-body caresses are a foundation of sizzling sex and help manage OA.
- **Use extra pillows.** Padding under achy joints may help.
- **Try a vibrator.** OA may stiffen fingers, interfering with loving touch. Vibrators may help.
- **Check in frequently.** Ask, *Is this okay?* Alert lovers to positions and moves that cause discomfort.
- **Consider sex coaching or therapy.** Therapists can suggest helpful adjustments.
- **Consider joint replacement.** In New York, Lenox Hill Hospital researchers surveyed 147 people with severe OA who reported sexual dissatisfaction. After joint replacement, 81 percent reported greater satisfaction.

Sex and Diabetes

Diabetes affects twenty-six million Americans—11 percent of US adults. In addition, prediabetes ("metabolic syndrome") affects eighty million Americans, one-third of adults.

Diabetes has two manifestations, type 1 and type 2. The former is an autoimmune condition that usually develops during childhood. It destroys the pancreatic cells that produce the hormone insulin. Type 1 diabetics must inject insulin daily. But type 1 accounts for just 5 percent of diabetes.

The rest—95 percent—is type 2. The pancreas makes sufficient insulin, but the body becomes "insulin resistant" and can't use it, usually because of obesity. Type 2 diabetes can be controlled or reversed with diet changes, exercise, weight loss, medication, and possibly insulin.

Diabetes prevents the body's main food, blood sugar (glucose), from entering the cells. Blood sugar rises abnormally high.

If you spill a sugary drink on the floor, it gets sticky. The same thing happens in blood vessels. The extra sugar makes blood sticky, which gums up the vessels and causes diabetic complications, including possible blindness, amputations, heart attack—and sex problems.

However, diabetics are *not* fated to suffer sexual impairment. Risk of all complications can be minimized by adopting a healthy lifestyle and maintaining blood sugar as close as possible to normal. Work closely with an endocrinologist and diabetes educator.

Still, many diabetics develop sex problems. Diabetes interferes with the nervous system's ability to mediate arousal and the circulatory system's ability to deliver the extra blood to the genitals and enable erection, clitoral sensitivity, and erotic responsiveness.

Diabetic Erectile Dysfunction

Men diagnosed with diabetes hear dire warnings about their high risk of erectile dysfunction (ED). This may become a self-fulfilling prophecy.

Diabetes may impair erection, but ED is not inevitable, and if it occurs, several safe, effective treatments are available—not to mention that *men don't need erections to enjoy sizzling sex and orgasms.*

Syracuse University researchers reviewed twenty-three studies of diabetic ED. Compared with the general population, men with diabetes have about twice the risk. But many diabetic men maintain their erections.

Risk factors for diabetic ED include:

- **Duration.** As time with diabetes increases, so does ED risk.
- **Complications.** Diabetes-related cardiovascular disease and nerve damage (neuropathy) raise risk of ED.
- **Obesity.** Increasing weight aggravates diabetes and raises risk of ED.
- **Smoking.** Tobacco accelerates the progression of diabetic cardiovascular disease.

If you suffer diabetic ED:

- **Quit smoking.** Arterial damage heals.
- **Maintain tight control.** Keeping blood sugar in the normal range reduces risk of complications.
- **Consult your doctor and pharmacist.** List all your medications, including supplements and over-the-counter drugs. Ask if any—or their interactions—might contribute to ED. If so, ask if you might switch to lower-risk alternatives.
- **Consider erection medication.** The drugs work best in men whose ED results from cardiovascular disease, less well in those with nerve damage. But if you take nitroglycerin for angina, you *cannot* take erection drugs. The combination might prove fatal. You might also ask your doctor about drugs derived from the bark of the West African yohimbe tree: Yohimbine, Yocon, Testomar, and Erex. They've received much less publicity than Viagra, Cialis, and Levitra, but they're FDA approved and may help.
- **Try a vacuum constricting device (VCD).** These appliances create a partial vacuum around the penis that draws blood into the organ, causing temporary erection. They include a squeeze-bulb pump attached to a plastic cylinder closed at one end that fits over the penis. Squeezing the bulb evacuates air from the tube, drawing blood into Mr. Happy.

    Studies of VCDs have produced wildly disparate findings, from 35 percent satisfaction to 95 percent: Iranian researchers taught 1,500 men with ED to use VCDs. When their wives were supportive, 95 percent were able to raise erections sufficient for intercourse. At Cleveland Clinic, seventy-nine men learned to use VCDs. Half were happy with them. And at Cornell, 129 men tried VCDs. Only one-third felt satisfied.

    Satisfaction was most closely linked to the amount of training the men received, their wives' support, and continued use over time.

    Sex toy catalogs offer several models, but for best results, consult a urologist for a custom-fitted VCD.
- **Consider sex therapy.**

Diabetic Vaginal Dryness and Orgasm Problems

Compared with diabetic ED, the condition's impact on women has been less researched and publicized. Fortunately, in recent years, a clearer picture has emerged:

- **Vaginal dryness.** With arousal, vaginal capillaries open (dilate) and some blood fluid (plasma) diffuses into the vagina as natural vaginal lubrication. Diabetic women's capillaries don't dilate normally, which contributes to dryness.
- **Orgasm difficulties.** Diabetic nerve damage may reduce clitoral sensitivity, impairing women's ability to enjoy erotic touch and work up to orgasm. Iranian researchers surveyed 150 type 2 women. Eighty percent reported sex problems: low desire, 50%; arousal difficulties, 47%; vaginal dryness, 50%; and orgasm problems, 42%.

Fortunately, diabetic women can minimize sexual dysfunction with:

- **Healthy lifestyle.** It may even eliminate type 2 diabetes.
- **Lubricants.** They help with both dryness and loss of genital sensitivity.
- **Vibrators.** Vibes intensify erotic sensation.
- **Sex therapy.**

Sex after Heart Attack

In the 2003 movie *Something's Gotta Give*, a sixty-something heart attack survivor (Jack Nicholson) hopes to bed an older hottie (Diane Keaton), but wonders if his damaged heart can take the strain. His doctor (Keanu Reeves) says, "If you can climb two flights of stairs without chest pain or feeling winded, you're good to go."

Hollywood rarely provides authoritative medical information, but this advice is correct. Lovemaking and orgasm are not taxing. A few months after a heart attack, if you can ascend two flights of stairs comfortably, you can get it on:

- **Ask your doctor.** The vast majority of heart attack survivors can make love without fearing recurrence, but your individual situation might differ, for example, if you also have moderate to severe congestive heart failure.
- **Adopt a heart-healthy lifestyle.** It's never too late to get healthier.
- **Make love regularly.** Stress is a risk factor for heart attack. Satisfying sex reduces it.
- **Consider sex therapy.** It can reassure you about returning to lovemaking.

Sex after Prostate Cancer

The myth is that prostate cancer treatment destroys erections. The truth is more complicated.

Men facing treatment for this disease should prepare emotionally for total, permanent, untreatable ED. But after prostate cancer, ED is *not* inevitable. And if it develops, sizzling sex and satisfying orgasms are still possible.

These days, most prostate cancer is diagnosed early and prognosis is excellent. Early-stage prostate cancer can be treated with:

- **Surgery.** Removal of the gland (radical prostatectomy).
- **External beam.** Conventional radiation.
- **Brachytherapy.** Also known as seed implantation, this involves injection of radioactive pellets into the gland.

All three are equally effective, with five-year survival around 80 percent. However, surgery is somewhat more likely to leave men with ED:

- National Cancer Institute researchers followed 1,187 men for five years—901 had surgery, 286 radiation. Sexual function declined in both groups, but ED was more likely after surgery, 79 versus 64 percent respectively.
- Harvard investigators followed 987 men for two years after treatment. After surgery, 65 percent developed ED; after external beam, 63 percent; and after seed insertion, 57 percent.
- Other studies have reported ED rates ranging from 60 to 82 percent.

After surgery, most men experience sudden erection loss, but over time, some recover partial function. After radiation, fewer men report immediate ED. But it often develops over time.

In addition to type of treatment, ED after prostate cancer also depends on:

- **Age.** Men under sixty are more likely to maintain erections.
- **Prostate-specific antigen (PSA).** The prostate produces this compound. Several studies show that the lower PSA is before treatment, the greater likelihood of erections after.
- **Pretreatment sexual function.** Compared with men who reported infrequent, unsatisfying sex before treatment, those who had regular, enjoyable sex usually show better erection capacity after.
- **Morning wood.** Young men often wake with morning erections and some older men wake with partial firmness. Compared with men who don't, those who do are more likely to recover at least partial erection function.

Prostate cancer treatment causes ED because erection nerves run adjacent to the gland. Surgery often severs them and radiation may damage them.

For years, surgeons have striven to reduce postsurgical ED by leaving erection-related nerves intact. If the tumor develops near a nerve line, this might be impossible. If nerve-sparing surgery is possible, it helps somewhat. However, even with nerve-sparing surgery, outcomes vary tremendously based on the definition of "erection." If the criterion is:

- Any firmness, success rates are high
- Erections sufficient for intercourse, rates are lower
- Firmness equal to baseline before treatment, even lower

As a result, published outcomes are all over the map:

- Among 140 men one year after nerve-sparing surgery, University of Michigan researchers found that 74 percent could raise erections sufficient for intercourse.
- English scientists asked 531 men if nerve-sparing surgery returned them to presurgical firmness. Among men under sixty, 35 percent said yes, but in men over sixty, only 24 percent.
- One year after nerve-sparing surgery, Danish scientists asked 210 men if they'd returned to presurgical firmness. Only 21 percent said yes.

Several studies have assessed nerve-sparing surgery plus erection medication, particularly Cialis. Again, results have varied considerably:

- In the Danish study just mentioned, 21 percent said they'd returned to presurgical erections, but with the addition of daily erection medication, the figure rose to 33 percent.
- Two years after nerve-sparing prostatectomy, researchers at Memorial Sloan Kettering in New York surveyed 180 men. Without erection drugs, 22 percent said they'd returned to baseline; with drugs, 43 percent.
- Turkish researchers followed fifty-five men who could raise firm erections before nerve-sparing surgery. Six months later, with daily Cialis (5 mg), 72 percent reported presurgical firmness.
- Finally, men who regain their erections may still suffer sex problems. In the Memorial Sloan Kettering study just mentioned, many of those who regained their erections reported poor sexual satisfaction.

With so many studies showing such different outcomes, anything can happen, from minimal impairment to total ED. Every man treated for prostate cancer should prepare emotionally for the latter. But many men retain some function.

A small proportion of prostate cancer survivors opt for penile implants. However, implant insertion may deform the penis. And mechanical implants may malfunction, necessitating repair surgery.

Finally, several studies show that after prostate cancer treatment, Kegel exercises may improve firmness.

Meanwhile, all the attention on post–prostate cancer erections obscures this key truth: *Men don't need erections for satisfying sex and marvelous orgasms.* Different nerves control erection and orgasm. Even when treatment damages erection nerves, those involved in orgasm usually remain intact.

To have orgasms without erections, it helps to have:

- An alluring partner motivated to provide pleasure
- An erotic context: candlelight, music, lingerie—whatever turns you on
- Vigorous, sustained penile stimulation by hand, mouth, sex toy, or some combination

Orgasm with a flaccid penis requires adjustments. But among couples who make the effort, after a year or so, most men call their lovemaking satisfying. If not, sex coaching or therapy usually helps.

Sex after Breast Cancer

Breast cancer can wreak havoc with women's sexuality. But by a year after treatment, coupled survivors in supportive relationships usually adjust and enjoy lovemaking as much as ever—sometimes more.

Most studies paint a depressing picture of breast cancer's sexual impact, including "long-term" sexual impairment. Actually, things aren't always that dire.

Any cancer may impair sexuality. But sex after breast cancer is particularly problematic because women's breasts are so intimately connected with sexual attractiveness and lovemaking.

Unfortunately, most studies have explored only the problems of sex after breast cancer, not their resolution. And most "long-term" studies report findings at only six to twelve months after treatment, not very long term. Fortunately, some research has focused on couples' return to lovemaking. Those studies show that in supportive relationships:

- Sexual frequency and satisfaction usually return to prediagnosis levels within a year.
- Men's sympathy for women's emotional distress plays a significant role in women's sexual recovery.
- Among women who opt for mastectomy, reconstruction hastens return to satisfying lovemaking.

University of Southern California researchers surveyed 863 survivors two years after treatment. All were sexually active at diagnosis and all had surgery, with some opting for radiation and/or chemotherapy. Compared with cancer-free controls, the participants' libidos, responsiveness, orgasms, and sexual satisfaction were pretty much the same.

However, survivors who had mastectomies without reconstruction often reported extended discomfort with:

- Showing lovers mastectomy scars
- Having lovers touch affected areas
- Having sex in the nude and in daylight

Women dissatisfied with their relationships were most likely to report lingering posttreatment sex problems. But two years after treatment, few women who rated their relationships supportive and satisfying complained of sexual dissatisfaction. In fact, women in the happiest relationships often said their sexual satisfaction had improved.

In a UCLA survey of 139 married breast cancer survivors twenty months after diagnosis, sexual satisfaction depended on couples' mutual emotional support. When the men listened to their mates and also discussed their own feelings, the women returned to prediagnosis sexual comfort. But when the men were distant and clammed up, the women typically reported continuing sexual dissatisfaction.

My wife is a long-term breast cancer survivor. Like other relationship shocks, coping depends on spousal willingness to face the situation, discuss it, and provide generous emotional support. In addition:

- Don't expect genital sex during treatment and for a few months afterward. But kissing, cuddling, and massage, particularly foot massage, help many women feel loved and cared for.
- Reassure them often that you still find them desirable.
- If they have mastectomies, they may feel more sexually restored with reconstructions. But some women don't want reconstruction. Support whatever the woman decides.
- When you return to lovemaking, use lubricant.
- Finally, cancer survival brings a deeper appreciation of life's fragility, which can make sex feel more precious than ever.

For individualized assistance, consider sex coaching or therapy.

Does Hysterectomy Affect Women's Sexuality?

Hysterectomy, the removal of the uterus, is America's leading gynecological surgery—six hundred thousand a year. One in four American women has one.

Possible reasons for hysterectomy include uterine fibroids, uterine prolapse, pelvic pain, and uterine cancer. Most are performed to treat fibroids—noncancerous growths in the uterine wall that cause heavy and/or prolonged menstrual periods and possibly severe abdominal, pelvic, and back pain. Most fibroids resolve by themselves at menopause, which makes fibroid-related hysterectomy controversial. Critics charge that many are unnecessary. Compared with the US, European women are much less likely to have hysterectomies.

Equally controversial is hysterectomy's impact on women's sexuality.

The conventional wisdom is that the procedure *improves* sex. Freed from fibroid symptoms, many women enjoy increased desire, pleasure, and satisfaction. But many women complain of posthysterectomy sex problems.

During hysterectomy, surgeons sever some pelvic nerves, so it's reasonable that the operation might impair sexual function. However, most studies support the conventional wisdom—either no sexual impact or enhancement:

- Dutch researchers surveyed 352 married women before and six months after hysterectomy. Overall, their sexual satisfaction improved. Before surgery, 68 percent were sexually active; afterward, 83 percent.
- University of California, San Francisco, researchers tracked sixty-three fibroid sufferers before and six months after surgery. Most reported increased desire and improved function.
- Northwestern University investigators surveyed seventy women before and six months after hysterectomy. Seventy percent said it either had no sexual impact or increased satisfaction.

However, all three studies also contained some bad news:

- In the Dutch trial, 40 percent reported sex problems: loss of lubrication, difficulty with arousal, and feeling less sensitive and responsive.
- In the San Francisco study, many women experienced sexual difficulties.
- And in the Northeastern study, if 70 percent experienced no sexual impact or improvement, then 30 percent suffered impairment.

Dutch researchers described how hysterectomy might interfere with women's sexuality:

- It reduces blood engorgement of the vaginal wall, possibly reducing sexual responsiveness and lubrication.
- It may shorten the vagina, possibly causing discomfort during intercourse.
- The uterus contracts during orgasm. Without one, orgasm loses its uterine component and possibly some intensity.

The Dutch group criticized studies of hysterectomy outcomes for bias toward good-news conclusions.

If you have problematic fibroids, treatments other than hysterectomy are possible, notably uterine artery embolization. Ask about it. If your gynecologist suggests hysterectomy, understand that it might cause sexual impairment. Consider living with your fibroids until menopause, when they'll probably go away.

For Better Sex, Stop Snoring

A Mayo Clinic study of 827 men shows that snorers reported two contradictory findings—no loss of libido or sexual function, but significantly reduced sexual satisfaction. Huh? Turns out that men's snoring irritated the *women* in their beds, disturbing *their* sleep and reducing their sexual energy to the point that men's satisfaction suffered.

Anyone can "sleep out loud" but men do it considerably more than women. Bedmates typically respond with nudges that coax the offender from a supine position, which promotes snoring, to side sleeping, which doesn't.

To stop snoring:

- **Lose weight.** Snoring may be caused by excess throat tissue. Breathing makes it vibrate audibly. With less throat tissue, you're less likely to snore. However, plenty of thin people snore as well.
- **Use earplugs.** If your partner snores, consider earplugs. Cheap ones are available at pharmacies. Custom plugs cost more but work better. Ask your physician.
- **Needle and thread.** Sew a golf or tennis ball into a closed pocket on the back of the snorer's pajamas. This prevents supine sleeping.
- **Treat allergies.** Hay fever makes throat tissue swell and vibrate.
- **Stop alcohol within four hours of retiring.** Alcohol relaxes throat tissue and promotes snoring.
- **Avoid sedatives.** Sedatives are similar to alcohol.
- **Don't smoke.** Smokers develop chronically swollen throat tissue, which increases snoring.
- **Raise your head.** Adding a pillow may help. Or, if you can tolerate a slightly tilted bed, place small blocks under the head of your bed.
- **Consider minor surgery.** Some otolaryngologists claim good results implanting small flexible bands in the throat like the stays sewn into shirt collars. Cost: Around $4,000, usually out of pocket.
- **Sleep separately.** If one of you sleeps somewhere else, activities when you share the bed are likely to benefit.

Sex and Disability

In the 1978 film *Coming Home*, a paraplegic Vietnam veteran (John Voight) is a bitter wreck—until a chance reunion with an old high school acquaintance (Jane Fonda) becomes romantic. They discover how to enjoy lovemaking. In one scene, Fonda goes down on Voight and asks, "Can you feel this?" He replies, "I can see it and I love what I see."

According to census data, 19 percent of Americans—fifty million people—suffer disabilities. The many challenges they face include toxic myths about their sexuality:

MYTH: Disabled people are not sexual.
TRUTH: Everyone has handicaps. Some are just move visible and limiting than others. Except

for the asexual 1 percent, everyone is sexual and enjoys erotic pleasure. Even severe handicaps don't negate sexuality. Disabled people often face serious obstacles *expressing* their sexuality. But they're as sexual as everyone else.

MYTH: Disabled people are not desirable.
TRUTH: Everyone is attractive to someone.

MYTH: Disabled people have so many problems, they don't have the time or energy for sex.
TRUTH: Sex is not a luxury some can't afford. It's one of life's greatest pleasures. Disabilities don't change that.

MYTH: Disabled people can't have "real" sex.
TRUTH: Some disabilities make vaginal intercourse difficult or impossible. But there are other satisfying ways to make love. Even those who have no genital sensation can enjoy erotic pleasure from nongenital touch and, with sufficient stimulation of unfeeling genitals, even orgasms. When there's a will, there's always a way.

MYTH: Sex is private and disabilities preclude privacy.
TRUTH: People with severe disabilities may need round-the-clock attendants and may not have the privacy able-bodied folks take for granted. But that doesn't cancel their sexuality. Attendants or lovers can position the disabled to masturbate or for partner sex.

MYTH: Disabled sex can't be sizzling sex.
TRUTH: Actually, after a few years, some people who suffer disabling injuries report *improved* sex. Compared with able-bodied sex, disabled lovemaking requires much more discussion of what feels good and coaching to accomplish it. That deepens intimacy and enhances sex.

Of course, disabled sex is no bed of roses. Many disabled people feel undesirable. Disabilities complicate finding partners. Mobility limitations may interfere with solo sex and partner love-making. Many disabilities cause chronic pain and/or fatigue and interfere with sexual energy and responsiveness. Many disabled people take medications, notably antidepressants, which may cause sex-impairing side effects. Some disabilities, for example, spinal cord injuries, inter-fere with genital sensation and orgasm. And disabled people who require attendants may have difficulty negotiating the assistance they need to masturbate and enjoy partner sex. But with sufficient stimulation, many men with spinal injuries can raise erections and around half of all people with spinal injuries can have orgasms.

Some suggestions for those with disabilities:

- You can be as sexual as you have the energy to be.
- Focus on your *abilities*, the pleasure you can enjoy and provide.
- If chronic fatigue is an issue, schedule sex when you have the most energy.
- To whatever extent possible, enjoy masturbation. Solo sex does not require much mobil-ity or genital sensitivity. Self-sexing is not second-best sex. It's the foundation of sexuality. When you have physical challenges, it becomes even more central to erotic satisfaction.

For many people with disabilities, shower massagers can be great boons to masturbation. Water can be directed at nipples, genitals, or other spots you enjoy. For those who need attendants, shower massagers may also allow privacy. Attendants can set up in the tub and direct the spray, then leave.

- Solo sex can be enjoyed with others. Partners can masturbate in each other's presence or by phone.
- Orgasm is not necessary for erotic enjoyment. If it happens, great. But try not to view sex without orgasm as a "failure." The goal of sex is not orgasm, but pleasure—and any sustained, gentle touch can provide it.

For more, I recommend *The Ultimate Guide to Sex and Disability* by Miriam Kaufman, MD, Cory Silverberg, and Fran Odette.

Surrogate Partners for People with Disabilities

In conjunction with sex therapists, surrogate partners can bring joy to those with disabilities. For more, see the film *The Sessions* with Helen Hunt and John Hawkes. He's quadriplegic. She's his surrogate partner. And with her help, he enjoys sex. Visit the International Professional Surrogates Association (IPSA, surrogatetherapy.org).

CHAPTER 27:
Sex and Drugs: Many Spoil Lovemaking, Some Enhance It

THREE DRUGS ARE notorious for causing sex problems: alcohol, tobacco, and antidepressants. But they're just the tip of the iceberg. Many widely used drugs might impair libido or sexual function, and few doctors or pharmacists mention it.

The key word is "might." The drugs discussed here *might* have sexual side effects, but users are not fated to experience them. Drugs' sexual effects are often idiosyncratic. Some people notice no problems while others can't function.

Beyond individual differences, drugs' sexual effects are dose related. As the dose increases, so does risk of impairment.

When people develop sex problems—especially older adults—few suspect drug side effects. Actually, sexual side effects are common and many medications may cause them.

If you suspect drug-related sexual impairment, consult your physician and/or pharmacist. Perhaps a less problematic drug can be substituted.

Alcohol
Alcohol is the world's leading cause of drug-related sexual impairment. From Shakespeare's *Macbeth*, alcohol "provokes the desire, but takes away the performance." How true. The first drink is disinhibiting. Prospective lovers are easier to coax into bed. But if people of average weight drink more than two beers, cocktails, or glasses of wine in an hour or so, alcohol becomes a central nervous system depressant that interferes with erection in men and sexual responsiveness in women.

Meanwhile, many people lose their virginity drunk, then continue to rock 'n' roll intoxicated through young adulthood into maturity. Alcohol is also a key risk factor for sexual assault. Drunk sex is often lousy sex, and that's the only kind many people have ever known. Try making love sober or after just one drink. You may be pleasantly surprised.

Tobacco
Kissing a smoker is like licking an ashtray. Smoking makes lovers taste unpleasant. It also fouls the flavor of semen.

Smoking narrows the blood vessels, including the arteries that carry blood into the genitals. Male smokers face a substantial risk of erectile dysfunction (ED). In women, smoking reduces clitoral sensitivity and limits blood flow into the vaginal wall, decreasing natural lubrication.

But when smokers quit, arterial damage subsides and after a few years, most ex-smokers recover from tobacco-related sex problems.

Over-the-Counter Drugs

A few common OTCs have been linked to sex problems:

- Aleve (naproxen, pain reliever): Erection problems, reduced vaginal lubrication, orgasm delayed
- Antihistamines (hay fever, hives): Erection impairment, reduced vaginal lubrication
- Tagamet (cimetidine, heartburn): Libido loss, erection loss, decreased vaginal lubrication
- Zantac (ranitidine, heartburn): Libido loss, erection problems, reduced vaginal lubrication

Cannabis/Marijuana

Most drugs' sexual effects are reasonably predictable, but cannabis is an exception. Some lovers say it ruins sex by pulling them deep inside themselves, isolating them from partners. Others swear it increases intimacy, boosts desire, heightens erotic sensuality, and enhances satisfaction.

A 1975 study showed that cannabis reduces testosterone sufficiently to impair libido. Damning headlines ensued. Many subsequent trials debunked it, showing no cannabis-related testosterone suppression and no loss of libido or sexual function even among frequent, heavy users. Nonetheless, some discussions still cite that lone discredited study as proof that cannabis is a sex killer. Meanwhile, recent studies have shown that weed is more likely to enhance lovemaking than destroy it:

- Kansas City researchers interviewed ninety-seven stoner adults. Two-thirds said cannabis increased emotional closeness and sexual pleasure and satisfaction. But one-third said it had no sexual impact or reduced pleasure.
- St. Louis University investigators surveyed 289 women before routine gynecologic exams. One-third (ninety-six) had used marijuana prior to lovemaking. Of that group, 65 percent called it sex enhancing, 11 percent said it reduced their pleasure, and 24 percent said it had no sexual impact.
- Finally, Stanford researchers tracked 51,119 adult marijuana users for fourteen years (28,176 women, 22,943 men, average initial age of thirty). Some reported enhancement, others impairment, but overall, cannabis was mildly libido-boosting—one extra roll in the hay per month.

When I've blogged about sex and cannabis, most comments have called it enhancing. Some have said it's a turnoff. And some have said its effects depend on the dose, the strain, or their mood.

If you wonder how marijuana affects you sexually, try some and see.

Blood Pressure Medications (Antihypertensives)

A generation ago, many blood pressure medications caused substantial risk of sexual side effects. Today, that's no longer the case. Nowadays typical first-line treatments include angiotensin converting enzyme (ACE) inhibitors or angiotensin II receptor blocker (ARB) drugs, neither of which carry much risk of sexual side effects.

The only sexually problematic blood pressure drug still widely prescribed is hydrochlorothiazide (Esidrix, Hydrodiuril, Oretic). It may cause erection problems and loss of vaginal lubrication.

If you develop sex problems soon after starting a blood pressure medication, suspect a drug side effect. Ask your doctor and see if you can switch to something else.

Antidepressants

The most popular antidepressants are the selective serotonin reuptake inhibitors (SSRIs): Celexa, Cipralex, Lexapro, Lustral, Luvox, Paxil, Prozac, Seroxat, Trintellix, Viibryd, and Zoloft. SSRIs often cause sexual side effects:

- Celexa: Libido loss, erection loss, less vaginal lubrication, delayed or no orgasm
- Cipralex: Libido loss, erection impairment, delayed or no orgasm
- Lexapro: Libido loss, erection problems, reduced vaginal lubrication, delayed or no orgasm
- Lustral: Libido loss, erection problems, decreased vaginal lubrication, delayed or no orgasm
- Luvox: Libido loss, erection impairment, decreased vaginal lubrication, delayed or no orgasm
- Paxil: Libido loss, erection loss, less vaginal lubrication, delayed or no orgasm
- Prozac: Libido loss, erection problems, reduced vaginal lubrication, delayed or no orgasm
- Trintellix: Libido loss, erection difficulties
- Viibryd: Libido loss, erection loss, ejaculation problems
- Zoloft: Libido loss, erection problems, decreased vaginal lubrication, delayed or no orgasm

Other antidepressants may also cause sexual impairment:

- Effexor: Erection impairment, less vaginal lubrication, delayed or no orgasm
- Tofranil: Erection problems, reduced vaginal lubrication, delayed or no orgasm
- Trazodone: Priapism, delayed or no orgasm

If you experience sexual side effects from these or other antidepressants, ask your doctor if you can switch to Wellbutrin or Remeron. Occasionally, they cause sexual side effects—libido loss, erection problems—but compared with the medications above, they're much less problematic.

In addition, the medicinal herb ginkgo may mitigate antidepressant-induced sexual impairment (page 267).

Tranquilizers, Antianxiety, and Psychiatric Drugs

Like alcohol, when drugs alter mood, they often impair sexuality:

- Anafranil: Libido loss, erection problems, decreased vaginal lubrication, delayed or no orgasm
- Eskalith: Erection impairment, less vaginal lubrication
- Lithonate: Erection loss, reduced vaginal lubrication
- Mellaril: Erection problems, decreased vaginal lubrication, delayed or no orgasm
- Prolixin: Libido loss, erection problems, decreased vaginal lubrication
- Trilafon: Delayed or no orgasm
- Xanax: Libido loss, delayed or no orgasm

Seizure Medications

The most likely to cause sex problems include:

- Diamox: Libido loss, erection problems, less vaginal lubrication
- Dilantin: Libido loss, erection problems, less vaginal lubrication
- Mysoline: Libido loss, erection loss, decreased vaginal lubrication
- Primidone: Libido loss, erection problems, less vaginal lubrication
- Phenobarbitol: Libido loss, erection problems, reduced vaginal lubrication
- Tegretol: Libido loss, erection impairment, reduced vaginal lubrication

Other Prescription Drugs

Dozens of other medications may also cause sexual impairment:

- Atromid (lowers cholesterol): Libido loss, erection problems, decreased vaginal lubrication
- Danocrine (endometriosis): Usually, libido loss, but some reports of libido increase
- Digoxin (Digitek, Lanoxin, congestive heart failure): Libido loss, erection loss, reduced vaginal lubrication, breast enlargement in men
- Dutasteride (prostate enlargement): Ejaculation problems
- Estrogen (hormone replacement therapy): Libido loss, breast tenderness
- Finasteride (prostate enlargement and male pattern baldness): Erection loss, ejaculation difficulties
- Ketoconazole (antifungal): Libido loss, erection problems, reduced vaginal lubrication
- Methadone (narcotic addiction): Libido loss, erection loss, less vaginal lubrication, delayed or no orgasm
- Mintezol (antiparasitic): Erection problems, reduced vaginal lubrication
- Niacin (high dose for lower cholesterol): Libido loss, erection impairment, decreased vaginal lubrication
- Nizoral (antifungal): Libido loss, erection loss, less vaginal lubrication
- Valium (antianxiety, muscle relaxant, anticonvulsant): Libido loss, delayed or no orgasm

Narcotics, Cocaine, Amphetamines

There's a good reason why narcotics are called downers. That's what happens to users' sexual desire and function. But uppers are no better. Cocaine and amphetamines (including meth-amphetamine, meth) stimulate sexual desire, but often eliminate orgasm. With regular use, desire also fades.

Testosterone Replacement: New Male Vigor? Or Overprescribed Hazard?

Advocates of testosterone replacement call the hormone a fountain of youth. They claim it restores older men's flagging libidos and erections, returning them to lean, muscled, youthful vigor. But in 2014, an expert panel of the Food and Drug Administration (FDA) overwhelmingly urged the agency—by a vote of nineteen to one—to impose strict limits on prescribing it. Their arguments:

- No evidence suggests any recent spike in testosterone deficiency (low T). But since 2000, the number of men taking the hormone has quadrupled to more than two million.

- In men who are truly deficient, supplemental testosterone restores libido and erection function. But in men who are within the normal range, extra testosterone has little impact on libido and less on erection.
- Audits show that many physicians have written prescriptions without blood tests sufficient to establish low T diagnosis.
- Consequently, many men taking testosterone don't need it, subjecting them to potentially serious health risks.
- Low T may develop at any age but is most likely in men over sixty-five. Currently, younger men account for 60 percent of prescriptions.
- The debate over testosterone replacement bears eerie similarity to the controversy decades ago surrounding estrogen hormone replacement therapy (HRT) in older women—also initially proclaimed to restore youthfulness, then later shown to increase risk of heart disease and breast cancer.

Testosterone is produced in the testicles. For decades, scientists have known that unusually low blood levels cause fatigue, depression, libido loss, ED, weight gain, and muscle atrophy. Supplementation provides quick relief.

But supplemental testosterone also thickens the blood, a risk factor for heart disease and most strokes. It also accelerates atherosclerosis, the arterial narrowing that causes those two problems. Finally, the hormone may spur the growth of prostate cancer—as common and deadly in men as breast cancer in women. During the late twentieth century, concerns about the hormone's potentially serious downsides limited prescriptions.

But after 2000, a few researchers argued that testosterone does not increase risk of prostate cancer or cardiovascular disease, at least in short-term studies. Increasing numbers of physicians have been prescribing it to more middle-aged men complaining of fatigue, libido decline, and erection problems.

Many of those prescriptions appear unnecessary and ill advised. The Endocrine Society recommends testosterone supplementation *only* for men with unequivocally low T, a finding that requires several blood tests because testosterone fluctuates throughout the day. Men who appear low in one test often look normal in others.

Meanwhile, researchers at the University of Texas (UT) Medical Branch in Galveston have found that 25 percent of the men taking testosterone had just one blood test prior to receiving prescriptions, suggesting that many doctors have prescribed it irresponsibly.

Even if multiple blood tests show clear deficiency, the Endocrine Society recommends against supplementation unless men report libido collapse. No credible evidence indicates a recent plague of low T, but the quadrupling of prescriptions since 2000 suggests the hormone is overprescribed.

Finally, low T is a late-life condition, but the UT study shows the fastest growing group taking supplements are men in their forties, another indication of overprescribing—hence the FDA panel's near-unanimous recommendation that the agency reduce prescribing.

Traditional Aphrodisiacs: Some Stimulate More than Just the Imagination

What do these have in common: ginseng, chocolate, oysters, coffee, powdered rhinoceros tusk, a pulverized Mediterranean beetle, and the bark of a West African tree? They're just some of the many items people have ingested through the ages to enhance lovemaking. For almost as long, scientists have dismissed traditional aphrodisiacs as worthless—and sometimes dangerous.

But old beliefs die hard when they promise sizzling sex. The rhinoceros has been hunted almost to extinction partly because of the mistaken belief that its powdered horn boosts virility. And the reputed libido booster Spanish fly, made from Mediterranean *Cantharis* beetles, can be poisonous.

Most scientists say that nothing ingested can boost libido and sexual performance beyond a placebo effect. Nonetheless, belief in aphrodisiacs runs deep. It's embedded in the very term we use to describe sexual attraction. Why do people fall in love? *Chemistry.*

Science has not identified anything guaranteed to charm reluctant love interests into disrobing. But a surprising number of herbs, drugs, and foods have physiological effects that just might make reluctant paramours more receptive to erotic invitations.

Note: All the herbs discussed below are considered safe in recommended amounts, but side effects are possible. Follow package directions. If problems develop, reduce your dose or stop.

Coffee, maté, guarana. These plants all contain the powerful stimulant caffeine. Throughout history, all stimulants have been considered lust boosters. There may be something to this. University of Michigan researchers surveyed 744 married couples, age sixty or older, and discovered that women who were daily coffee drinkers were more likely to call themselves sexually active—62 percent versus just 38 percent of the women who abstained.

Most coffee drinkers consume one to two cups a day and become tolerant to that intake. For an aphrodisiac buzz, a higher dose is necessary. But that may cause jitters, irritability, and insomnia.

Cocoa, chocolate. Cocoa and its derivative, chocolate, contain caffeine, but less than coffee. Both stimulate release of endorphins, the body's own mood-elevating compounds. Endorphin-related mood enhancement might pique libido.

Cocoa and chocolate also contain phenylethylamine (PEA), a natural antidepressant amphetamine. Sexual attraction boosts PEA blood levels, but after heartbreak, PEA plummets. Cocoa and chocolate contain high levels of PEA. The broken-hearted sometimes binge on chocolate—perhaps to raise their PEA.

Damiana. The ancient Mayans used this herb as a sex enhancer. Botanists dubbed it *Damiana aphrodisiaca*. With a name like that, you'd think scientists would have flocked to research it, but oddly, only a few studies have. Italian and Mexican research has shown that damiana increases copulation by male rats. Damiana is also an ingredient of the sex supplement ArginMax. In two University of Hawaii studies, ArginMax enhanced women's libidos, reduced vaginal dryness, improved clitoral sensitivity, and boosted sexual satisfaction.

Ginkgo. Ginkgo has no historical reputation as an aphrodisiac, but since the 1980s, many studies have shown that it improves blood flow through the brain, slowing progression of Alzheimer's disease. Ginkgo also boosts blood flow through the genitals.

At the University of California, San Francisco, researchers gave ginkgo (240 mg/day) to sixty-three men and women suffering sexual side effects from antidepressants (page 267). The herb provided relief in 76 percent of the men, and 91 percent of the women.

Unfortunately, this study had no placebo group. Placebos usually benefit around one-third of users. The response rate in this study was two to three times higher, which suggests real benefit.

If Anything Hurts, Pain Relievers Help

Pain can destroy erotic focus. Many people of all ages have chronic aches and pains that interfere with lovemaking. Check with your doctor if, an hour before sex, you might take pain medication: aspirin, ibuprofen (Advil, Motrin), acetaminophen (Tylenol), or naproxen (Aleve). High-CBD cannabis, a natural pain reliever, may also help.

Ginseng. This root, revered in Asia, subtly enhances vitality. It's only a short step from this to sex enhancement. In addition, ginseng increases synthesis of nitric oxide, a compound essential to sexual function.

Korean researchers gave forty-five ED sufferers either a placebo or ginseng (900 mg three times/day). After eight weeks, the ginseng group experienced significant improvement. Another Korean study corroborated these findings. But the effective dose (2,700 mg/day) is expensive and may cause jitters and irritability.

Maca. When Spanish conquistadors reached the high Andes, their livestock had difficulty breeding. The Incas showed them a cure, this Andean ground cover. Eventually, maca's folk reputation grew from fertility drug to sex enhancer.

Chinese researchers treated male rats with either a placebo or the herb for twenty-two days, then paired them with sexually receptive females. Compared with females mated with control rats, those paired with maca-treated males were more than twice as likely to show sperm in their vaginas, demonstrating that the herb stimulated copulation.

Maca might also boost horizontal romps in humans. Peruvian researchers gave men a daily placebo or maca (1,500 or 3,000 mg). After eight weeks, both herb groups reported increased sexual desire. Peruvian doctors also recommend it to men with ED.

Muira puama. Locals call this Amazonian shrub "potency wood." French researchers surveyed the sexuality of 202 healthy women troubled by low libido, then gave them a combination of muira puama and ginkgo. Two-thirds reported increased libido, more intercourse, and more and better orgasms. A UCLA study showed that Revactin, an herbal blend containing muira puama, improved erection function in half of men who took 500 mg/day.

Yohimbine. For centuries, the bark of the West African yohimbe tree was reputed to restore faltering erections. Scientists laughed—until the 1980s, when several studies showed that a compound in the bark, yohimbine, increases blood flow into the penis. Years before Viagra, the FDA approved yohimbine as a prescription treatment for ED. Brand names include yohimbine, Testomar, Aphrodyne, and Yocon.

Yohimbine may also boost women's sexual arousal. University of Texas researchers gave twenty-five arousal-challenged women either a placebo or a combination of yohimbine and the amino acid L-arginine, which the body converts into sex-supporting nitric oxide. The women then viewed erotic videos. Compared with the placebo group, the women who took the herb reported greater arousal.

Yohimbine drugs are prescription medications, but many preparations are available over the counter. Unfortunately, according to an FDA analysis, many OTC products contain only traces of yohimbine, nowhere near enough to have sexual impact. If you're interested in yohimbine, ask your doctor for a prescription.

Zestra. A topical fluid applied to the clitoris and vulva, Zestra is an OTC blend of herbal oils (borage seed, coleus, evening primrose, and angelica root), plus vitamins C and E. In traditional herbal medicine, all these plants' oils have prosexual reputations. In addition, Zestra is a lubricant, and lube enhances lovemaking. Two studies by University of Minnesota researchers suggest it's sex enhancing. In one, twenty women used Zestra—ten sexually functional and ten with sex problems. Both groups reported improved lovemaking. In the other, 256 women with sex problems, age twenty-one to sixty-five, used a placebo or Zestra. After four months, the Zestra group reported significantly enhanced desire, arousal, and satisfaction. However, in both studies, some women reported burning. Zestra is available at some pharmacies and on the internet.

Tribulus terrestris: A Sex Booster for Both Women and Men

Tribulus terrestris, commonly called puncture vine, is becoming better known as evidence mounts that a leaf extract helps treat sex problems. Not all studies show benefit and scientists still aren't sure how it works, but *Tribulus* is safe in recommended amounts and the weight of current evidence suggests the plant is a sex booster.

Native to Asia, *Tribulus* grows in temperate locales worldwide. Its seed shells bristle with sharp thorns, hence puncture vine. Indian and Chinese herbalists have long considered it an aphrodisiac. Western scientists scoffed—until they tested it.

Several studies show that *Tribulus* extract (7.5–750 mg/day for one to four months) enhances women's sexual function:

- Brazilian researchers gave a placebo or *Tribulus* (750 mg/day) to thirty-six postmenopausal women complaining of low libido. After four months, the placebo group reported modest improvement, but those taking *Tribulus* reported greatly increased desire, arousal, and lubrication, and more and better orgasm.
- Another Brazilian team gave a placebo or *Tribulus* (750 mg/day) to sixty postmenopausal women with sexual complaints. After four months, the herb group reported significantly greater desire, arousal, and lubrication, more comfortable intercourse, and more orgasms.
- A third Brazilian group gave the herb (250 mg three times a day) to 120 women with low libido. One hundred six (88 percent) reported significant improvement.
- Iranian scientists gave sixty low-libido women a placebo or *Tribulus* (7.5 mg/day). A month later, the women reported significantly enhanced desire, lubrication, and satisfaction.

Tribulus also shows promise for men. In a three-month trial, Bulgarian researchers gave a placebo or the herb (750 mg/day) to 180 men with mild to moderate ED, some of whom also complained of low desire. The herb group reported significantly more desire, better erections, and improved sexual satisfaction.

In addition, several studies show that *Tribulus* (750–1,500 mg/day) improves sperm motility and quality. It might help treat infertility.

Tribulus raises levels of the male sex hormones that govern libido in all genders. It also increases synthesis of sex-boosting nitric oxide. *Tribulus* is safe in recommended amounts, but some study participants have dropped out because of side effects, typically stomach upset. If you try it, take 750 mg in divided doses (250 mg three times a day) after eating. If you experience intestinal upset, reduce your dose or stop.

Tribulus is an ingredient in many "sexual health" supplement blends, but usually at doses much lower than those in the studies just discussed. If you're interested in this herb, steer clear of combination products and go with 100 percent *Tribulus*. It's available at health food stores and herb shops, and on the internet.

CHAPTER 28:
How Men Can Support Women through Menopause

MANY MEN THINK menopause is a brief interlude around women's fiftieth birthdays. Actually, it's a long, slow process that often lasts a decade.

Menopause marks the end of women's fertility. Synthesis of the female sex hormone estrogen gradually declines and ovulation (egg release) and menstrual periods become less regular and eventually cease.

As recently as 1900, women's life expectancy was forty-eight years, so only a minority experienced extended postmenopausal living. Today, it's about eighty, so most women live several decades beyond menopause.

As life after menopause became the norm, physicians mistakenly decided it was an illness requiring drug treatment. But women's health activists advised celebrating the Change as a normal transition that opens doors to new productivity, wisdom, and fulfillment. In recent years, drug treatment of menopausal discomforts has waned.

For women and the men who love them, the passage through menopause may be easy or challenging. Gentlemen, if you familiarize yourself with the transition and help your partner through it, her process should be easier for both of you—with your sex life less disrupted and possibly even enhanced.

A Long, Slow Process

Most menopausal discomforts occur from forty-five to fifty-five, but they may begin as early as women's late thirties and may last into their sixties.

Around forty, estrogen typically begins to decline, and women develop menstrual irregularity—skipped periods or unusually heavy, frequent, or extended flow with possible spotting between periods. During their early forties, many women notice the beginnings of the three hallmark menopausal complaints: hot flashes, vaginal dryness, and mood changes. After fifty, women may also develop vaginal atrophy, tissue thinning that might make intercourse uncomfortable or impossible.

However, every woman is unique and experiences menopause individually. Around 20 percent hardly notice it. About half experience mild discomforts. And around 30 percent suffer considerable distress from:

- **Hot flashes.** These sudden feelings of heat occur without warning and last thirty seconds to several minutes. Hot flashes typically affect the face, neck, and chest, and cause sweating. They can strike any time, day or night. At night, women may kick off blankets and lose sleep.

- **Vaginal dryness.** With age, genital blood flow declines. In men, this causes erectile dysfunction (ED); in women, decreased vaginal lubrication.
- **Emotional upsets.** The myth is that menopause makes women irritable. Actually, emotional reactions vary tremendously. Some women experience few if any mood changes. Others become grouchy, anxious, and/or depressed. Any woman may experience menopausal emotional challenges, but those with histories of premenstrual syndrome and/or postpartum depression are at greatest risk.

Some women experience chemical or surgical menopause, sudden cessation of estrogen synthesis due to cancer chemotherapy or surgical removal of the ovaries (oophorectomy) during hysterectomy or ovarian cancer treatment. Sudden menopause often causes more severe discomforts.

- **Vaginal atrophy.** The mucous membrane that lines the vagina thins, which may aggravate irritation from vaginal dryness.
- **Pain during intercourse.** Dryness and atrophy may cause pain with vaginal fingering, toy insertions, and intercourse.
- **Reduced libido.** In many women, menopausal discomforts reduce sexual desire. This is most likely from age forty-five to fifty-five. But as women adjust to postmenopausal living, many experience some libido rebound.
- **Sleep problems.** Trouble falling or staying asleep.
- **Difficulty concentrating.** Many women complain of "brain fog," problems with memory, focus, and attention.

How Men Can Help

Menopause varies so greatly that men have only one way to discover how it affects the women they love. Ask and keep asking. Show you care. Discussions of her passage deepen intimacy at a time when many women feel emotionally fragile and need reassurance that you still love and desire them.

Take initiative. Don't wait for her to announce hot flashes. If she's over forty, raise the issue. As menopause unfolds, ask for updates about her feelings and reactions. Menopause marks a significant transition, which may change your relationship. Be there for her. Ask how she's faring. Listen, then continue to ask and listen.

Gently correct misconceptions. Men aren't the only ones in the dark about menopause. Some women are also poorly informed. Just because women's friends had rough passages doesn't mean they will.

Minimizing Hot Flashes

Some doctors prescribe estrogen for hot flashes. It works, but it's also problematic (below). Fortunately, there are other safe, effective treatments.

Soy foods. Compared with most Americans, Chinese and Japanese women experience fewer, milder hot flashes. The reason? Their diets are rich in soy foods, notably tofu. Soy foods—but not soy sauce—contain plant estrogens (phytoestrogens), chemically weaker versions of the hormone that reduces hot flashes. A few studies show soy foods useless for hot flashes, but most trials support soy's effectiveness:

- Harvard researchers analyzed ten large, rigorous trials of soy foods for hot flashes. Seven showed significant benefit.
- Japanese researchers analyzed thirteen rigorous trials. Women who consumed the equivalent of one serving of tofu three times a week for at least six weeks reported significant relief.

Men can encourage women to eat more soy foods—and join them. Tofu is almost tasteless but acquires the flavor of anything cooked with it. Add it to soups, pasta sauces, casseroles—almost anything. In addition, many meat substitutes are made from "textured vegetable protein," another name for soy.

More fruits and vegetables, less meat and junk food. Soy is particularly rich in phytoestrogens, but all plant foods contain them. Many studies have shown that compared with omnivores, near-vegetarian women usually have fewer menopausal complaints, with committed vegetarians, especially vegans, reporting even fewer.

- Australian researchers followed 6,040 midlife women for nine years. As their fruit and vegetable consumption increased, they suffered fewer, milder hot flashes. Meanwhile, those consuming the most meat and sugar reported the most frequent and severe problems.
- Researchers with the Kaiser-Permanente health plan in Oakland, California, surveyed 17,473 menopausal women. As their fruit and vegetable consumption increased, they suffered fewer, milder hot flashes.

Men can encourage women to eat more fruits and vegetables—and join them. Have fruit with breakfast. Keep a fruit bowl for snacking. Add fruits and vegetables to meat dishes. Eat more salads and vegetable soups. Go meatless at least one day a week.

Take vitamin E. Many studies show that vitamin E (800 IU/day) minimizes hot flashes. German investigators analyzed twenty-two reports. Their conclusion: it helps.

Vitamin E also reduces risk of heart disease, the leading killer of postmenopausal women. Men can purchase the vitamin and encourage women to take it.

Relax deeply. Emotional stress aggravates hot flashes. Deep relaxation minimizes them:

- Harvard researchers surveyed hot flashes in thirty-three women, then divided them into three groups. One maintained routines. The second read a novel. The third listened to deep relaxation audio daily. After seven weeks, only the women in the audio group reported hot flash reductions.
- University of Washington investigators gave 427 menopausal women a placebo pill, or told them to continue their daily routines, or enrolled them in a relaxing yoga class. After three months, the yoga group reported fewer, milder hot flashes.

Men can buy "visualization" or "guided imagery" audio and encourage women to meditate or do yoga—and join them.

Exercise. The more women sweat, the fewer hot flashes they're likely to experience.

- South Korean researchers asked 631 menopausal women how much they exercised. As it increased, their hot flashes decreased.
- Finnish researchers surveyed 159 largely sedentary menopausal women, then encouraged them to work up to walking a mile a day. After six months, they reported significantly less discomfort from hot flashes. Four years later, daily walking maintained the benefit.
- University of Washington researchers surveyed a dozen menopausal women, then enrolled them in a weekly hour-long yoga class with fifteen minutes of daily yoga at home. After ten weeks, they reported significantly fewer, milder hot flashes.

Men can encourage women to exercise. Better yet, exercise with them: take walks together. Go for bike rides. Garden. Swim. Take yoga or dance classes. Join a gym. Exercise also helps prevent osteoporosis and heart disease, both major health issues for older women.

Try herbal medicine. A Native American herb, black cohosh (*Cimicifuga racemosa*), contains phytoestrogens. Like soy, it minimizes hot flashes. A commercial extract, Remifemin, is available at most health food stores. Men might buy it.

Coping with Vaginal Dryness

Phytoestrogens—soy, other plant foods, and black cohosh—help replace lost estrogen and preserve natural vaginal lubrication. In addition, if you don't already use a sexual lubricant, try one. Lubes usually eliminate discomfort from dryness. For some, saliva is sufficient. But many menopausal women prefer commercial lubricants. The latter are available at pharmacies near the condoms.

Beyond lubricants, doctors can prescribe topical estrogen creams, which don't cause the problems linked to hormone replacement therapy (below).

Goodbye Contraception

With menopause, birth control becomes unnecessary. But don't rush it. Women who still have periods, however infrequently, are still ovulating, might get pregnant, and need contraception. Continue to use it until women haven't had periods for several months. When in doubt about terminating contraception, consult a physician.

The Hormone Replacement Controversy

Starting in the 1970s, doctors urged menopausal women to replace lost estrogen with supplements (hormone replacement therapy, HRT). Initially, it looked miraculous. HRT minimized hot flashes and dryness, and reduced risk of diabetes, osteoporosis, heart disease, stroke, dementia, and several cancers. Doctors pushed HRT and millions of older women took it.

But questions remained. To resolve them, in 1991 the National Institutes of Health launched the Women's Health Initiative, which tracked 160,000 women age fifty to seventy for fifteen years. In 2014, the results showed that HRT did, indeed, reduce hot flashes and risk of osteoporosis and colorectal and uterine (endometrial) cancers.

But contrary to the hype, HRT *increased* risk of heart disease, stroke, breast cancer, and dementia. Heart disease is the leading killer of older women and most women fear breast cancer and dementia. Some doctors still recommend HRT for those at high risk of osteoporosis who have low risk of heart disease, breast cancer, and dementia. But most women stopped HRT.

Women should ask their physicians about their personal risk profiles and the wisdom of HRT. Men can help by becoming informed and accompanying women to doctor visits to discuss it.

Soy foods and other phytoestrogens do not cause the problems associated with HRT.

CHAPTER 29:
No One Is Ever Too Old
for Sizzling Sex

FOR THE FIRST fifty years of modern sex research (1948–98), investigators largely ignored older adults. As recently as 1994, when University of Chicago researchers produced one of the largest and most cited studies of American sexuality, they interviewed no one over fifty-nine—implying that sex ends at sixty.

Then, four years later in 1998, Viagra took the world by storm. Since then, despite lingering beliefs that people age out of sex, a tremendous amount of research has shown that no one ever becomes too old to enjoy erotic touch, pleasure, and orgasm.

Crones, Hags, Dirty Old Men?

The biblical prescription, sex only for procreation, continues to haunt us. Around age fifty, menopause marks the end of women's fertility, making them too old for procreation and, biblically speaking, "too old" for sex. Historically, older women became "crones," stock characters in folk tales. Some were benevolent, such as the fairy godmother who aids Cinderella. But most crones, from the Old Anglo-French for *carrion*, were sinister: the evil queen in Snow White, and the hag who abuses Hansel and Gretel—"hag," from the Old English for *witch*.

Elderly men have fared no better. A few escaped desexualization, for example, Moses, who Deuteronomy says retained his "vigor" at 120. But sometime after fifty, most men lose the ability to raise erections sufficient for intercourse. They, too, were traditionally considered too old for sex. Older gents who remained sexual in defiance of the supposed age limit were dismissed as "dirty old men." And older couples who remained lovingly sexual in the face of sex-negative stereotypes were considered sweet but odd rarities.

Erotic Pleasure: No Expiration Date

The success of Viagra, Cialis, and Levitra, the latter two approved in 2003, show that people never grow too old for sex. But traditional beliefs persist. In 2010, a dozen years after Viagra's approval, the cultural bias against late-life sex prompted *Bloomberg News* to run this headline: "Sex After 70? Not Much." The article began: "According to a new report in the *British Medical Journal*, the average person's sex life ends by seventy. . . ." That assertion represented a complete misreading of the study, which actually concluded that, if older adults have lovers and remain in reasonably good health, most retain interest in partner lovemaking and pursue and enjoy it.

Meanwhile, sexologists blasted the previously mentioned Chicago study's implication that sex ends by sixty. In 2007, the Chicago investigators returned with a study of lovemaking among a representative 3,005 coupled Americans age fifty-seven to eighty-five, many of whom reported the bedroom tango at levels some younger lovers might envy. Among couples age fifty-seven to seventy-four, two-thirds reported sex two or three times a month. And more than half of couples over seventy-five (54 percent) reported that same frequency. Older couples might not have vaginal intercourse, but there are several other satisfying, orgasmic ways to play (below).

Subsequently, the Chicago group expanded their sample to 6,037 older men and women and asked about sex during the previous six months:

- Partner sex at least weekly—24 percent
- Those calling their sex "good"—men 71 percent, women 51 percent

Indiana University researchers used different parameters in a study of 5,865 adults and confirmed late-life sexual resilience:

Men over seventy during the past year
- 46 percent admitted masturbating.
- 19 percent said they'd received fellatio.
- 24 percent reported providing cunnilingus.
- 43 percent stated they'd had vaginal intercourse.

Women over seventy during the past year:
- 33 percent admitted masturbating.
- 8 percent reported receiving cunnilingus.
- 7 percent said they'd provided fellatio.
- 22 percent stated they'd had vaginal intercourse.

Herbenick, D., et al. "Sexual Behavior in the United States: Results from a National Probability Sample of Men and Women Ages 14–94." *Journal of Sexual Medicine* 7, suppl. 5 (2010): 255.

Aging and Body Anxiety

Throughout life, most people feel self-conscious about their bodies. But as Joan Price relates in *The Ultimate Guide to Sex after 50*, with age, body anxiety can turn into self-loathing as wrinkles, flab, and sagging take their toll.

No matter how you look, some folks are sure to find you sexually alluring. Amateur porn featuring real men and women over fifty (grannies, grandpas) is quite popular and not just with older adults, but with viewers of all ages.

To minimize body anxieties:

- Maintain good health and fitness.
- Make love with lights low. Older eyes are less likely to see imperfections.
- Suggest playing with blindfolds.
- Wear loose-fitting clothing in bed: nightgown, pajamas, lingerie. As things heat up and garments fall, aroused lovers are less likely to balk at what they find underneath.
- Laugh. There you are being sexual at your age. Try to see the humor.

All these figures probably understate elder sex. The participants were born before World War II and came of age in an era when masturbation was heavily stigmatized and most people believed older adults retired from sex.

Compared with the reproductive years, sexual frequency declines in later life, but most elders want to remain sexual and a substantial proportion succeed, solo and/or with lovers. No one is ever too old for sex.

In addition, the conventional belief that sexual quality declines with age appears mistaken. University of Minnesota investigators surveyed 6,278 adults up to age ninety-three. While sexual frequency declined with age, sexual satisfaction did not. The researchers concluded that older lovers cope in ways that provide erotic enjoyment even as they experience physical decline.

No Bed of Roses

Some men in their seventies can raise erections sufficient for intercourse without drugs, and some women twenty years past menopause have no difficulty with vaginal dryness or atrophy. But they're the lucky few. For most older adults, starting as early as the late forties, sex becomes increasingly problematic:

MEN	Age 57–64	65–74	75–85
Little or no interest in sex	28%	29%	25%
Performance anxiety	25%	29%	30%
Erection problems	31%	45%	43%
Premature ejaculation	30%	28%	22%
Unable to orgasm	16%	23%	33%
Sex not pleasurable	4%	7%	5%
Sex painful	3%	3%	1%
WOMEN	Age 57–64	65–74	75–85
Little or no interest in sex	45%	38%	49%
Trouble lubricating	36%	44%	44%
Sex painful	18%	19%	12%
Unable to orgasm	35%	33%	38%
Sex not pleasurable	23%	22%	25%
Performance anxiety	11%	13%	10%

Laumann, E. O., et al. "Sexual Dysfunction among Older Adults: Prevalence and Risk Factors from a Nationally Representative U.S. Probability Sample of Men and Women 57–85 Years of Age." *Journal of Sexual Medicine* 5 (2008): 2300.

Among older men, premature ejaculation and orgasm/ejaculation issues continue to be problematic, and erection difficulties and libido loss become more prevalent. And among older women, orgasm difficulties and loss of desire and lubrication become challenges. But even in the oldest group, those over seventy-five, 95 percent of men and 75 percent of women call their lovemaking pleasurable.

How could this be?

- The fundamentals of lovemaking—kissing, cuddling, whole-body massage, oral sex, novelty, and fantasy—can be great fun at any age.

- Problems don't necessarily trump pleasure. I'm a homeowner. My house requires constant repairs. It's always something. But overall, I love my home. Sex is similar. One can have sexual complaints but still enjoy lovemaking.
- Finally, if men have alluring partners who provide the caresses that turn them on, even those who can't raise erections can still enjoy thrilling orgasms.

Shrinking Penises, Less Semen, and Retreating Little Heads—But Better Orgasms

On the Q&A site I publish, GreatSexGuidance.com, many older men have complained, *My penis has shrunk!* This is possible. Causes include arterial narrowing (atherosclerosis) and/or replacement of penile smooth muscle tissue with collagen, a protein found in connective tissue (penile fibrosis).

Flaccid or erect, penis size depends on blood flow through the organ. The more blood, the larger your stick shift. But aging, high cholesterol, high blood pressure, a high-fat diet, few fruits and vegetables, and sedentary lifestyle cause cholesterol-rich deposits to form on artery walls, narrowing them and reducing blood flow. In the heart, this causes heart disease; in the penis, possibly some loss of length—but not much. German researchers measured 143 penises, some attached to male teens, the rest to men forty to sixty-eight. The latter's were shorter—but only an eighth of an inch.

Many older men also notice that they produce less semen, sometimes hardly any. This is normal. Sperm production continues throughout life, but with age, the prostate and adjacent glands produce less fluid. This can be disconcerting, but it also offers advantages: less messiness and fewer objections to coming in the mouth.

Older circumcised men also complain that the heads of their penises retreat into what's left of their foreskins. The medical literature is silent on this, but I surmise the cause is reduced genital blood flow.

Finally, some older men say their orgasms feel more intense. Yes. The reason is prostate enlargement. With age, the prostate expands and pinches the urine tube (urethra). To empty their bladders, older men must increasingly contract the muscles between their legs. These same muscles contract during orgasm. As men work them to void, they inadvertently perform Kegel exercises. Their pelvic floor muscles grow stronger—and orgasms feel more intense.

Orgasms *without* Erections: The Joy of "Outercourse"

How can men with severe ED still enjoy earthquake orgasms? Simple: different nerves control erection and orgasm. Men can have porn-star erections and not climax. They can also have convulsive orgasms *without* erections. Many men with spinal cord injuries can't raise erections but can still come. The same applies to older men with ED. Satisfying sex involves more than just intercourse. There are many other equally enjoyable ways to play.

Meanwhile, many older women develop vaginal dryness and atrophy. Even with lubricant, the old in-out may become uncomfortable or impossible.

Older lovers who remain happily sexual generally jettison intercourse in favor of what sexologists call "outercourse," the many ways to enjoy lovemaking without penis-vagina insertion: kissing, cuddling, bathing together, mutual whole-body massage, fellatio, cunnilingus, sex toys, and perhaps some kink, for example, blindfolds and light spanking. Outercourse allows older adults to eliminate the one element that no longer works while still enjoying everything else.

A tip for older couples who still want intercourse: assuming the man can become somewhat firm, here's a way to slip it in. She lies on her back, legs spread, knees by her armpits so her vulva points up at the ceiling. He kneels between her legs, positions his partial erection at her opening, and one of them gently pushes it inside. Lube helps.

Arousal: A Lifelong Issue for Many Women Becomes an Increasing Problem for Older Men

Across the lifespan, desire and arousal problems are big issues for women. Depending on the survey, one-quarter to half of women of all ages report little or no libido and/or difficulty becoming aroused.

Meanwhile, for young men, arousal is rarely an issue. An old joke asks, What single word can women say to sexually excite young men? *Hello.*

But after around fifty, for many men, arousal becomes increasingly challenging. They may feel as erotically interested as ever, but when opportunity knocks, they have trouble shifting the classic car out of neutral. Some try erection medications. The drugs aid erection in men who already feel aroused but do nothing to pique arousal.

Arousal difficulties help explain the demographics of pornography (part VII). Many people assume that most porn consumers are either wide-eyed adolescent boys or single men. Actually, almost half the porn audience (45 percent) is men over forty, and most are married. Men of all ages use porn as a masturbation aid, but many older men also use it to goose flagging arousal and convince themselves they can still get turned on.

Older gentlemen, you can still become aroused—if you're patient and embrace the suggestions in chapters 1–10.

Dating after Fifty: Are Condoms Still Necessary?

AARP asked thousands of older singles if they used condoms to prevent sexually infections (STIs). Only 22 percent—one in five—said they used them every time, 32 percent of the women, 12 percent of the men. Most older adults believe they're no longer at significant risk for STIs. They're *almost* right.

Older adults cite three reasons for dispensing with condoms:

- No risk of pregnancy
- Compared with young adults, STI risk after fifty is 90 percent lower
- Less likelihood of vaginal intercourse

Public health authorities feel differently. Older adults' STI risk is low, but as fifty has become the new thirty, rates have risen. Since 2005, risk of syphilis among retirees has jumped 67 percent, chlamydia 40 percent. Health officials exhort lovers of all ages to use condoms every time unless both are monogamous and test STI-free.

Blame Evolution

Late-life erection changes are disconcerting but totally normal. Live long enough and pretty much every man goes softer, if not limp (chapter 34).

Blame it on the energy efficiency of evolution. During men's reproductive years, the body invests considerable energy in maintaining its sperm-injection system. But after the reproductive years, the elderly body retreats from enabling procreation. The nervous system loses some of its erotic excitability. Fantasies and touch that produced firm erections at twenty-five may do little, if anything,

Before PSA Testing, Don't Ejaculate for Four Days

For early detection of prostate cancer, prostate-specific antigen (PSA) testing is controversial, but millions of older men get tested annually. If PSA is high, invasive, unpleasant prostate biopsies are the next step. Unfortunately, few doctors tell men that orgasm/ejaculation raises PSA. To avoid erroneously high PSAs, men should abstain from ejaculation—solo or partnered—for four days before PSA testing.

at sixty-five. And blood levels of testosterone decline, possibly causing libido loss.

After sixty or so, even the healthiest men usually notice erection softening. Those taking erection drugs find they need higher doses, and as the years pass, even those may stop working. As arousal fades and erections decline, some decide they've reached the end of their erotic ropes and "retire" from sex, often to their partners' chagrin.

Solo versus Partner Sex

Most studies of elder sexuality focus on partner sex and ignore masturbation. That's a shame. As shown on page 24 [Herbenick chart], more late-life adults admit masturbating than say they have partner sex (except for those who have just fallen in love, this is true in every age group).

Single or coupled, solo sex provides lifelong pleasure. An Australian study provides insights into elder self-sexing. The researchers surveyed 3,274 independent-living men age seventy-five to ninety-five, average age eighty-two:

Problem	Whole Group (3,274 men)	Partnered (857)
Lack of interest	48%	24%
Sexual anxiety	20%	37%
Erectile dysfunction	49%	66%
Premature ejaculation	15%	26%
Difficulty ejaculating	39%	43%
Low testosterone	7%	not tabulated

Hyde, Z., et al. "Prevalence and Predictors of Sexual Problems in Men Aged 75–95 Years: A Population-Based Study." *Journal of Sexual Medicine* 9 (2012): 442.

Having lovers works wonders for older men's libidos. Compared with single seniors, those in relationships were only half as likely to report lack of interest. But compared with solo sex, partner play is more complicated. You have two people to please, not just one, and that may cause sex-impairing stresses. The partnered men were more likely to report sexual anxiety, ED, premature ejaculation, and difficulty coming. Self-sexing is less fraught.

Note that in this sample, only 7 percent suffered low testosterone. Deficiency was associated with only one issue, libido loss. In men with normal testosterone, supplementation had no impact on other difficulties.

Widowed Women:
Lengthening Odds and Unrecognized Sexual Grief

In their 1963 hit "Surf City," the Beach Boys sing of a mythic town with "two girls for every boy." That actually happens—at age eighty-eight.

In every age group, more men than women die. Testosterone encourages risk-taking, so men are more likely to attempt death-defying feats—and sometimes perish. Men also are more likely to die on the job, in war, in motor vehicle (often motorcycle) accidents, and by suicide. Consequently, the aging population becomes increasingly female, and unattached older women face increasing competition for partners:

Age	US population of men	US population of women	Ratio of women to men
65–69	5.8 million	6.6 million	1.14
70–74	4.2	5.0	1.20
75–79	3.2	4.1	1.28
80–84	2.3	3.4	1.48
85–89	1.3	2.3	1.77
90+	0.5	1.4	2.80

Figures from the 2010 census.

When mates die, in addition to widows' general grief, many (both female and male) also specifically grieve their loss of partner sex, usually in isolation because friends and family rarely raise the issue. In one survey, 76 percent of widows said they mourned lost sex but didn't discuss it.

If the subject comes up, many well-meaning friends and family members invoke unsupportive myths about sex after grieving:

- *You don't miss sex, just touch. Get a massage.* Of course you miss touch. But if you're a sexual person, chances are you also miss partner play.
- *Wait at least a year.* Forget the calendar. Return to partner lovemaking when you feel ready.
- *Sex with a new lover betrays your departed mate.* Spouses swear fealty "till death do us part." After one dies, the other is free to move on.
- *Wait until you stop grieving.* You never completely get over any significant loss. When you return to partner sex is up to you.
- *Enough already. It's time you dated again.* Widows are adults. They can decide for themselves when to seek new relationships.

For more, I recommend *Sex after Grief* by Joan Price.

How Older Adults Maintain Sizzling Sex

Researchers at Sonoma State University in California invited coupled adults over fifty to complete a survey posted on the NBC News website. More than nine thousand people participated.

The researchers divided responses into four groups:

- Low frequency, low satisfaction (3,985 respondents)
- Low frequency, high satisfaction (1,065)
- High frequency, low satisfaction (951)
- High frequency, high satisfaction (3,163)

Low frequency and low satisfaction were strongly associated with desire differences, boredom, little or no coaching, no mood setting (music, candlelight, etc.), rushing into intercourse, chronic relationship tensions, and one partner's invocation of the myth, "I/we are too old for sex."

Meanwhile, high frequency and high satisfaction were strongly associated with the ten ingredients of sizzling sex discussed in part I, notably mutual coaching, novelty, mood setting, frequent relationship discussions, mutually agreed frequency and repertoire, extended whole-body outercourse before attempts at intercourse, and a mutual commitment to remain sexual together.

Elder Sex Just Might Be the Best of Your Life

Aging changes sex, but for those with partners, a few adjustments usually make late-life lovemaking feel as good as ever—possibly better:

- After divorce or widowhood, some seniors find new relationships and experience erotic resurrections.
- Older lovers are more sexually in sync. Many young men are all finished before their lovers have even warmed up to genital play. In addition, young women tend to be less genitally focused than young men and more interested in mutual whole-body massage. But after fifty, men's and women's erotic sensibilities usually converge. Men need more time to become aroused, and as erection and intercourse become more challenging, most men who remain sexual warm up to the kind of lovemaking most women prefer throughout life, sex based on whole-body massage.
- Most older men become less fixated on their own pleasure and more interested in their partner's. Couples whose lovemaking evolves in this way just might enjoy more fulfilling sex at seventy-five than they had at twenty-five—even without erections and intercourse.
- Women are more likely to get the sex they want. As older men learn to enjoy a slow pace and playful whole-body mutual massage, many older women enjoy sex more. This increases their erotic responsiveness, which, in turn, boosts men's.
- Older men don't need erections to experience marvelous orgasms.
- Concerns about pregnancy and contraception disappear. Freedom from contraception allows deeper relaxation, which boosts erotic pleasure.
- The kids are probably gone. Empty nests allow couples to turn up the music, whoop it up, and play in any room of the house.

Of course, it's not easy adjusting to the sexual changes of older adulthood. Change is challenging, especially when it involves sexual losses. But older lovers who transition from intercourse to outercourse often discover that late-life lovemaking can be great fun, possible the most sizzling sex of their lives.

Aches and Pains?

Pain distracts from erotic focus. If you have chronic aches and pains that interfere with lovemaking:

- **Add pillows.** Extra padding under achy spots may help.
- **Change positions often.** Frequent movement minimizes aches, soreness, and stiffness.
- **Consider pain medication.** Unless your doctor says otherwise, an hour before lovemaking, try aspirin, ibuprofen (Advil, Motrin), acetaminophen (Tylenol), or naproxen (Aleve). High-CBD cannabis, a natural pain reliever, may also help.

The New Erotic Frontier: Sex in Nursing Homes

Nursing homes once frowned on sex. Now, most smile. When eighty-five-year-old Audrey Davison met a special guy at the Hebrew Home at Riverdale, the Bronx, New York, they did more than just sit together at meals. He invited her to his room and hung a Do Not Disturb sign on the door. In the morning, they arrived at breakfast giggling.

Of the home's 870 residents, around 5 percent, forty or so, are coupled. The staff wish there were more. Relationships make people happier. Happiness reduces stress and irritability. It improves mood, appetite, sleep, sociability, and immune function. Sex also provides exercise, and at a stage of life when many people feel chronically cold, a bedmate provides warmth.

The Hebrew Home does more than just tolerate elder lovemaking. It holds regular happy hours and dances and has even organized a dating service for residents.

Until the 1990s, nursing homes ran like the military. Staff woke everyone at the same time, marched them to meals, shepherded them to activities, and put them to bed. No longer. Today, most nursing homes have embraced individualized care. Within logistical constraints, residents arrange their own schedules and increased self-determination has led some to sexual involvements.

Hebrew Home CEO Daniel Reingold was a pioneer in sex-positive care. In 1995, a nurse walked in on two residents in the throes and ran to Reingold asking what to do. "Tiptoe out," he replied, "and close the door quietly." Today, most nursing homes have sexual-expression policies that instruct staff to respect residents' privacy and decision-making and inform incoming residents and their families that sex among residents is fine—except in public.

This new sexual tolerance has provoked pushback. Some families view sex as appropriate only for procreation or inappropriate for the very old. Others object to relationships involving nursing-home residents who are still married to nonresidents. But the trend is clear—sex is part of life, even in nursing homes.

Institutional objections may be fading, but demographics remain cruel. The typical nursing home population is largely female, meaning that many women compete for the few men. Staff must contend with jealousy, hurt feelings, and awkward breakups. That's sad, but that's life, and people should be free to live it in all of its glory and rancor—at any age.

But when does elder sex become elder abuse? What if one person is deep into dementia and can't give clear consent? In 2014, at age seventy-eight, Donna Rayhons had to be placed in an Iowa nursing home dementia unit. Her husband, Henry, also seventy-eight and a former Iowa state legislator, visited frequently and was charged with sexual abuse when staff discovered the couple making love. It was the first such case in the nation.

The prosecutor said Donna was incapable of legal consent. The defense countered that despite her dementia, she welcomed sex with her husband and often initiated it.

Rayhons was acquitted. The verdict is unlikely to settle the issue, but these days, most nursing homes are moving from a policy of "no sex" to "no problem."

CHAPTER 30:
How to Approach Sex Problems: From Self-Help to Sex Coaching to Sex Therapy

SEX PROBLEMS ARE prevalent, but not necessarily debilitating. Two large studies spotlight the distinction:

- University of Chicago researchers surveyed a representative 3,160 Americans age eighteen to fifty-nine. Thirty-seven percent—43 percent of the women, 31 percent of the men—complained of sex problems.
- British researchers surveyed a representative 4,000 UK adults age eighteen to seventy-five. Three-quarters (75 percent) said they felt satisfied with their sex lives, and among those who made love weekly, satisfaction topped 80 percent.

But if 37 percent report problems, how could 75–80 percent feel satisfied? The apparent contradiction reflects how the researchers framed their questions. The Chicago group asked about specific sex problems: "During the past year have you experienced"—followed by a long list of possibilities. The English group asked more general questions: "Do you have problems with sex?" Specific questions skew results toward problems. General questions skew them toward satisfaction.

Consider your own sex life. You may have some complaints, but still feel pretty good about it. Depending on how you're questioned, your sex life might appear fraught or fine. People often report "satisfaction" even when they have issues researchers call "problems." Meanwhile, even chronic dysfunctions may not feel sufficiently severe or disruptive to negate overall satisfaction.

When do sex problems warrant treatment? Whenever they bother you enough to seek a remedy.

Do You Really Have a "Sex" Problem?
When couples experience relationship problems, sexual frequency and satisfaction usually suffer. Sex becomes collateral damage.

Many issues that challenge couples have little to do with sex. They typically concern money, children, family, communication, power, control, and decision-making—with those issues often complicated by anger, guilt, shame, and fear of breakups. Any issue may reverberate sexually. But when sex goes to hell, it's quite possible you don't have a "sex" problem. Ask yourself what you're really upset about. Just sex? Or other issues as well?

How can you know if your sex-related issues are best served by self-help, sex coaching, or sex therapy? That's subjective. My suggestion: try self-help first. If that doesn't resolve things, try sex coaching. And if you need more intensive psychological counseling, if the problem has festered and the issue is driving you or your partner crazy, proceed to sex therapy.

Sexual Self-Help Usually Works

As discussed in the introduction, many studies show that self-help approaches resolve about two-thirds of sex problems, notably those caused by lack of information, misleading ideas (for men, often about self-sexing to porn), or misconceptions about the elements of satisfying lovemaking.

Of the remaining third, three German analyses of fifty-four studies show that sex therapy helps about two-thirds (these studies predate sex coaching).

Which leaves around 10 percent of sexual issues resistant to treatment. If you're among them, try not to despair. As time passes, new insights may improve things. Even if your problem is intractable, when there's a will, there's always a way to enjoy erotic pleasure.

Sex Coaching: Well-Informed Direction

Sex therapy was invented in the 1960s, when pioneering sex researchers William Masters, MD, and Virginia Johnson (mostly Johnson) showed that a combination of sex education, whole-body massage ("sensate focus"), and specific sexual techniques could resolve many sex problems, even severe, chronic dysfunctions. Unlike today's sex therapists, neither Masters nor Johnson were mental health professionals. They were what today would be called sex coaches.

Contemporary sex coaching is an outgrowth of life and career coaching, which emerged during the late twentieth century. Coaching is based on the idea that many people who are basically okay—no significant emotional or personality problems—can benefit from discussions with experienced, well-informed counselors who can answer questions, challenge faulty assumptions, and provide supportive guidance.

Sex coaching emerged as an occupation in the 1990s when distinguished Southern California sex educator Patti Britton, PhD, MPH, launched the first training program. In 2005, Britton published *The Art of Sex Coaching*. In 2010, she and colleagues created Sex Coach University (sexcoachu.com) to train and certify sex coaches. Training takes one to two years and involves both counseling skills and thorough grounding in the kind of sexological information presented in this book.

Coaching usually involves weekly discussions that may continue for up to a few months. Cost varies depending on the practitioner, but expect $75 to $200 an hour. Health insurers do not cover it. Some coaches discount their fees for low-income clients. Many coaches offer remote sessions so they can work with clients anywhere. When coaches discern their clients have significant emotional problems—personality issues, chronic relationship resentments, severe stress from sex-negative upbringing, and so forth—they are trained and ethically obligated to refer them to psychotherapists or sex therapists.

To find a certified sex coach near you, visit the World Association of Sex Coaches (WASC, worldassociationofsexcoaches.org).

An Intimate Guide to Sex Therapy

Sex therapists are mental health professionals certified by the American Association of Sex Educators, Counselors, and Therapists (AASECT). They have broad training in psychology and couple counseling, and extensive additional training in sexual issues. Certification requires adherence to a strict code of ethics and involves hundreds of hours of clinical work supervised by AASECT-accredited mentors.

Early sex therapists counseled many women unable to have orgasms and many men eager to gain ejaculatory control. Sex therapists still treat these problems, but today, premature ejaculation and orgasm difficulties can usually be resolved with self-help resources and/or sex coaching.

The issues most couples bring to sex therapists include:

- **Desire differences.** Chronic desire differences can poison relationships. Once things have turned toxic, many couples need professional help. Chapter 22 presents a self-help version of the treatment program sex therapists have developed.
- **Erection problems.** Mention erection wilting, and doctors are quick to prescribe medication. But several studies show that the drugs work best when combined with sex therapy. In some cases, sex therapy alone provides relief.
- **Low or no libido.** This may be caused by antidepressants, low testosterone (in women, low androgens), or relationship frustrations. Self-help resources often resolve the problem, notably *A Tired Woman's Guide to Passionate Sex* by Laurie B. Mintz, PhD; *Wanting Sex Again* by Laurie J. Watson, PhD; and *The Return of Desire* by the late Gina Ogden, PhD. But many people with low or no libido benefit from sex therapy.
- **Sexual aversion or virginity after thirty.** People in these situations either fear sex or feel so shy and awkward that friendships never progress to sexual relationships. Sex therapy can help, possibly with the help of a surrogate partner.
- **Women's sexual pain.** Possible causes include vaginismus, endometriosis, birth control pills, relationship stress, reproductive infections, or a history of sexual trauma.

University of Pennsylvania researchers tracked 365 couples who consulted sex therapists for a variety of problems. In two-thirds (65 percent), sex therapy resolved things. Treatment success was unaffected by the presenting problem(s), the gender of the person with the main complaint(s), or the partners' history of sexual trauma. Among couples who did not respond to sex therapy, the reasons often involved chronic illness, for example, heart disease or diabetes, both of which can impair sexual functioning. The researchers concluded, "Sex therapy is effective in the real world."

Some wonder if therapists' gender affects the quality of therapy. People may have personal preferences, but the study just mentioned and others show that the therapist's gender doesn't matter. Men and women respond equally well to male and female therapists. What matters most is the rapport between clients and therapists, and clients' commitment to the process.

What if one partner refuses to go? Even when one person voices the complaint(s), the problem is the *couple's,* and the solution involves both. Sex therapy isn't torture. The spouse who wants it should say it's likely to help them both by improving their lovemaking and strengthening their relationship in and out of bed. But if one partner flatly refuses, the one who wants therapy can go solo. That person can vent frustrations, gain information and perspective, and take home new insights that might help. Eventually the other might join the process.

Sex therapy is similar to talk psychotherapy, but with "homework." Clients *never* have sex with or in the presence of their therapist. For a light-hearted but realistic look at the process, see the 2012 film *Hope Springs* with Meryl Streep, Tommy Lee Jones, and Steve Carell.

For most problems, sex therapy takes a few one-hour sessions to a few months of weekly sessions. Homework may include conversations to gain experience with new communication skills or hands-on assignments to practice massage or new lovemaking techniques.

Depending on the location and therapist, sex therapy typically costs $150 to $250 an hour. Some therapists discount their fees for low-income clients. Some health insurers cover it, others don't, and some that offer coverage limit the number of sessions, after which you pay out of pocket.

Sexually Informed Medical Practitioners

Few medical training programs emphasize sexual medicine. Fortunately, nurses, physician assistants, and doctors who specialize in sexual medicine can be found through the Sexual Medicine Society of North America (sexhealthmatters.org/resources/find-a-provider).

PART III:
A Guide to Resolving Men's Sex Problems

CHAPTER 31:
Penis Size: Look Your Largest— Safely and Inexpensively

FOR A DOZEN years, I worked with a company that marketed sex toys. I answered customers' sex questions and weighed in on new products. One pitch came from a man hawking penis-enlargement pills.

"What's in them?" we asked.

"Flour, some herbs, other things . . ."

"So it's a fraud."

"I prefer to call it a placebo."

"We call it a fraud."

"Call it what you want—but it's a super-high-profit item that sells like crazy and buyers are too embarrassed to request refunds."

The catalog's owners declined it.

Most men have received junk email touting penis-enlargement miracles. *Three inches in a month!* No one knows the size, as it were, of the penis-enlargement industry, but in 2003, *Wired* magazine reported that hackers had mined a month of one company's sales. During those four weeks, the outfit sold six thousand bottles of enlargement pills at $50 a pop, grossing $300,000. Who bought? Not just the totally clueless, but a cross-section of American men (and a few women).

Attention, gentlemen, there is no pill, potion, traction device, or exercise regimen that can permanently enlarge your dick. None. All products that make permanent enlargement claims—100 percent—are cynical frauds, and the miscreants behind them belong in prison. However, you *can* make the most of what you've got safely and inexpensively.

Most men who want huge ones believe jumbo bratwurst increases their attractiveness and women's pleasure. Actually, if you want to please most women, what hangs between your legs—no matter what size—is almost always less important than how you use your fingers, lips, and especially your tongue.

Men's Leading Sexual Insecurity

In 2015, data analyst Seth Stephens-Davidowitz tracked one month of Google searches dealing with sexual worries and discovered—no surprise—that men were by far most anxious about guess what. *Why is mine so small? How can I make it larger?*

Does Shoe Size Predict Penis Length?

Some people believe that big feet mean a big penis. English urologists documented the shoe size of 104 men and then measured their penis length. The former had nothing to do with the latter. "The supposed association of penile length and shoe size has no scientific basis."

Why are men so stressed? They're convinced women want phone poles. But for every gal who searched "penis size," men searched it *170 times*. And when women searched, 40 percent of their queries dealt with pain during intercourse because their man was *too large*.

During four decades of answering more than twelve thousand sex questions, I can't recall a single woman complaining that her man was too small. When women have raised the issue, they usually want to know how they can persuade their partners to stop obsessing about size.

How Women Feel about Penis Size—Really

Whenever I've written that size doesn't matter to the large majority of women, I've received pushback from some gals who insist it matters a great deal to them. Yes, just as breast size matters to some men, penis size matters to some women—to be exact, 14 percent of women, one in seven.

This figure comes from researchers at UCLA and Cal State Los Angeles. They posted a survey on MSNBC.com and heard from 26,437 women age eighteen to sixty-five. Respondents were self-selected, which raises questions about validity. But as sample size increases, reliability concerns recede—and 26,437 is such a huge number that statistically, the results look valid.

Men also responded—25,594. Two-thirds rated their penises as "average," exactly matching what the women said about their partners. But women were only half as likely as men to call their man's "small" and more likely to call it "large."

- Men: I'm "small": 12%
- Women: He's "small": 6%
- Men: It's "large": 22%
- Women: He's "large": 27%

Seven out of eight women (84 percent) said they felt "very satisfied" with their man's size. One in eight (14 percent) wished it were larger and one in fifty (2 percent) wanted smaller. Hence, my assertion that the substantial majority of women are happy with their men as they are. Most women value warmth, caring, kindness, consideration, solvency, supportiveness, shared values, and a good sense of humor over baseball bats in men's pants.

Fifty Shades of Penis Size

With sales topping 150 million copies, the BDSM romance *Fifty Shades of Grey* became one of the all-time bestselling novels—after just five years in print. Written from a woman's perspective, it's filled with kinky sex between dreamboat billionaire Christian Grey and the naive young woman he can't resist, Anastasia Steele. Steele rhapsodizes about Grey's virility, but never alludes to his size, and never once pulls out a ruler. Instead, every time they embrace, she mentions feeling his penis pressing against her—and swelling. To Steele, Grey's size is irrelevant. All that matters is *her* ability to arouse *him*.

For the Record

"Penis size" usually implies length. Most studies measure on top from the pubic bone at the base to the tip of the head (glans)—without pushing the ruler into the gut or pulling on the shaft to stretch it.

English researchers measured fifteen thousand adult men:

- Average flaccid length: 3.6 inches
- Average flaccid girth/circumference: 3.7 inches
- Average erect length: 5.2 inches
- Average erect girth: 4.6 inches

Other studies agree to within two-tenths of an inch

- Flaccid size has little to do with erect size. Compared with large flaccid organs, small ones grow more to erection
- Only 2.5 percent of erections measure less than 3.8 inches long
- 13.5 percent are 3.8 to 4.5 inches
- 68 percent are 4.5 to 6.0 inches
- 13.5 percent are 6.0 to 6.8 inches
- And only 2.5 percent are longer than 6.8 inches
- Size may decrease slightly in elderly men

From Ancient Greece to Michelangelo to Porn

The ancient Greeks and Romans preferred *small* penises. In Aristophanes's play *The Clouds* (423 BC), an elder admonishes delinquent boys that if they continue to misbehave, as punishment, their penises will grow larger. But if they repudiate wickedness, their organs will remain blessedly small. What the Greeks wanted was a jumbo *scrotum*. A big nut sack suggested great potency. The Greeks considered penises incidental injection devices for what really counted, big ejaculations. Five centuries later, the Roman novel *Satyricon* (ca. AD 50) describes bathers at a public bath who ridicule one character's large penis.

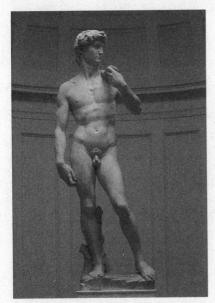

Michelangelo's *David*, 1501–4,
Galleria dell'Accademia (Florence)

The view that small is beautiful persisted through the Renaissance. Consider Michelangelo's *David*. His penis is surprisingly small.

Men's feelings about size changed during the nineteenth century as photography (1840) and motion pictures (1890) paved the way for modern pornography. Porn has always been primarily a masturbation aid for men. Stroking is all about erections. Porn spotlighted the penis, transforming it from an incidental syringe into the center of attention—and the bigger the better.

Why Men Think They're Too Small

Almost all men are much shorter than professional basketball players, but few become distraught. They know that NBA Goliaths represent only a tiny fraction of men, that the vast majority are Davids like them.

But penis size is different. Other than their own, most heterosexual men catch only brief glimpses of other men's willies and, unless they're doctors, never get to examine them closely. The only penises most heterosexual men view closely are those in porn. Recall that 2.5 percent of penises are longer than 6.8 inches. Men who audition for commercial porn usually come from this small minority. As a result, virtually every penis men see in commercial porn is significantly larger than theirs, so they're completely justified in believing they have one of the smallest penises they've ever seen.

In addition, men look *down* on their own, which makes them look smaller. In porn, cameras often shoot up from under, which makes them look larger.

For a dose of reality, check out amateur porn—search "Amateur" on aggregator sites (PornHub.com, ixxx.com). Like the vast majority of men, they have average endowments—yet still have great fun.

Surgical Enlargement: Don't

Some surgeons offer penis enlargement. The more popular procedure involves lengthening. It's based on the fact that men have more penis than what hangs between their legs. The organ extends into the abdomen. A ligament holds the internal penis in place. Cut it and much of the internal penis emerges, adding length. Surgeons claim men gain up to several inches, but Israeli urologists reviewed thirty-four studies and found that most gain only around half an inch.

Surgical lengthening has one significant downside: the ligament that gets cut makes erections stand up. When aroused, a surgically lengthened penis becomes as firm as ever, but no longer salutes. Instead, it hangs down between the legs. Men or their lovers must manually direct it into erotic openings.

The other surgical option is girth enhancement. The surgeon removes fat from the buttocks (liposuction) and injects it under the skin of the shaft and glans. Surgeons display before-and-after photos showing pencils turned into burritos. But fat injections may not "take," requiring additional surgery, and if they take unevenly, the result is a lumpy, deformed pleasure wand.

Perils of a Huge One

Most men in porn are huge, but one 1970s male porn star, stage name Richard Pacheco, was Mr. Average. He auditioned on a lark and, being average-sized, was surprised he kept getting cast. Back then, many producers allowed the women to choose their partners. They often chose Pacheco. His penis didn't hurt them. A huge one can bang into the cervix, causing pain, particularly during rear-entry (doggie) intercourse. Pacheco joked that he had "the smallest dick to ever hit the big time."

New York City sex educator Betty Dodson, PhD, is a veteran of group-sex parties. "Once in a blue moon, a guy would show up with a huge porn penis. The women would *oooh* and *ahh*—but nobody would let him near them. *No way you're sticking that monster in me.* Most wouldn't even suck huge ones. Talking with these guys, they all complained that their size was a burden."

Finally, a man with a huge one commented on my blog: "Women say I hurt them. I can't find gym shorts and bathing suits that fit. People treat me like a freak."

Gentlemen, be careful what you wish for.

The Israeli team found high rates of deformity from failed fat injections, along with unsightly scarring, postsurgical sex problems, and even penis *shortening*. Their conclusion: enlargement surgery "should be discouraged."

Health insurers don't cover enlargement. Most surgeons charge $8,000 to $10,000—plus travel expenses.

Be All You Can Be

Even if you're convinced your penis is fine, there's nothing wrong with looking your largest. To make the most of what the good Lord gave you:

- **It's all about blood inflow.** The penis is not a balloon. Flaccid or erect, blood continually flows in and out. Outflow fluctuates only a little. Size largely depends on inflow through the pudendal arteries. The more blood flowing in, the larger you look. Two factors affect inflow—stress and arterial narrowing (atherosclerosis).
- **Stop stressing.** Worrying about size *makes your penis shrink*. The arteries that carry blood into the penis are lined with smooth muscle tissue sensitive to stress. Anxiety releases the stress hormone cortisol, which constricts the arteries in the central body, including those in your joystick. Constricted arteries mean less inflow. Want to look your largest? Stop stressing about your size.
- **Stay warm.** Perhaps you've noticed that in drafty locker rooms, you look smaller, but after a hot shower, you appear better hung. Heat opens the penile arteries. More blood flows in and the organ grows larger.
- **Relax deeply.** Heat boosts size because it's relaxing. Other relaxation regimens also increase inflow: meditation, yoga, and regular moderate exercise.
- **Don't rush into intercourse.** Before attempting insertion, enjoy at least twenty minutes of mutual whole-body massage. It's deeply relaxing and opens the arteries so more blood flows into the penis.
- **Value a committed, loving, long-term relationship.** One-night stands can be fun and new relationships feel exciting, but they involve sex with women you don't know well, if at all. That may produce sufficient anxiety to reduce blood inflow. Sex with longtime partners may feel less sizzling, but familiarity fosters relaxation, which boosts size.
- **Quit smoking.** Smoking damages the arteries, spurring formation of fatty, cholesterol-rich deposits (atherosclerotic plaques). Plaques narrow the arteries, limiting inflow (smoking is also a major erection killer).
- **Engage in regular, moderate exercise.** Walk, run, cycle, garden, swim—any regular, moderate exercise reduces plaque formation and maintains arterial elasticity, increasing inflow. But exercising the penis itself is pointless. Some writers call it the "love muscle," implying that, like the biceps, targeted exercises can add bulk. No—the penis's smooth muscle tissue cannot be enlarged with exercise.
- **Eat more fruits and vegetables, and less meat and whole-milk dairy products.** A diet high in animal fat—meats, cheese, ice cream—raises cholesterol and narrows the arteries. Eat fewer animal foods. In addition, increase fruit and vegetable consumption from the average American's two or three half-cup servings a day to what nutritionists recommend, five to eight servings. Fruits and vegetables are high in antioxidant nutrients that help prevent arterial narrowing.

- **Lose the pot belly.** A big belly encroaches on the base of the penis, making it look smaller. Lose abdominal fat and you look larger.
- **Trim your pubic hair.** When less of the penis is obscured by hair, it looks larger.

Toys for Temporary Boosts

Two sex toys may produce modest temporary enlargement:

- **Cock rings.** These erection aids are either rubber donuts or small leather straps. Rings constrict the base of the penis. This has no effect on inflow. The arteries that control it run through the center. But one vein that carries blood out runs close to the top skin. Rings compress it, decreasing outflow somewhat. More blood remains inside, slightly increasing size.
- **Penis pumps.** These devices draw in extra blood. Models differ, but all include squeeze-bulb pumps and plastic tubes closed at one end. Squeezing the bulb sucks air from the tube, causing a partial vacuum that coaxes a little extra blood in. Fit is crucial. Without a good seal at the base, there's no vacuum. Urologists prescribe custom-fitted pumps to help men raise erections. They also boost size a bit.

Neither toy produces miracles. Any effect is modest and temporary.

Pleasing Women Involves Much More Than Just Your Penis

Men can enjoy great pleasure from any size penis. But women's pleasure and orgasms usually depend on your hands, lips, and especially your tongue—that is, how you caress them *without using your penis*. Porn star Ron Jeremy, famous for his huge one, has said, "More women have gotten off on my tongue than my cock."

No matter what men's size, only 25 percent of women are consistently orgasmic from vaginal intercourse alone. Vaginal stretching has little to do with most women's pleasure and orgasms. To come, the large majority need direct, gentle, patient clitoral touch with fingers, tongue, or toys.

Still, the penis is integral to lovemaking. To make the most of Mr. Woody:

- **Caress her all over.** Unless women specifically request genital play as soon as they disrobe, assume they want—and need—at least twenty minutes of kissing, cuddling, and gentle whole-body caressing from scalp to toe before any genital play. That's how long it often takes vaginas to relax, open, and self-lubricate sufficiently to comfortably accept any size penis. Men also benefit from extended whole-body massage. It increases size and helps prevent premature ejaculation and erection impairment.
- **Use lube.** Many women of all ages don't produce much natural vaginal lubrication. Even when they do, commercial lubricants boost the pleasure of hand jobs and intercourse.
- **Start shallow.** All parts of the vagina are erotically sensitive, but some men only want to plumb its depths. In fact, the vulva and vaginal lips are quite sexually excitable—and any size penis can arouse them. Use the head of your penis to tease them. Gently run your erection up the fleshy groove between them to her clitoris. Ask for coaching. Insert for a while, then withdraw and tease her vaginal lips and clitoris some more before reentering.
- **Enter slowly.** When men plunge in quickly, even women who feel highly aroused and well lubricated may experience discomfort or pain. Start with the woman-on-top position. It allows women to control the speed and depth of insertion. Lie still and allow

her to sit on your erection at her own pace. Don't start moving until she's comfortably seated. Then unless she requests otherwise, move slowly until you approach orgasm.

- **Discuss deep penetration.** Many women enjoy feeling filled up. Others don't care for it. Discuss this. If women enjoy it, deep penetration depends less on penis size than on position. The best fill-her-up positions are woman-on-top and rear entry (doggie). For deep filling in the man-on-top position (missionary), place a pillow under her hips and/or raise her legs. Note to the few men with unusually large penises: don't penetrate deeply. It's likely to hurt women.

- **Get rhythm.** An old blues tune goes: *It ain't the meat / It's the motion.* Unless women specifically request it, don't pump in and out furiously like the men in porn. Instead, adopt a slow grind: in, out, and around in circles. As women move their hips, move with them.

- **It ain't the meat, it's the clitoris.** "I wish men would get over their preoccupation with size," sex educator Betty Dodson says. "If you want to please women, focus on the clit. Fondle it gently and especially lick it. That's more enjoyable than feeling impaled on any size penis."

- **You're large enough.** Dodson tells men: "Make peace with your penis. It's fine. Enjoy what you've got and the pleasure it brings. Most women enjoy gentle, well-lubricated intercourse, but if you want to please women, focus on gentle, direct clitoral caresses. Personally, I don't care how large or small a man is—as long as he's enthusiastic about providing oral." In other words, gentlemen, eat more pussy. Feast on it every time.

Two Common Birth Defects May Slightly Reduce Size

Each affects around one man in 250.

- **Hypospadias (hype-oh-SPAY-dee-as).** In most men, the tube that carries urine and semen out of the body (urethra) opens dead center on the tip of the glans. In hypospadias, it opens somewhere along the underside. In 90 percent of cases, hypospadias is minor and requires no treatment. The rest are treated surgically, usually during infancy. Urethra reconstruction usually leaves men looking normal or nearly so and functioning fine, but the repair may reduce length a little.

- **Chordee.** During erection, the penis bends downward. Chordee develops during gestation when more erectile tissue grows on the top side of the penis than on the underside. Surgical correction may reduce erection length and girth a bit.

CHAPTER 32:
The Cure for Premature Ejaculation: How to Last Longer

G ENTLEMEN, NO MATTER how quickly you've ejaculated for no matter how long, you can almost certainly learn to last as long as you'd like.

This chapter presents a self-help version of the easy, enjoyable program sex therapists have developed to cure rapid, involuntary, premature ejaculation (PE). It teaches most men bomb-proof control in just a few months. It also offers a bonus benefit, enhancement of women's erotic pleasure—ironically, not because you last longer, but because the program promotes the kind of lovemaking most women prefer.

Self-Help Usually Works

At the University of Liege, Belgium, researchers produced a forty-page self-help booklet similar to this chapter. Then they recruited 487 PE sufferers, some of whom had wrestled with it for decades. The investigators placed 66 on a waiting list and gave the pamphlet to the other 392. After two months, the wait-list group reported scant improvement. But two-thirds of the self-help group declared themselves cured. A follow-up survey a year later showed that hardly any of them had relapsed into PE.

What about the third of men who don't gain reliable control with self-help? Two-thirds of them benefit from individualized sex coaching or therapy. And what about the 20 percent who continue to struggle despite professional help? Several alternatives are available.

Throughout Life, Men's Number One Sex Problem

Instead of "premature," I wish this problem had been dubbed "involuntary" ejaculation. That's a more descriptive term. Curing it involves learning voluntary control over a reflex that's been involuntary. Unfortunately, most physicians and sexuality authorities continue to use "premature." I use both terms and "PE." But whatever you call it, the large majority of men can learn to last as long as they'd like—usually without much difficulty.

Men's best-known sex problem is erectile dysfunction (ED). But few men develop it until well into their forties. Meanwhile, according to a University of Chicago study, throughout the lifespan, rapid, involuntary ejaculation ranks as men's leading sex problem. The myth is that it affects only young men. Actually, the Chicago investigators found that in every age group, one-quarter to one-third of men admit having it. Other studies agree, estimating prevalence at 20–30 percent of men (given reluctance to admit sex problems, true prevalence is undoubtedly greater).

Any man can suffer PE, but risk factors include:

- Performance anxiety—any concerns that cause stress and compromise men's sexual self-confidence.
- Genital infections that cause pain, particularly prostatitis.
- Iffy erections, particularly in middle-aged men. An Italian study of 57,229 men showed that the stress caused by middle-age erection changes causes a midlife spike in PE.
- Diabetes. Most diabetic men know the condition raises risk of ED. Stress about erection loss contributes to PE.
- Depression. It often includes severe anxiety. Sexual anxiety contributes to PE.
- Varicoceles. These varicose veins in the scrotum cause tenderness or pain—and sexual anxiety.
- Hyperthyroidism. An overactive thyroid gland makes the nervous system more excitable, which may trigger PE.
- Caffeine and other stimulants increase nervous-system excitability.

How Soon Is Too Soon?

Urologists typically diagnose PE if men ejaculate within two minutes of slipping it in. But in the Belgian self-help study just mentioned, many men who lasted well beyond two minutes insisted they had PE. How long did they want to last? To quote countless popular songs, "all night long."

The real issue is not how long you last in seconds, minutes, or even hours. It's feeling out of control, ejaculating *involuntarily*.

Toss your stopwatch. You have PE if you come before you want to, whether it's two minutes or two hours.

PE throughout History

Ejaculatory control issues have been documented for more than 1,500 years. The *Kama Sutra*, the fourth-century Indian sex guide, declares: "Women love the man whose sexual energy lasts a long time. They resent a man whose energy ends quickly. He finishes before they climax."

In the West, men were less concerned about women's sexual satisfaction. During the nineteenth-century Victorian era, male doctors declared that women were *incapable* of erotic pleasure. Women were viewed as little more than fleshy receptacles for men's lust. They endured leg locking only to have children and retain husbands. Of course, modern sex research has established beyond any doubt that all genders are equally capable of erotic pleasure and orgasm.

During the era when women were considered nonsexual, ejaculatory control was not an issue. If women could not experience erotic pleasure, men were under no obligation to last long enough to provide it. In fact, nineteenth-century authorities considered rapid ejaculation a sign of male *vigor*. Other mammals ejaculate quickly, prompting biologists to declare the trait was rooted in evolution.

By World War I, Victorian notions began to fade and some doctors decided premature ejaculation was a problem. One was psychoanalyst Sigmund Freud, who declared that PE sufferers harbored unconscious, neurotic hostility toward women. Rapid ejaculation satisfied them but punished their lovers. Freudians claimed PE could be cured with psychoanalysis. However, no credible evidence suggested that rapid ejaculators had unusual hostility toward women, and even years of psychoanalysis rarely taught men ejaculatory control.

Psychoanalysts' inability to help men delay ejaculation convinced early sexologists that PE was normal. In *Sexual Behavior in the Human Male* (1948), Alfred Kinsey noted that 75 percent of men said they ejaculated within two minutes. Kinsey saw no problem with this.

During the 1960s, William Masters, MD, and Virginia Johnson proved that all genders are equally sexual and urged men to provide as much pleasure as they received. Coming quickly interfered with this, prompting Masters and Johnson to declare it a problem.

But if PE wasn't neurotic, what caused it? Sexologists theorized that perhaps some men's penises were unusually sensitive to touch. But researchers have found no sensitivity differences between PE sufferers and men who can last forever.

Others suggested PE indicated anxiety or depression. But the Belgian researchers found PE sufferers no more likely than average to suffer anxiety problems or depression. Finnish researchers corroborated these findings in a seven-year study of 985 men. They found "no association between premature ejaculation and anxiety disorders or depression."

Actually, PE is usually caused by a combination of sex-specific worries, masturbation habits, and wham-bam porn-style sex.

How Most Women Feel about PE

Men with PE typically fear it distresses their lovers. They believe that women have orgasms during extended intercourse, and that when men come quickly, women can't come at all.

As I've discussed, only 25 percent of women are reliably orgasmic during intercourse—no matter how long it lasts. While most women enjoy the intimacy of joining genitals, intercourse doesn't provide sufficient clitoral stimulation for most women to come. Even when men last forever, to have orgasms, three-quarters of women need gentle, direct, sustained clitoral caresses by hand, mouth, or sex toy.

The Belgian group interviewed dozens of women involved with PE sufferers. As long as their men used their hands, mouths, or sex toys to provide the direct, gentle, sustained clitoral caresses that brought them to orgasm, the women were not bothered by their men's PE. Their main concern was the distress it caused their partners.

Usually Just an Unfortunate Habit

For the vast majority of men, involuntary ejaculation is little more than a habit—one that can usually be changed fairly easily.

The PE habit may begin in many ways. Some teens train themselves to come quickly during masturbation. The adolescent male nervous system is very excitable and primed to ejaculate. Many young men self-sex vigorously and climax quickly. Over time, this may become habitual. Some also fear getting caught in solo sex. To avoid detection, they work up to orgasm even more quickly.

Other men develop PE as they transition from solo to partner sex. Losing one's virginity is rite of passage, but it may cause sufficient stress to trigger PE. Once they've done the

Erection Drugs for PE

Several studies show that in older men stressed by iffy or failing erections, Viagra, Cialis, and Levitra not only restore firmness but also relieve PE caused by stressing over faltering erections.

deed, most young men consider themselves "experienced," but most remain unschooled about mutually satisfying lovemaking. They also have fears: they're too small. Someone might walk in. She might change her mind. Or get pregnant. Or transmit a sexual infection. Or tell friends someone's a lousy lover. These and other sex-specific anxieties often push men to come quickly and then cement the habit.

Start with a Checkup

Medical problems may contribute to PE. A doctor should review your medical history, including all the drugs you take; perform a physical exam; assess you for anxiety and depression; and check for prostatitis, STIs, varicoceles, and hyperthyroidism.

Unfortunately, few doctors are trained in sex counseling. Few are aware of the simple self-help program that teaches most men dependable ejaculatory control. Doctors are much more likely to offer medication that's usually unnecessary (page 204). After a doctor rules out physical causes, try self-help or sex coaching or therapy before drugs.

Don't Tune Out Your Body. Tune Into It.

Faced with rapid ejaculation, most men try to distract themselves by thinking of other things. *The Giants beat the Dodgers 3–1* . . . But distraction rarely helps.

Don't tune out your body. Tune into it, especially how you feel as you approach the moment you know you're about to climax. Once you become familiar with your "point of no return," it's pretty easy to make small adjustments that keep you highly aroused—without popping your cork.

In the vast majority of men, sexual arousal is a four-phase process: excitement, plateau, orgasm/ejaculation, and resolution. During excitement, breathing deepens, and arousal and erection begin.

Sobriety Helps

From the teen years on, many men combine sex with alcohol and/or other recreational drugs. While learning ejaculatory control, it helps to eliminate intoxicants—or cut way down. Alcohol and other drugs interfere with the self-awareness crucial to learning ejaculatory control.

Plateau involves increased arousal and erection firming—though with age and medical conditions, wood may wax and wane. Peak arousal triggers orgasm/ejaculation. Finally, during resolution, arousal and erection subside, and breathing and consciousness return to normal. Learning ejaculatory control involves extending the plateau phase without triggering orgasm/ejaculation.

How to Last as Long as You'd Like

During the late 1960s, Masters and Johnson demonstrated that minor lovemaking adjustments could cure PE. Subsequently, other sex therapists have refined their program, making it easier and more effective.

Get regular, moderate exercise. Deep relaxation is key to ejaculatory control. Exercise is relaxing.

- Turkish researchers urged 105 PE sufferers to engage in at least thirty minutes of daily exercise. Most noted improved control.
- Finnish investigators compared the lifestyles of men with and without PE. The PE sufferers reported significantly less exercise.

Breathe deeply. While in the throes, slow deep breathing calms the nervous system. Focus on exhaling slowly and fully. Many men are amazed how much this one little change improves things.

As you breathe deeply, add sound to create love moans. They reinforce deep breathing and often help with lasting longer. They also communicate arousal—which is contagious. It makes women feel desired, which turns most on.

Value whole-body massage. Mr. Happy loves to be stroked and sucked, but if he gets too much attention too quickly—wham!—PE. Many men think the penis is their only sexual part. That view is a one-way ticket to involuntary ejaculation. To gain reliable control, expand your definition of "sex" from just the penis to your whole body—hers, too.

Gentle caresses from head to toe are fundamental to hovering near your point of no return without ejaculating. Every square inch of the body is an erotic playground. Coach your lover to explore all of it and as she touches you everywhere, savor her caresses and return the favor.

This may be challenging for men who get their sex education from pornography. Porn depicts sex that's 95 percent genital and only 5 percent the rest of the body. To cure PE, do the *opposite* of what you see in porn. Emphasize mutual whole-body caresses.

It may feel odd to postpone genital play while you kiss, hug, roll around, and gently massage one another from scalp to feet. But a slower erotic pace offers a big payoff—reliable control.

Whole-body massage takes pressure off the penis. It releases tension and promotes deep relaxation—but not the kind that includes a recliner, a six pack, and *Monday Night Football*. Instead, it's what you feel after a hot shower. In fact, showering before lovemaking—alone or together—promotes relaxation and helps with control. If you're tense during sex, your body may have no way to release the stress other than ejaculating quickly. But when you embrace whole-body massage, arousal saturates the entire body. It takes pressure off your little pal and helps you last longer.

Finally, most women *prefer* lovemaking based on whole-body massage. They enjoy genital play, but before that feels good, most need considerable warm-up time. Many women complain that men push in before they feel ready. As you learn to enjoy being touched all over, treat your lover to that same gift. Compared with most men, most women take longer to warm up to genital play. Give them all the time they need. How long? A good rule of thumb is at least twenty minutes—if you make love with music playing, five or six standard songs. But everyone is erotically unique. Ask.

Adjust your fantasies. Some men's fantasies are so hot they have trouble maintaining control. Give your hottest reveries a rest, and focus on others that excite you but don't push you over the edge.

Self-sex with a dry hand. Once exercise, deep breathing, whole-body massage, and a slower pace have thoroughly relaxed you, it's time to stroke sausage. Masturbation is key to overcoming PE. But solo sex while learning ejaculatory control is different from what you may be used to.

Hurried yanking often trains men to come quickly. To change this, stroke slowly and vary your caresses. This teaches you to stay highly aroused for extended periods without coming.

When you approach your point of no return, breathe deeply, emphasizing exhalations, and release your grip. Stroke more gently or stop and simply hold your penis—while continuing to breathe deeply. You should notice that the urge to ejaculate subsides. Congratulations. You've successfully approached your point of no return, then retreated from it without coming. You're on your way to good control. When you no longer feel about to climax, return to more vigorous wanking. Practice approaching your point of no return and then backing away until you can reliably last thirty minutes—or as long as you'd like.

Over several weeks, repeat this exercise until you consistently last thirty minutes. Approach your point of no return, then back off, approach, and retreat again and again. For most men, it doesn't take long to develop good ejaculatory control solo with a dry hand.

In addition, while practicing, consciously relax your major muscle groups. Muscle tension contributes to triggering ejaculation. By deliberately relaxing your jaw, neck, shoulders, and especially your butt muscles, most men find it easier to maintain a high level of arousal without coming.

Note: accidents happen. As you approach your point of no return, you might not back off in time. Don't berate yourself. It takes time to learn new skills. If you ejaculate before you want to, figure out why your arousal got away from you. Then return to the program and keep practicing.

Stroke with a lubricated hand. Lubricants—saliva and commercial lubes—increase genital sensitivity. Consequently, it's more challenging to maintain ejaculatory control with a lubricated hand. Practicing that is the next step. With a lubed hand, stroke until you approach your point of no return, then back off. Repeat this over a few weeks until you can last thirty minutes or as long as you'd like.

Proceed to partner sex. The transition from solo to partner sex presents new control challenges. Partner sex is inherently more complicated. You must provide coaching about what pleases you and request coaching so you know what pleases your partner. Don't be surprised if you relapse into PE for a while.

Does your partner support the program? Many women are happy to help, but others believe that as long as men provide clitoral caresses sufficient for their orgasms, it doesn't matter how long men last. If your partner feels that way, explain that learning control matters a great deal to you and request her assistance.

With new lovers, you may feel embarrassed to ask for help and provide the coaching that gets you the caresses you need. Consider mentioning that you've been working to learn ejaculatory control but may not be quite there yet. Say you're so excited to get down that you might come before you'd like. Explain that you enjoy the best control with a slow pace and lots of whole-body massage. She probably prefers that, too. If you come quickly, laugh it off. *Whoa, you really excite me.* Don't worry about being judged harshly. As long as men provide the clitoral caresses that let women work up to orgasm, most women's main concern about PE is the distress it causes men. They usually feel flattered when men ask for their for help. And be sure to request coaching about the caresses that bring them pleasure and orgasms.

Longtime lovers present different dilemmas. They may slip into old patterns that contribute to the problem. If you haven't previously coached each other, it may feel awkward. And if your relationship is problematic—especially if you haven't provided the touch that brings her pleasure and orgasms—that history may cause stress that sabotages the program. Consider sex coaching or therapy.

Assuming your partner is on board . . .

She strokes your penis with a dry hand. First, arrange "stop" and "start" signals. You might use the words "stop" and "start," or nonverbal cues—one pinch for "stop," two for "start," whatever communicates your needs quickly and clearly.

You lie still and invite your lover to stroke your erection with a dry hand. As you approach the point of no return, signal her to stop. She should immediately suspend stroking and simply hold your erection, while you breathe deeply and focus on the sensations you feel as you back away from ejaculating. When you no longer feel about to come, invite her to resume stroking.

If you have trouble lasting, try the Squeeze. Masters and Johnson combined stop-start with squeezing the glans. During stops, one of you pinches the head of the penis with thumb and index finger, which helps suppress the urge to ejaculate. In recent decades, the Squeeze has fallen from favor, but it still helps some men.

How many stops and starts make a session? A half dozen over thirty minutes works well for most couples. Do what feels comfortable on the schedule that works for you and your relationship.

She strokes you with a lubricated hand. Lube should make her strokes feel more arousing. Using your stop and start signals, practice until you can last thirty minutes or as long as you'd like. Your partner should play with different grip tightness and stroke speeds during several sessions on a schedule that works for your relationship.

Stop-start with fellatio. At first, you should lie still. Coach her about the kinds of licks and sucks that keep you highly aroused but on the right side of the line. Once you've gained good control during fellatio while remaining still, feel free to move your hips, first slowly, then more vigorously.

Stop-start during intercourse. If you engage in vaginal intercourse, incorporate stop-start into it. When learning ejaculatory control, the best position is woman-on-top. It's among the most relaxing for men. You lie on your back. She straddles your hips. You stay still. She sits down on your erection and moves gently until you invoke your stop signal.

As you gain control, feel free to move with her and try other positions. However, the man-on-top (missionary) position presents ejaculatory control challenges. You have to hold yourself up and thrust your hips, which may trigger PE.

In every intercourse position, vary your pelvic movements. Many men imitate pornography, thrusting in and out furiously. This often threatens ejaculatory control. Embrace slow pelvic movements, which help you maintain control. Beyond in and out, try a slow circular grind while pressed deep inside. And keep breathing deeply, with slow, full exhalations.

Give it time. Chances are you can't wait to gain ejaculatory control. Be patient. With regular practice, most men learn to last as long as they'd like in a few months. Try to maintain a sense of humor about any setbacks.

New partner? You may have to start over. New partners change things and those differences might cause sufficient anxiety to flip you back into PE. With any new lover, discuss your situation, and ask for her help with the program.

Note: During the couple program, the focus is on your learning process. Your partner might feel ignored. Don't forget her needs. Ask if she'd like you to make any erotic adjustments for her pleasure. Invite her to coach you about the kind of touch she enjoys.

Affairs? Sex workers? *I have great control with my wife. Why can't I last with my girlfriend?* Affairs and commercial sex may cause sufficient stress to trigger PE. Other women may be willing to work the last-longer program with you, but unless you patronize a sex worker regularly, don't expect help.

Why PE often recurs around age fifty. Some men complain that their once-reliable control falters in middle age. Several studies document a spike in PE around age fifty and usually a return to better control by sixty. Usually, the cause is age-related erection changes. At some point in most men's late forties to early sixties, erections become less reliable and lose their youthful firmness. This may cause sufficient anxiety to trigger PE. Italian researchers reviewed eighteen studies involving 57,229 men and found that erection concerns were strongly associated with PE. But as time passes and men adjust to living with iffy erections or flaccid penises and outercourse instead of intercourse, the stress usually resolves and most men regain their control. If this is a challenge, rework the program.

If self-help doesn't work. Sex coaching or therapy help most men who can't learn control with the self-help program.

If She's Reluctant to Help

Many men want to learn ejaculatory control so badly they can't imagine their partners not wanting to help. Actually, that's quite possible:

- **Desire difference?** If a significant desire difference plagues your relationship and you have the greater libido, she might fear that when you gain ejaculatory control, you'll want sex even more. If so, negotiate a mutually acceptable sexual frequency and pledge you won't pressure her for more.
- **She might not want sex all night long.** Negotiate how long you last. You can enjoy lasting longer without going all night.
- **Extended intercourse may cause discomfort.** Many women of all ages don't produce much natural vaginal lubrication. Extended intercourse may chafe. Commercial lubricants usually help. But even with lube, few women want sex to last hours.
- **She might fear you'll have affairs and leave her.** If so, the two of you might consider couple counseling or sex therapy.

Other Ways to Treat PE

I don't recommend them, but here they are:

- **Masturbating beforehand.** This works for young men who can raise new erections shortly after ejaculating. After coming solo, the next time they usually last longer. But as the years pass, men need more time to raise subsequent erections. After forty, it may take several hours. Chances are you can learn good control without self-sexing beforehand.
- **Low-dose antidepressants.** Few PE sufferers are seriously depressed, but the most widely prescribed class of antidepressants, the SSRIs (Prozac, Paxil, Zoloft, etc.), share

a side effect of delayed ejaculation. Tinkering with the dose allows some men to last as long as they'd like. Drug treatment means doctor visits. It may be costly and involve medication for the rest of your life. And if you stop taking the medication, PE usually returns. You can probably learn reliable ejaculatory control without drugs. Finally, even when antidepressants help, several studies show that drug treatment plus self-help or sex therapy work better than drugs alone.

- **Topical anesthetics.** PE sufferers' penises are not unusually touch sensitive, but several anesthetic "delay" ointments numb the penis and studies show modest benefit. Men who ejaculate in less than a minute can often last for two or three. However, anesthetics don't teach ejaculatory control. They dull sensitivity, which interferes with both pleasure and self-awareness as you approach your point of no return. They must be applied shortly before intercourse, which may interrupt lovemaking. And some women complain that delay ointments taste bad and ruin fellatio.
- **Acupuncture, supplements, and medicinal herbs.** A few studies suggest that various combinations of acupuncture, supplements (tryptohan, zinc, folic acid), and herbs (among them, *Tribulus terrestris*) help some men last longer. But most men can learn good control without them.

Women Also Benefit—But Not Because Men Last Longer

Recall that only 25 percent of women are consistently orgasmic during intercourse no matter how long it lasts. For the other 75 percent, sex with men who can last all night might be fun, but it's unlikely to bring them to orgasm.

When researchers have surveyed women about how they prefer to make love, most endorse the sexual style that helps men learn ejaculatory control—leisurely, playful, whole-body massage that eventually includes the genitals but is not preoccupied with them. Women often complain that men try to imitate porn, that they're too eager for intercourse, have sex too mechanically, and fixate on women's breasts and genitals. Most women consider the whole body an erotic playground and can't understand why so many men explore only a few corners. The last-longer program teaches men to jettison porn-style sex for the moves most women prefer.

Rushed, mechanical, penis-obsessed, porn-style sex stresses the penis and contributes to involuntary ejaculation. But when men make love the way women prefer, whole-body arousal takes the pressure off the penis and men last longer. It's a win-win. Men get what they want, reliable ejaculatory control. And women get what they want—leisurely, playful, whole-body, massage-based lovemaking.

Premature Orgasm in Women?

Reports of it pepper the internet and one Portuguese study has documented it. Otherwise, at this writing, little is known. If you're a woman who comes before you'd like, try the program in this chapter. If you need more help, consult a sex therapist.

CHAPTER 33:
Trouble Climaxing? How to Resolve Orgasm/Ejaculation Problems

PROBLEMS WITH ORGASM/EJACULATION (O/E) are the flip side of premature ejaculation. Men with PE come too soon. Men with O/E problems have trouble coming at all.

Orgasm is not the goal of lovemaking any more than dessert is the goal of dinner. Many people can eat delicious dinners, skip dessert, and feel fine, even virtuous. Some people can't have orgasms because of pain, disabilities, or neurological conditions. For others, fatigue or major stress—job loss, grieving—might put orgasm beyond reach.

Orgasm, per se, doesn't prove your love, intimacy, or sexual responsiveness. Nor can it redeem sex that's boring, fraught, or abusive. But assuming enjoyable sex—solo or partner—orgasm feels wonderful, and many people believe lovemaking is incomplete without it—dinner without dessert.

Surprisingly Common, Especially after Fifty

O/E issues are men's secret sex problem. Unlike premature ejaculation and erectile dysfunction, no drugs treat it, so doctors, the drug industry, and the media have largely ignored it. But in two surveys involving 2,865 men age eighteen to eighty-five, University of Chicago researchers found that O/E problems occur throughout men's lives, with older men at greatest risk. The two studies show that from age eighteen to sixty, around 10 percent of men experience O/E difficulties. After sixty, prevalence steadily rises. By eighty, one-third of men report the problem.

Men Fake It, Too

The myth is that only women fake orgasm. Depending on the study, up to two-thirds of women say they've pretended to come at least once. Why? To stoke partners' egos, avoid hurting their feelings, sidestep interrogations—*What's wrong with you?*—and dodge accusations of being a lousy lay.

Men also fake orgasms, and for the same reasons. University of Kansas researchers surveyed 180 college men. Those who said they'd faked it at least once—28 percent.

It's not difficult for women to fake it. They just have to moan and thrash. But ejaculation can't be faked, so how can men pretend they've come? Some use condoms and remove them before women notice they're empty. Others explain, *I don't come much when I've been drinking.* . . . And some women have sex so drunk they don't notice.

Many Possible Causes

Orgasm and ejaculation usually occur simultaneously. But different nerves control them. It's possible to come without ejaculation (dry orgasm) and to ejaculate without orgasm (numb come). This discussion assumes that orgasm and ejaculation happen as they usually do, together.

Causes of O/E problems include:

- **Masturbation style.** Some men develop idiosyncratic solo-sex styles, inadvertently training themselves to come only in one particular way. They grip their erections tighter and/or yank harder than most women would without coaching.
- **Alcohol.** Drinking is usually associated with ED, but in some men, it causes O/E problems.
- **"Delivery boy" attitude.** Many men feel chastened by accusations that they just "take" sex from women. Some men overcompensate, developing a "delivery boy" attitude that sex is all about pleasing women. Berkeley, California, sex therapist Bernard Apfelbaum, PhD, says most young to midlife men with O/E problems believe that sex has little to do with their own pleasure, just women's. Preoccupied with their partner's satisfaction, they ignore their own. Washington, DC, sex therapist Barry McCarthy, PhD, explains that many men with this problem don't understand that erection and arousal are different. Men may raise firm erections, but not feel particularly turned on. Erection medications may aggravate this. The drugs increase the likelihood of erection, but may leave men insufficiently aroused to experience O/E.
- **Stress.** Just as emotional stress causes headaches in some men and stomachaches in others, sexual stress may cause PE or ED in some men and O/E difficulties in others. However, sex therapists cite several stressors as frequently associated with O/E problems: anger, relationship problems; unusual fear of PE, ED, or unwanted pregnancy; sexual infections; and fundamentalist upbringing that condemns recreational sex.
- **Infections.** Prostate infection (prostatitis) and STIs may cause pain or other symptoms that inhibit O/E.
- **Depression and antidepressant medication.** The sex problem usually caused by depression is libido loss. But sometimes, it causes O/E problems. In addition, many antidepressant medications cause O/E impairment.
- **Other drug side effects.** Beyond antidepressants, many other medications may impair O/E (chapter 27). If you develop difficulties within a month of starting any new drug, consult the prescribing physician. It might be possible to substitute a less problematic medication.
- **Neurological problems.** Diabetes, multiple sclerosis, paraplegia, and other conditions might damage the nerves that control O/E. But having any of these conditions doesn't doom men to this problem.
- **Aging.** Many men who, when young, struggled to last longer find that, as they age, they last too long. With age, the nervous system becomes less excitable. After fifty or so, increasing numbers of men notice that they need more vigorous and extended self-sexing, fellatio, or intercourse to come. Aging is also associated with a gradual loss of tone in the pelvic floor muscles, the ones involved in O/E. As pelvic-muscle tone wanes, semen may dribble out instead of spurting and orgasms may produce less pleasure. To restore orgasmic intensity, practice Kegel exercises.
- **Surgery for prostate enlargement.** Surgical transurethral resection of the prostate (TURP) doesn't affect orgasm; however, it leaves men with "retrograde ejaculation." Semen no longer spurts from the penis, but backfires into the bladder (dry orgasm).

Semen leaves the body during urination. This causes no ill effects, but the presence of semen may change urine's color and consistency.

Many Women Assume It's *Their* Fault

German researchers surveyed 240 women. Half said men's O/E was "very important" to their sexual satisfaction. But few women understand that O/E problems are quite prevalent. When it develops, they often blame themselves: *I must be unattractive.* Ladies, unless you have serious, chronic relationship issues, his O/E problem probably has nothing to do with you. If you want to help him, support the program in this chapter.

How to Cure O/E Problems

The biological purpose of life is reproduction. For men, that means ejaculating. Your body is hardwired to come, but some men need help learning how. The main teacher is masturbation. Most men with O/E problems have little difficulty self-sexing to climax. If you can't, consult a sex therapist. Assuming you can masturbate to O/E, the key to resolving this problem involves expanding that ability to partner lovemaking.

Sex therapists advise:

- **Start with a checkup.** Tell your doctor about your O/E difficulty. Bring a list of all the drugs you take, both over-the-counter and prescription. Ask if any might contribute to the problem. Ask your pharmacist, too. And check the internet.
- **Don't drink alcohol for an hour or two before lovemaking.** Alcohol may contribute to the problem and interfere with treatment.
- **Masturbate with your pelvis, not just your hand.** Men who masturbate to porn typically sit still, with only one hand moving. Try lying on your side. Keep your hand still and move your pelvis back and forth. This more closely approximates intercourse. Over time, hip thrusting to O/E helps train men to come in the vagina.
- **Get the stimulation you need.** You're more than a delivery boy. You deserve pleasure—and it's okay to be a little selfish to get it. Many young men can have orgasms and ejaculate under any circumstances. But many older men discover that without particular caresses, they may develop O/E problems. Don't insert your erection into erotic openings unless you feel highly aroused. To become highly aroused, you may well need whole-body massage, vigorous penile stroking, extended fellatio, certain intercourse positions, and possibly receptive anal sphincter massage or fingering. If your partner doesn't provide what you need, coach her or consult a sex coach or therapist.
- **Show her how you self-sex.** This often helps men with idiosyncratic masturbation styles. Try polishing pipe with your lover watching. Show her the specific strokes you need to get off. Of course, this may be problematic. You may never have tickled your pickle in front of anyone else. Both of you may feel awkward or embarrassed. If so, admit it—and try to laugh. Remember, you're working together to resolve a problem. Demonstrating how you masturbate shows her what you need.

  It also deepens intimacy through self-revelation. What's more revealing than displaying how you self-sex? Masturbating in front of your partner is a win-win. You're more likely to get what you need to come and you both gain a more intimate relationship.

When wanking for your partner, explain what works for you—the strokes, pressure, and pace that excite you. Pay particular attention to the sensations that bring you to your point of no return when O/E becomes inevitable. Show her what gets you to the edge—and over it.

To heighten arousal, lubricant usually helps. Place some on your hand as you masturbate for her and urge her to use lube as she strokes you.

After she's watched you, place her hand on your penis, cover hers with yours, and show her exactly how you like to be caressed. Physically guide her to provide everything you've demonstrated.

Close your eyes and revisit hot fantasies that have previously helped you climax. They need not include your partner. If she's amenable, you might also watch some porn that excites you. Gently guide her hand with yours several times over a few weeks until she understands how best to help you to get to O/E.

- **She strokes you.** Then withdraw your hand and turn things over to her. She should stroke you in the way(s) you've guided her. She might also use a penis sleeve, a sex toy designed to simulate a woman's vagina or mouth (Fleshlight). Your lover should use lots of lubricant. You coach her as necessary while breathing deeply and enjoying hot fantasies. Do this until she's brought you to O/E several times over a few weeks. If you enjoy receptive anal fingering, that, too, may help trigger O/E. Use lots of lube.
- **Guided fellatio.** Once she can consistently bring you to O/E by hand, experiment with oral sex. Some men find fellatio very exciting by itself. Others need oral with simultaneous shaft stroking and perhaps scrotum fondling and/or anal fingering. Coach her. Tell her exactly what you need to trigger O/E.

  During fellatio, she might also try the "little lick trick." It involves sucking the head for a while, then lightly licking the underside directly below the glans. This area is often highly sensitive. Little licks may help trigger O/E.
- **Tell her which intercourse position(s) provide(s) what you need.** For O/E problems, the man-on-top (missionary) position is usually better than woman-on-top. Sexuality authorities often recommend the latter for lasting longer. It's usually more difficult for men to delay O/E in the man-on-top position, so it's often a good one for men working to resolve O/E difficulties.

For extra stimulation in the missionary position, after insertion, ask your lover to close her legs so you lie atop her thighs, not between them. That way, her inner thighs squeeze your shaft, which may help. If you feel inclined, the man-on-top position also allows the woman to gently massage or finger you anally.

For Yourself

Men with O/E problems may also benefit from a classic self-help book for women who have trouble with orgasm: *Becoming Orgasmic: A Sexual and Personal Growth Program for Women* by Julia Heiman, PhD, and Joseph LoPiccolo, PhD.

Its basic message is that each of us is responsible for our own sexual satisfaction. Lovers can create an erotic context, but no one "gives" anyone else an orgasm. Orgasms come from deep within us. Like laughter, they emerge when we allow ourselves to experience sufficient relaxation and arousal to release them. By all means, shower your lover with erotic generosity. But also ask for the specific caresses *you* need.

You have every right to pleasure—including at times doing nothing but receiving it. Sizzling sex involves give and take. Chances are you've been giving generously, but not receiving enough of what really arouses you. If this situation has persisted for a while, you may also feel resentful, which can aggravate O/E problems.

If you've been so preoccupied with providing pleasure that you haven't allowed yourself to receive it, don't be hard on yourself. Many men come of age believing it's their responsibility to orchestrate sex. That's what you've been doing—only you've gone a bit overboard.

It's not your partner's fault that she hasn't provided you with enough of the stimulation that gets you off. Explain what you need and show her how to provide it.

Happy resolution of O/E challenges hinges on figuring out what you really need, not what you think you "should" need, and not what you think your lover wants to provide, but what actually turns you on, whatever that may be.

If this chapter doesn't provide sufficient relief after a few months, consult a sex therapist.

CHAPTER 34:
The Man's Guide to Firm Erections, and How to Treat Erectile Dysfunction

DURING THE TWENTIETH century, the term was *impotence*, literally powerlessness. Then in 1998, the Food and Drug Administration approved Viagra, and physicians adopted the less pejorative "erectile dysfunction" (ED).

What is ED? Definitions vary, but practically speaking, it's the inability to produce firmness despite vigorous, sustained, fantasy-fueled self-sexing.

Pre-Viagra, ED was poorly researched and little discussed. Today, studies abound. TV commercials tout erection drugs. And ED has become men's most widely publicized sex problem.

Viagra (sildenafil) has competition. Cialis (tadalafil) and Levitra (vardenafil) were approved in 2003, Staxyn (a different formulation of Levitra) in 2010, and Stendra (avanafil) in 2012.

This may come as a surprise, but only a small fraction of older men use erection medication, and fewer than half of those who obtain first prescriptions ever refill them. Most older couples move away from intercourse toward outercourse, the many other ways to make love: mutual whole-body massage, hand jobs, oral sex, toys, and perhaps some kink. If couples jettison intercourse, men don't need erections—but can still enjoy earthquake orgasms.

What Fraction of Men?

It's not clear how many men have ED. Many don't admit it. And definitions of *erection* range from any firming to sufficient turgidity for penis-vagina intercourse. Consequently, prevalence estimates vary. It's confusing—until we analyze the studies.

Let's begin with two oft-cited surveys by University of Chicago researchers. In 1992, they asked a representative 1,410 US men, age eighteen to fifty-nine, if they suffered ED. In 2006, they surveyed another 1,455 men, age fifty-seven to eighty-five. From age eighteen to forty-nine, men admitting ED increased with age from 7 to 11 percent. After fifty, the proportion continued to increase gradually until after sixty-five, when it reached 45 percent.

Now consider the two groups below. In the slightly younger group, 18 percent admitted ED, in the older, 31 percent, substantially more. Why the big difference?

Age	Men admitting ED
50–59	18%
57–64	31%

For ages 18–59: Laumann, E. O., et al. "Sexual Dysfunction among Older Adults: Prevalence and Risk Factors from a Nationally Representative U.S. Probability Sample of Men and Women 57–85 Years of Age." *Journal of Sexual Medicine* 5 (2008): 2300.

Perhaps men suffer a sudden substantial ED increase during their early sixties. However, ED usually develops gradually. No other studies show a big jump during men's early sixties.

Here's the most likely reason for the disparity. The younger men were interviewed in 1992, six years *before* Viagra's approval, when "impotence" was stigmatized and rarely admitted. The older men participated in 2006, eight years *after* approval, when ED was more accepted and more likely to be admitted.

Meanwhile, in 2002, Australian researchers launched the Florey Adelaide Male Aging Study (FAMAS), whose several hundred participants, age sixty-five to eighty-five, have been interviewed repeatedly over many years. The Chicago subjects spoke to researchers just once. The Australian men talked with FAMAS researchers regularly for years. Subject men became comfortable with them and over time presumably more candid. A dozen years after Viagra's approval and many interviews into the study, the FAMAS researchers broached the subject of ED:

Men admitting . . .	Percentage
Any ED ever	91%
Mild chronic ED	54%
Moderate to severe chronic ED	37%

Martin, S., et al. "Clinical and Biopsychosocial Determinants of Sexual Dysfunction in Middle-Aged and Older Australian Men." *Journal of Sexual Medicine* 9 (2012): 2093.

In the Chicago studies, 44 percent of men sixty-five to eighty-five admitted ED, in the Australian group, 61 percent.

Which figures should we believe? I go with the Australian findings. The FAMAS interviews took place more recently, with ED least stigmatized. And by the time the Australian researchers asked about it, the participants felt sufficiently comfortable to open up.

Older men's actual rate of ED probably surpasses the Australian findings. I bet some FAMAS participants felt reluctant to admit it or its severity. But even if we accept the Australian numbers, nine out of ten men over sixty-five appear to have some ED, with more than one-third experiencing moderate to severe problems.

When I've blogged about this, some men over sixty-five have insisted they could still raise firm reliable erections without drugs. *I'm the same as I was at thirty.* I don't doubt them. Nine percent of the Australians reported no ED at all. But they appear to be outliers. It seems safe to say that by sixty—and often earlier—most men suffer some impairment.

Most men's erections start to change during their forties. They stop rising effortlessly from just erotic thoughts. It starts taking work to get hard—active fantasizing with generous fondling and fellatio. This is *not* ED. Sex therapists call it "erection dissatisfaction" and say: *What young men want to do all night takes older men all night to do.* But when men over forty experience anything less than instant porn-star firmness, many fear their erections are history—which may generate enough stress to become a self-fulfilling prophecy.

Why is ED Age Related?

Blame evolution's energy efficiency. The evolutionary mission of life is to perpetuate the species. During the procreative years, the body invests considerable energy in reproduction—in men, erection and ejaculation, and in women, the menstrual cycle, pregnancy, and childbirth.

But after around forty, the body invests less and less energy in reproduction. Women's fertility declines. By their midforties, even with twenty-first century technology, pregnancy is unlikely and after menopause, impossible. And sometime after forty, most men develop iffy erections and, eventually, some manifestation of ED.

Boner Basics

Erections require erotic arousal and healthy nervous and cardiovascular systems (the heart and blood vessels). Few men under forty have problems with arousal or erection. Many young men are almost constantly horny and can get hard spontaneously or from erotic fantasies. But this fades. By men's forties, most men need fondling. During most men's fifties, raising wood takes greater effort, and arousal often becomes an issue. Even when playing with alluring women, men may not feel especially turned on.

Arousal spurs the nervous system to open (dilate) the penile arteries, allowing extra blood to pour in. Problems with the nerve system may derail this, including diabetic neuropathy and sex while drunk.

Assuming arousal and a healthy nervous system, more blood flows into the penis than its veins can drain. Excess blood pools in the spongy tissues of the shaft (the corpus cavernosum and corpus spongiosum) and erections rise hydraulically. As erections develop, the veins that carry blood out of the penis become somewhat compressed, which limits outflow and helps maintain firmness.

The penis is not a balloon with erection knotting the open end. Flaccid or erect, blood flows in and out. During erection, more enters than leaves—unless emotional stress or nerve or arterial damage restrict inflow.

Morning Wood: Why Do Younger Men Wake with Erections?

Almost all young men raise erections while sleeping (nocturnal penile tumescence). Many have several a night. With age, morning erections fade, but many middle-aged and older men continue to notice some morning fullness. Why? That's not clear, but speculation abounds:

- **Sexual arousal?** Possibly, but imaging studies show that male fetuses develop erections in utero when they're presumably presexual.
- **Dreaming?** Deepest sleep is associated with dreaming and spontaneous nighttime ejaculations (wet dreams). Deep sleep may produce erotic dreams that raise morning erections. But many men who wake with wood and remember their dreams don't recall anything sexy.
- **Need to urinate?** Many men wake with full bladders. The penis contains a valve that allows urine to flow when it's flaccid but prevents urination when it's erect. Perhaps the body raises morning wood to prevent bed-wetting. But many men wake with morning wood and feel no need to urinate.
- **Oxygen?** It's possible that the extra blood involved in morning wood delivers extra oxygen to the penis and contributes to the health of its cells. But as men age and morning erections subside, there's no evidence that penile tissue suffers.

Scientists aren't sure why morning erections develop and then fade away. Loss of morning wood is nothing to worry about. But what if you're used to waking with morning erections and they suddenly disappear? First, check your stress load. Severe stress—job loss, financial reversals, serious family or relationship problems, or the death of a loved one—may flood the bloodstream with the stress hormone cortisol, which constricts the arteries in the penis, limiting blood inflow and impairing erection. In that case, stress management may help: meditation, exercise, or professional counseling.

If you're not suffering unusual stress and morning firmness disappears, schedule a checkup, especially if you smoke, are overweight, or have high cholesterol or blood pressure. Loss of morning erections may be an early symptom of diabetes, depression, or heart disease.

ED Risk Factors

Until the 1980s, the vast majority of erection impairment was considered psychological in origin. Today, sexologists understand that it's more likely to develop for medical reasons:

- **Emotional stress.** Anxiety releases cortisol, which constricts the penile arteries, reducing blood inflow. Causes of erection-deflating stress include performance anxiety, relationship turmoil, family problems, job, money, or legal woes, and the stress caused by other sex problems, notably premature ejaculation. Italian scientists analyzed eighteen studies involving 57,229 men. Chronic PE tripled risk of ED.
- **Acute illness or injury.** Don't expect your penis to stand up if you can't. Illness and injury cause stress, fatigue, pain, and other challenges that may impair erection. Decreased sexual interest and function are the body's ways of focusing on healing.
- **Depression.** At some point in life, one American in eight—around 12 percent—suffers debilitating depression. In men, it may cause the classic symptoms: deep melancholy and feelings of helplessness and hopelessness. But male depression may also present with anxiety, anger, insomnia, alcohol or drug abuse, and/or self-harm. Chinese researchers pooled forty-nine studies involving several thousand men. Compared with mentally healthy individuals, men with depression had three times the ED risk.
- **Antidepressants.** Many antidepressant drugs are as erection killing as depression itself. The most popular mood elevators are the selective serotonin reuptake inhibitors (SSRIs), among them: Prozac, Paxil, Zoloft, Luvox, and Celexa. Around 10 percent of male users suffer ED as a side effect. Fortunately, another antidepressant is equally effective, but less likely to cause ED—Wellbutrin (bupropion). If you develop erection trouble within a few weeks after starting an antidepressant, ask your physician if you might switch to Wellbutrin.
- **Atherosclerosis.** Once called hardening of the arteries, atherosclerosis involves the growth of fatty, cholesterol-rich deposits (plaques) on artery walls. Atherosclerosis narrows the penile arteries, reducing blood inflow. It's also the cause of heart disease.
- **Tobacco.** Smoking accelerates atherosclerosis. Smokers have twice nonsmokers' risk of heart disease and substantially greater risk of ED before sixty. But within five years after quitting, the arteries recover, and erections may, too (lung cancer risk remains high much longer.)
- **More than two alcoholic drinks a day.** Alcohol is a leading erection saboteur. A few drinks may not deflate young men, but after fifty, even one beer, glass of wine, or cocktail may hit below the belt. Alcohol impairs arousal and depresses nerve function.

Chronic overindulgence raises blood pressure, damaging the arteries and accelerating atherosclerosis.

- **Sitting.** Sedentary lifestyle is strongly associated with obesity, diabetes, high blood pressure, and heart disease. They all damage the arteries and reduce blood inflow.
- **Meats, cheeses, ice cream, fast food, and junk foods.** They're all high in animal (saturated) fat, the type that's dirtiest for atherosclerosis. However, fruits and vegetables contain no saturated fat and are high in antioxidant nutrients that help maintain arterial health.
- **Obesity.** It takes energy to drag extra weight around, energy the body might otherwise invest in libido and erection. Obesity is also strongly associated with diabetes, high blood pressure, and heart disease, all contributors to ED.
- **Diabetes.** Ninety-five percent of diabetics have type 2 disease, usually caused by a combination of obesity and sedentary lifestyle. Diabetes greatly accelerates atherosclerosis. Compared with healthy men, diabetics face three times the risk of heart disease and considerably greater risk of ED.
- **Obstructive sleep apnea.** Apnea is often caused by excess tissue in the throat, typically the result of obesity. Its hallmark is loud snoring punctuated by choking silences when the extra tissue momentarily blocks the throat, interrupting breathing. This sets off biological alarms that rouse apneics, restoring breathing. But frequent nightly rousings destroy sleep and raise blood pressure. Apnea is a major—and underappreciated—ED risk factor.
- **Prostate cancer treatments.** These include removal of the gland (prostatectomy), hormone therapy, and radiation. All usually impair erection. "Nerve-sparing" surgery is somewhat less likely to leave men with ED, but it's no guarantee of firm erections or sexual satisfaction.
- **Neurological disorders.** Multiple sclerosis, spinal cord injuries, and other conditions may damage erection nerves.
- **Anabolic steroids.** Some athletes and bodybuilders take these drugs to increase muscle mass. Over time, they suppress testosterone, raising ED risk.
- **Significant prostate enlargement before sixty.** As men age, their prostates grow larger (benign prostate hyperplasia, BPH). As the gland expands, it pinches the urine tube (urethra), causing weak stream, trouble getting started and finishing, and the need to get up at night to urinate. Both BPH and ED affect older men, but until this century, physiologists considered them unrelated. Since the early 2000s, a growing body of research has linked early-onset BPH with early-onset erection dissatisfaction and ED.
- **Drugs prescribed for BPH.** Finasteride (Proscar, Propecia) and dutasteride (Avodart) are both associated with increased ED risk. Italian researchers analyzed seventeen studies involving 46,733 men. The two drugs raised risk 50 percent. Unfortunately, few physicians mention this when prescribing them.
- **Gum disease (periodontitis).** Chronic inflammation impairs the body's ability to raise blood levels of nitric oxide, a compound critical to erection. Chronic gum disease causes persistent inflammation. Ten percent of American adults have it. Several studies show that periodontitis is associated with ED, and that as gum disease becomes more severe, so does ED.
- **Vitamin D deficiency.** Several studies show that low vitamin D is associated with ED. Some foods contain this vitamin: mushrooms, tofu, and soy and almond milks. But the skin produces most on exposure to sunlight. Unfortunately, many Americans spend

little time outdoors, and when outside, they slather on sunscreen, which suppresses vitamin D synthesis.

Few men appreciate ED's many risk factors. Swiss urologists surveyed 126 men who complained of erection trouble. Half could not name a single one.

Healthy Lifestyle Helps Preserve Erections

Reducing risk factors helps maintain firm erections. Even an exemplary lifestyle doesn't guarantee wood for life, but healthy living usually postpones ED.

- **Don't use tobacco.** If you smoke, ask your doctor for help quitting. Chinese researchers tracked the sexual function of 719 men intent on quitting. Among those who succeeded, erection function improved significantly within six months.
- **Don't imbibe more than two alcoholic drinks a day.** Don't drink shortly before sex. Don't make love drunk.
- **Get regular moderate exercise.** Health authorities recommend the equivalent of a daily, brisk, thirty- to sixty-minute walk. Don't obsess about the "best" exercise. Just move your body any way you enjoy for at least a half hour every day.
- **Eat more fruits and vegetables.** The typical American man eats only two to three half-cup servings a day. Nutritionists recommend five to nine. A diet high in plant foods reduces risk of atherosclerosis, high blood pressure, stroke, and many cancers. Canadian researchers report that with each daily serving of fruits and vegetables, ED risk drops 10 percent. It's not difficult to eat five a day: one or two servings of fruit at breakfast, a salad with lunch, a salad and vegetable with dinner, and fruit snacks between meals.
- **Eat less animal fat.** That means less beef, pork, lamb, and poultry, and fewer whole-milk dairy products: butter, cheeses, and ice cream. These changes reduce risk of atherosclerosis, obesity, diabetes, and high blood pressure.
- **Eliminate deep-fried and junk foods.** They're high in erection-impairing fats and largely devoid of erection-supporting nutrients.
- **Maintain healthy weight.** This helps prevent atherosclerosis, obesity, diabetes, and high blood pressure. People who lose weight usually report more energy, greater libido, and better sexual functioning.
- **Practice stress management.** Effective approaches include exercise, gardening, meditation, yoga, prayer, tai chi, hot baths, music, and social connections. Deep relaxation contributes to whole-body health, including healthy erections.
- **Get evaluated for obstructive sleep apnea.** If your bedmate says you snore with intermittent silences, ask your doctor to refer you for a sleep study. If you sleep alone and feel drowsy during the day, a sleep study might also be indicated. Sleep apnea can be effectively treated with a device that gently pushes air down the throat, a continuous positive airway pressure machine (CPAP). Swedish researchers prescribed CPAPs for 401 men with apnea and ED. Their sexual function improved significantly. A Chinese study of 207 men with apnea and ED showed similar results.
- **Floss your teeth daily and see a dentist regularly.** This helps prevent gum disease.
- **Take vitamin D.** Discuss dosage with your doctor. Supplements are widely available.

Attention Cyclists: Sit on Wide Seats

Exercise is good for sex. But cycling more than three hours a week on a narrow "banana" seat may cause ED. Fortunately, men can enjoy cycling without erection problems—if they use wide seats.

Starting in the 1980s, case reports appeared describing erection problems in healthy young men who had no risk factors—except a devotion to bicycling. Danish researchers surveyed eight hundred healthy, young adult bike racers. More than three hundred (38 percent) reported difficulty raising erections for a few days after races.

Researchers with the Massachusetts Male Aging Study analyzed cycling among 1,709 men. Less than three hours a week caused no difficulties. In fact, short-duration riding *reduced* ED risk. But bicycling more than three hours a week on banana seats raised risk in all age groups.

While seated, the buttock bones (sit bones, ischial tuberosities) bear your weight. But cyclists using banana seats bear weight on the soft tissue between the scrotum and anus (perineum). Over time, this injures the nerves and arteries involved in erection. The first sign of trouble is numbness or tingling in the groin after riding.

Since researchers noticed the banana seat-ED link, bike manufacturers have developed wider seats that prevent this problem. Use a seat wide enough to bear your weight on your sit bones. Also, tilt your seat down and handlebars up. This deters leaning forward, which compresses the penile nerves and arteries. And periodically, ride standing.

Women should also opt for wide seats. Stanford researchers surveyed 178 women cyclists. More than half reported genital pain, numbness, and sex problems.

Erection Impairment throughout the Lifespan

According to the American Urological Association (AUA), ED involves "the inability for at least three months to achieve or maintain erection sufficient for satisfactory sexual performance."

That's vague. If you define "erection" as the pipe you see in porn and "satisfactory performance" as porn sex—instant erections that last forever, never wilt, and come on cue—then it's a rare man who *doesn't* have ED. Erections change throughout the lifespan, and so do difficulties with them.

Men under forty. The myth is that young men don't develop ED. Actually, some do—usually because of injury, illness, or less-than-healthy lifestyle—smoking starting in their teens, obesity, early type 2 diabetes, or other risk factors (above). Or they may be superanxious about their penis size or other issues, for example, so-called "sex addiction."

Men forty to sixty. Around 10 percent of men notice no middle-age erection changes, but from forty to sixty, most erections change. After decades of reliable firmness from erotic thoughts alone, that ability fades, and men need fondling. When midlife erections rise, they may not become sufficiently firm for intercourse. And minor distractions may deflate them—a phone ringing, an ambulance siren.

As ED risk factors increase in number and severity, midlife men are likely to develop erection changes closer to forty than sixty.

When middle-aged men develop erection changes, some decide it's the end of sex, often to their partners' chagrin. But most can still raise erections solo, so technically the problem is not erectile dysfunction, but erection dissatisfaction. Whatever the term, few men are prepared for midlife erection changes, and many jump to the mistaken conclusion that they have ED.

Men over sixty. Even if they have healthy lifestyles, older men face increasing likelihood of ED. Fortunately it's often treatable (below).

If men over sixty have partners, they are likely to be postmenopausal. They may suffer vaginal dryness and/or atrophy that may make intercourse uncomfortable or impossible even with lubricant. Consequently, most older couples evolve their lovemaking away from intercourse to outercourse. If couples no longer do the deed, men don't need erections.

In addition, many men over sixty develop arousal difficulties. Trouble getting turned on complicates erection issues. *I'm not even interested, so why hassle with erection?* Fortunately, with deep relaxation and whole-body massage, arousal difficulties usually resolve.

Erection Myths—and Truths
Several fallacies mislead many men (and women)—and may cause sufficient stress to contribute to ED.

MYTH: Men "achieve" erections. Recall the AUA's definition: "inability to achieve erection." But how exactly do men "achieve" them? Most take erections for granted until midlife, then strain for the little guy's cooperation. The struggle to "achieve" erection is counterproductive. It generates stress that constricts the very blood vessels you want to dilate. Forget "achieving" erections. You can't will or force them. Instead, do the *opposite* of achieving—relax deeply and enjoy extended loveplay.

MYTH: Sex is a performance. The AUA definition also mentions "sexual performance." But "performance" may have pernicious implications. It makes men feel they're being watched and judged. Actually, viewing sex as a performance invites what sex therapists call "spectatoring." Instead of feeling fully present, sex becomes an out-of-body experience. Part of the man is making love, while the rest of him is a spectator at a show, observing and criticizing.

Spectatoring is distracting and stressing. Sizzling sex is not a theater full of critics. It's *play*. It works best when lovers focus on giving and receiving pleasure. There's no audience, no reviews, no booing. It's just the two of you playing together.

MYTH: Men are sex machines. This assumes men are so easily aroused that any female attention triggers trouser bulges. That may be true for teens and young adults, but when stiffies become iffy, when arousal is no longer automatic, like most women, most men develop conditions that must be met before they can feel sufficiently turned on to get hard.

Men's conditions for erection vary, but typically include privacy, comfort, safety, deep relaxation, an alluring partner, a romantic setting, no distractions, specific erotic moves, and perhaps toys and some kink (parts V and VI).

It's perfectly normal to have preconditions for sex. It's unusual not to. Many men love to attend major league baseball games—but not in driving rain. If conditions aren't inviting, penises may rebel, especially those attached to men over forty.

MYTH: You get just one shot at erection. If you wilt, sex is over and you're a failure. During lovemaking after forty, erections may subside. Try not to think, *It's all over. I failed.* Instead, breathe deeply, ask your lover for caresses you enjoy, and focus on arousing fantasies. You'll probably refirm.

Many women also believe that men "should" remain hard throughout shagging. If erections soften, they may doubt their desirability. Ladies, it's perfectly normal for erections to soften in the midst. When men deflate, what most usually need is more massage all over and vigorous penis caressing by hand or mouth.

MYTH: I blew it last time. I'll never get it up again. When professional baseball players strike out, are their careers kaput? It's disconcerting to be anything but rock hard. But it's a mistake to overgeneralize a single letdown to a lifetime of ED. Analyze what caused your deflation. Work to correct it—see Risk Factors (page 255).

MYTH: If men can't raise erections, women can't be satisfied. Men who believe this myth put tremendous pressure on themselves. The stress can wreak havoc on little buddies. Most women's satisfaction depends less on firm erections than on men's creative use of their tongues.

MYTH: If men can't raise erections, they can't come. Actually, different nerves control erection and orgasm. Men can have earthquake orgasms *without* erections. Most paraplegic men can't raise erections, but with sufficiently vigorous penile stimulation by hand, mouth, or toy, they can still have orgasms. Ditto for prostate cancer survivors.

Men and Women Often View ED Differently

Men tend to view ED as a mechanical problem and look for quick fixes, for example, drugs. Women usually view it as a relationship problem. They want to discuss it, then despair if men withdraw into silence.

Gentlemen, whether or not medication helps, don't clam up. Silence makes women feel abandoned and undesirable. For most women, erection difficulties are usually less problematic than men's reactions to them.

Instead of moping, discuss your feelings, and ask about hers. Do you have ED risk factors? If you have sexual issues or relationship problems, discuss them. Consider sex coaching or therapy.

Women involved with ED sufferers should not say, *Oh honey, it doesn't matter.* Assuming he provides generous clitoral caresses that help you to orgasm, his ED may not matter much to you. But it matters a great deal to him. Don't blame yourself. The two of you may have sexual or relationship issues, but his problem is not your fault. Reassure him that his ED doesn't cancel your love or make him less of a man. Help him assess his risk factors. Accompany him to doctor visits. Offer to contact a sex coach or therapist. And if his ED can't be treated, outercourse still offers you both pleasure and orgasms.

Women, Porn, and Erections

Over the decades, I've received many distraught inquiries from women complaining that their midlife men prefer yanking to porn over lovemaking with them. Part VII discusses porn in detail, but I'll correct one common misconception here—the notion that porn appeals only to horny boys and lonely single men. Actually, most men of all ages, single and coupled, watch regularly, with one hand in motion. PornHub.com, among the world's largest porn sites, attracted 33.5 *billion* views in 2018, more than 100 million a day. The site analyzes its audience by age. Among US viewers:

Age	Percentage of PornHub audience
18–24	21%
25–34	31%
35–44	20%
45–54	14%
55–64	9%
65+	5%

PornHub statistics, 2018.

One-third of viewers are over forty. Older men want reassurance that they can still become aroused and get it up. That's easiest solo with visual aids.

Most older coupled men love their partners and don't want to hurt them. But partner sex is more complicated than solo play, especially for those with erection concerns. So they find solace in masturbation, which requires erotic fantasies. Their own get stale, so they turn to porn.

Their partners confront them. *Don't you want me anymore?* Many midlife women fear loss of desirability and can't comprehend men's attraction to porn. To midlife men, women's anguish is regrettable but largely beside the point. They wank because they always have. Porn makes it more enjoyable. And in midlife, solo play provides reassurance that they're still functional.

I'm not for a moment excusing men who unilaterally withdraw from partner sex. Spouses must negotiate sexual frequencies both can live with. But even when older couples agree on frequency, erection worries impel many older men to stroke to porn. I wish more women understood that the reason usually has less to do with their desirability than with their spouses' erection anxieties.

Coping with Age-Related Erection Changes
Fortunately, men with iffy midlife erections and ED can still enjoy sizzling sex:

- **Forget quickies and spontaneous sex.** Unless you've just fallen madly in love, sex after forty usually takes time and planning. Schedule it. This may require adjustments, but once couples adapt, scheduled sex usually feels marvelous and helps midlife men make the most of remaining erection function.
- **Before making love, enjoy quality nonsexual time together.** Absence makes the heart grow fonder. Presence does, too. Before you boink, have fun together—whatever you both enjoy.
- **For several hours before sex, don't drink alcohol.** Or at least limit consumption. Alcohol is a major erection killer.
- **Bathe or shower together beforehand.** It's deeply relaxing, therefore erection enhancing.
- **Be patient with your penis.** It's fine to be flaccid when you hit the sheets. Breathe deeply. Kiss and cuddle. Touch each other all over. Ask for the touch you enjoy. Use lube. Go down on each other. Savor novelty. Enjoy vivid fantasies. Most women prefer leisurely extended loveplay. After forty, it also helps most men's erections.
- **Feather your love nest.** Young men can have sex almost any time anywhere. But most older men benefit from privacy, comfort, clean sheets, no distractions, and possibly candles, music, lingerie, and toys.

- **Consider erection medication.** When men over forty complain of balky erections, doctors are quick to offer drugs. If you can take them safely and tolerate their side effects, fine. But erection drugs don't guarantee happy humping (below).
- **Erection dissatisfaction may *enhance* lovemaking.** Young men typically become aroused faster than young women, and often finish before their ladies have even warmed up to genital play. Men who successfully adjust to midlife erection changes slow the pace, allowing sufficient time to become aroused and firm. Slower pace matches most women's preferences, increasing older couples' erotic compatibility.

If you become chronically distraught about balky midlife erections or ED, consider sex coaching or therapy.

ED? Or a Lengthening Refractory Period?

After orgasm/ejaculation, erections subside, and it takes men a while to raise new ones (refractory period, RP). In teens, RPs may last only minutes, but from the twenties on, duration steadily increases. Among men over forty, RPs may last several hours; over fifty, as long as a day. Some men want a second go before their RPs have run their course. They have trouble getting it up or can't, leading many to decide they must have ED when the real culprit is lengthening RP.

Use masturbation to assess your RP. Once you know its duration, schedule self-sexing and partner sex so they don't interfere with each other. Your erections should improve.

At Your Doctor's Office

For suspected ED, start with a checkup. Unfortunately, when men say "erection," some physicians prescribe drugs without thorough workups.

Medical conditions cause a substantial proportion of ED—see Risk Factors (page 255). Erection trouble may be the first sign of cardiovascular disease. You should be worked up for all medical possibilities.

Bring a list of every medication you take: over-the-counter, prescription, and recreational. List dosages. Be honest about your drinking and use of other recreational drugs.

Doctors should:

- **Ask for specifics.** When did the problem start? How? What else has been happening in your life? Can you raise erections solo? Do you ever wake with morning wood? Do you have problems with all women? Or just some?
- **Review your medical history.** Relevant items include your age, weight, cholesterol, blood pressure, smoking, drinking, medications, recent illnesses, BPH, and history of diabetes, heart disease, prostate problems, chronic pain, high blood pressure, and hormonal or neurological conditions.
- **Review your psychological history.** Anxiety? Depression? Relationship problems?
- **Order tests.** The doctor should take your blood pressure and order tests for cholesterol, blood sugar, thyroid function, and possibly others.
- **Measure testosterone at different times of day.** Many men believe ED suggests testosterone deficiency. Review the discussion of testosterone (page 204). Levels fluctuate markedly during the day. One reading may suggest deficiency, but what counts is the

average of several readings taken at different times. No evidence suggests that testosterone deficiency has increased in recent years. But since 2000, prescriptions have more than doubled. This suggests overprescribing. In men in the normal range, extra testosterone does *not* boost erections.

A Brief Guide to Erection Medications

Erection medications relax the smooth muscle tissue surrounding the arteries that carry blood into the penis. The arteries dilate, increasing inflow.

Advantages:
- **Reasonably effective.** The drugs produce at least semifirm erections in half to three-quarters of users.
- **Private.** Women don't know.
- **Easy to use.** Just swallow a pill.
- **Fast acting.** Stendra starts working within fifteen to thirty minutes, Viagra, Levitra, Cialis, and Staxyn within an hour or so.
- **Duration.** Cialis works for thirty-six hours—just one pill before weekend getaways. The others last around four hours.
- **Most causes.** Most ED results from atherosclerosis, nerve damage, and/or severe psychological stress. The drugs help with ED caused by everything except nerve damage.
- **Fondling necessary.** No walking around with an embarrassing trouser bulge. To work, the drugs require loveplay.
- **Reasonably safe.** Some men should never take erection drugs (see sidebar), but for men who can take them, serious problems are unlikely. Common side effects include headache (16 percent of users), flushing (10 percent), upset stomach (7 percent), nasal congestion (4 percent). Rare but possible side effects include persistent painful erections (priapism) and hearing and vision loss (largely in diabetics).
- **Cost.** If covered by health insurance, they're reasonably affordable. Check your plan. As patent protections expire and generics become available, prices should drop.

Disadvantages:
- **Not all men can take them.** In men taking nitrate medication, erection drugs may prove fatal (see sidebar).
- **Best on an empty stomach.** If you take them after big meals, they may not work as well.
- **Often ineffective.** They don't work for 25–50 percent of users. As ED severity increases, effectiveness decreases. Even in men with mild balkiness, they may not work if you feel ill, fatigued, stressed, or turned off by the woman or the sex.

In Some Men, Erection Drugs Can Be *Fatal*

Since Viagra's approval, more than 1,800 users have died while using it. Most were also taking nitrate medication—the party drug amyl nitrate ("poppers") or nitroglycerine to treat angina. The combination of erection medication and nitrate drugs may cause a rapid, fatal drop in blood pressure. If you take nitrate medication, *never* take erection drugs.

- **Nerve damage.** If penile nerves become damaged—by diabetes, paraplegia, or prostate cancer surgery—the drugs may not work.
- **Porn erections unlikely.** Even when they work, the drugs may not produce superfirm erections.
- **Not aphrodisiacs.** Erection medications don't boost sexual desire or arousal.
- **Side effects.** Though usually mild, side effects may be problematic. Rising dosage increases their likelihood and severity.
- **Slightly increased risk of heart attack and stroke.** Erection drugs may increase risk of the internal blood clots that trigger heart attacks and most strokes. If you're at high risk for either, you doctor might advise avoidance or an anticoagulant.
- **Over time, higher doses.** University of Alabama researchers tracked 150 men who took Viagra regularly for at least two years. One-third had to increase their dose from 50 to 100 mg. The same is presumably true for the other drugs.

The Most Popular Erection Drug: *Not Viagra*

Viagra ranks among the world's most recognized brands, up there with Coca-Cola. But users prefer Cialis. In a dozen studies, men tried both and preferred Cialis three to one. In studies that included Levitra, Cialis was substantially more popular than either competitor.

Women also prefer Cialis. In four studies, couples sampled all three drugs. In every trial, the women strongly preferred Cialis.

Why? Cialis lasts longer. The others are effective for around four hours, but Cialis lasts thirty-six. Both men and women say Cialis allows them to take their eyes off the clock.

Cialis is advantageous for new lovers still in the hot-and-heavy period who value spontaneity. But it's also the choice of long-term spouses who are more likely to schedule sex. The larger window of opportunity makes for friendlier negotiations. *Tonight?* No, I'm exhausted. *Tomorrow?* Sure.

Surprise: Few Older Men Use Erection Drugs

Viagra's 1998 approval triggered the most frenzied new-drug launch in history. Analysts forecast sales of $5 billion a year. However, by a decade later, sales of all brands reached only half that, $2.5 billion annually. Today, they still remain far below original projections. Of course, billions a year is real money. But older men haven't flocked to erection medication in anywhere near the numbers pundits initially predicted.

The fact is, older men just aren't that into erection drugs. German researchers surveyed 3,124 men over fifty. Forty percent admitted ED. Of that group, 96 percent could name at least one erection medication, but only 9 percent had ever tried one. Cornell scientists surveyed 6,291 older men. Almost half—48 percent—reported some ED. But only 7 percent had tried a drug. And when men filled prescriptions, fewer than half ever refilled them.

Reasons men don't refill:

Effectiveness exaggerated. In preapproval studies of three thousand men, manufacturers claimed significant benefit for 70 percent of users. But a review of fourteen postapproval trials involving eighteen thousand men tells a different story. Some confirmed the 70 percent finding, but several showed success rates closer to 50 percent. The surprisingly low rate of refills suggests the drugs are less effective than advertised.

What does "effectiveness" mean? Manufacturers consider the medications effective when users are able to stuff semifirm erections into well-lubricated vaginas. But many men expect porn-star poles—and feel disappointed.

No instant erections. In porn, men unzip and out pops pipe. Because of porn, many men believe that erections should rise instantly to full firmness. In young men, they might, but with age, this becomes increasingly less likely. To work, the drugs require loveplay. Men expecting instant erections might decide they don't work.

Not aphrodisiacs. Many users get hard, but don't feel especially aroused. The drugs aid erection, but that's all. They neither pique libido nor stoke arousal. Men who expect an aphrodisiac are likely to feel disappointed.

Side effects underestimated. In preapproval trials, Viagra's manufacturer claimed side effects were rare. Some postapproval trials agree, but others show that as many as 40 percent of users also experience headache, flushing, upset stomach, and nasal congestion. The drugs may also produce serious side effects. In addition to the nitrate issue, an analysis ten years after Viagra's approval linked it to 2,500 nonfatal heart attacks and more than 25,000 other problems, notably ministrokes and, among diabetics, possible hearing and vision loss.

No help for damaged relationships. If relationship problems ruin sex, firm erections don't fix things. The couple needs therapy. The combination of drugs and sex therapy works better than drugs alone:

- University of California investigators gave eighty-three ED sufferers Viagra or the drug plus one ninety-minute class on erection preservation. After six months, those in the class showed significantly greater improvement.
- University of Washington investigators worked with forty-four couples struggling with ED. The men took Viagra and half the couples also received eight weeks of sex therapy. The combination group enjoyed better erections and greater satisfaction.
- Researchers at the Center for Sexual Health in San Jose, California, gave fifty-three couples either Viagra or the drug plus eight weeks of sex therapy. Using the drug alone, 38 percent expressed satisfaction, but in the combination group, 66 percent.
- At the University of Sao Paulo, Brazilian researchers analyzed eleven studies comparing Viagra alone versus the drug plus sex therapy. In every trial, combination treatment worked significantly better.

While many reasons explain the low rate of prescription refills, another question is more intriguing: Why have so many older men—around 90 percent—never tried erection drugs?

One reason is cost. If not covered by health insurers, they start at $50 per dose. But the main reason reflects the sexual changes of later life. Most older couples who remain sexual decide they'd rather play without intercourse, so who needs drugs?

Erection medications will, no doubt, continue to generate sales in the billions—in part because many men in their thirties and forties use them. But the drugs were developed for men over fifty—and surprisingly few are interested. Ironically, it has taken drugs focused exclusively on erections and intercourse to show the world that most older lovers move beyond erections and intercourse.

"Viagra-Vation:" Revived Erections May Cause Strife

When the drugs work, they may upset the status quo. If ED allowed men to avoid sex, the drugs eliminate that excuse. The drugs may also exacerbate desire differences. And when men's erections return, women may fear infidelity. Finally, if men with resurrected erections are involved with postmenopausal women with vaginal dryness and atrophy, intercourse may feel uncomfortable or impossible.

Couples returning to sex after ED should proceed slowly. Don't rush into intercourse. Review chapters 5–10. Erection restoration is no guarantee of sizzling sex. For Viagra-vation, consider sex therapy.

Other Treatments

Think of ED treatment as a ladder, with drugs the highest rung. Before you get there, consider trying the following.

Healthier lifestyle. Review chapter 2 and the information earlier in this chapter.

Reach out. Tell your lover how you feel. Ask how she feels. If you have relationship or sexual issues, work on them, perhaps with professional help. ED treatment is a team effort.

Ask for the touch you need. Review chapter 6. If you like to be caressed in particular ways, say so. Take turns giving and receiving pleasure. When it's your turn to receive, relax and enjoy it.

New fantasies. Over time, men's own erotic fantasies get stale. Try dreaming up hot new ones.

Penis rings. These sex toys—plastic donuts or leather straps—circle the penis tightly. The arteries that carry blood into the penis run through its central shaft, so rings don't reduce it. But one of the veins that carries blood out lies close to the skin. Rings compress it, reducing outflow. Rings also reassure some men, which aids relaxation. The main risk is bruising if rings are too tight. Some are adjustable.

Penis pumps/vacuum constriction devices. These appliances include plastic tubes that fit over the penis and squeeze-bulb pumps. Working the bulb evacuates air from the tube drawing blood into the organ. Once erect, you roll on a penis ring. Stop pumping, and erections last from five to twenty minutes. Possible side effects include penile numbing or a feeling of cold. Pumps are available from sex toy catalogs.

The key to pump success is a tight seal around the base of the penis. If sex toy pumps don't provide it, urologists can prescribe custom-fitted pumps (vacuum constriction devices, VCDs). After couples adjust, most studies show considerable effectiveness, even in men with nerve damage. The AUA endorses VCDs.

Penis extenders or prosthetic penis attachments (PPAs). Extenders are penis-shaped dildos with hollow bases. Insert a semi-erect penis inside, and the toy enables intercourse.

Strap-on dildos. In porn, only women use strap-ons—almost always on other women. But men with ED may also use them. Strap-ons include harnesses worn around the waist or hips and a front piece that sits over the base of the pelvis. A special dildo attaches to the base, allowing the user to enjoy the hip movements of intercourse.

Kegel exercises. Some studies suggest that Kegels help treat ED.

Professional help. Sometimes, sex coaching or therapy is sufficient. Australian sex therapists worked with thirty-two men suffering moderate to severe ED. After just ten sessions, half reported significant benefit—without drugs.

Yohimbine. Review chapter 27. In 1988, ten years before Viagra, the FDA approved yohimbine for ED—brand names yohimbine, Testomar, Aphrodyne, and Yocon. Yohimbine is not as effective as the Viagra family of drugs, but it may help. Possible side effects include increased heart rate and blood pressure, fluid retention, nervousness, irritability, headache, dizziness, tremor, and flushing. Yohimbine is available over the counter where supplements are sold, but supplements rarely contain therapeutic doses. If you're interested, obtain a prescription.

L-arginine. The amino acid L-arginine is the precursor of nitric oxide, a compound crucial to erection. Several studies show that supplementation helps treat ED. University of Hawaii researchers gave a placebo or ArginMax, a supplement containing L-arginine, ginseng, and ginkgo (below), to fifty-two men with ED. A month later, 24 percent of the placebo group reported improvement; in the ArginMax group, 84 percent.

ArginMax may also improve the effectiveness of erection drugs. Researchers at University of California, Davis, told ED sufferers disappointed with Viagra to try the drug with either a placebo or ArginMax. After four weeks, 22 percent of those taking the placebo reported improvement; among ArginMax users, 60 percent. L-arginine is available at supplement outlets.

South Korean researchers analyzed ten studies of arginine (1,500–5,000 mg/day). Compared with placebo treatment, supplementation "significantly improved ED."

Ginkgo. This medicinal herb improves blood flow throughout the body, including the penis. University of California, San Francisco, researchers gave ginkgo (209 mg/day) to thirty men with antidepressant-induced ED. After one year, 76 percent regained their erections. Other trials agree.

Ginseng. For centuries, Asians have considered ginseng a sex enhancer. Some evidence suggests it promotes release of nitric oxide. Korean researchers gave forty-five ED sufferers a placebo or Korean red ginseng, the root peeled, steam heated, and sun dried (900 mg three times a day). The ginseng group experienced significantly greater improvement. Ginseng is safe for most men. However, this study used a large dose that may cause nervousness and restlessness. Ginseng also has blood thinning (anticoagulant) action. If you take anticoagulant drugs, or regularly use aspirin, garlic, or vitamin E, you may experience bruising or bleeding. Consult your physician.

Maca. The Incas used this Andean ground cover to boost livestock fertility. Spanish conquistadors dubbed it a sex enhancer. Italian investigators gave fifty men with mild to moderate ED either a placebo or maca (1,200 mg of powdered root twice daily). After twelve weeks, the maca group reported greater firmness.

Saffron. Three Iranian studies suggest that saffron helps treat ED. Saffron is expensive, but in these studies, a daily pinch (15–30 mg) helped.

Alprostadil (prostaglandin E1). Used ten minutes before intercourse, this compound is a powerful, natural artery dilator that produces hour-long erections. Two formulations are available—MUSE and intracavernosal injection (ICI). MUSE involves inserting a pellet into the urethra. ICI involves self-injecting the compound into the penile shaft. Numerous studies confirm effectiveness, but few men can imagine doing what's required. Seventy percent of men who try alprostadil stop within two years. Men most likely to continue are diabetics used to self-injecting insulin. Many alprostadil users combine it with erection medication. Consult your physician.

Low-intensity shockwave therapy (LIST). For fractures and heart disease, LIST coaxes the body to produce new blood vessels that aid healing. LIST also improves erections in some men with ED:

- Israeli researchers tested LIST on twenty-nine men with moderate to severe ED, average age sixty-one. Seventy-two percent reported erections firm enough for intercourse.
- Chinese and University of California, San Francisco, researchers analyzed fourteen LIST/ED studies with 833 participants. "The evidence showed improvement."

LIST takes around twenty minutes. Doctors apply a gel to the penis then press a wave-generating probe into the gel, moving it around the shaft. Treatment causes no pain, just a tingling sensation. No significant side effects have been reported.

LIST is not available everywhere. Talk to your physician or urologist.

Penile implants. Implants require surgery. Two types are available: flexible rods and nested hydraulic cylinders.

Rods are the simpler option. The surgeon opens the penile shaft, removes erectile tissue, and inserts a flexible plastic rod. Afterward, recipients have permanent erections. Ordinarily, men bend them down so firmness is inconspicuous. During sex, they bend them up for fellatio or intercourse. However, the surgery may cause infection, scarring, and disfigurement. And the rod may cause embarrassment if you wear tight clothing or undress in a locker room.

The hydraulic approach produces more natural looking results, but mechanically it's more complicated. The surgeon inserts three elements: nested cylinders into the penile shaft, a saltwater reservoir into in the lower abdomen, and a squeeze pump into the scrotum. The flaccid penis usually looks normal. For erection, the man squeezes the bulb and fluid from the reservoir fills the cylinders, producing erection. After ejaculation, a release valve returns the fluid to the reservoir. Hydraulic implant surgery may cause infection and deform the penis, and implants may malfunction, necessitating corrective surgery. Researchers at the University of California, San Diego, reviewed the experiences of 7,666 men who'd opted for prostheses. Within ten years, 16 percent—one in six—required additional surgery to fix problems.

Few men opt for penile implants—and the proportion who do has fallen. Using Medicare records, Cornell researchers discovered that from 2001 to 2010, the proportion choosing implants fell by half.

If you want to know more about these surgeries, contact a urologist and your health insurer. Few policies cover implant surgery.

Never Buy Erection Drugs on the Internet

Most men have seen the internet ads: *Generic Viagra! No prescription needed!* Don't reach for your credit card. Researchers bought purported erection drugs from twenty-two websites. Chemical analysis showed 77 percent were counterfeit.

- Most pills looked genuine, but more than three-quarters contained less than half the dose the label claimed.
- Erection drugs are available only by prescription. No site asked to see one.
- No site warned that taking the drugs in combination with nitrate medications can prove fatal.
- No site included FDA-required package inserts with information about dosage, safety, and side effects.
- Almost all sites (91 percent) claimed to sell "generic Viagra." But at the time of the study, there was no generic Viagra.

If you want erection medication, obtain a prescription and buy from a pharmacy.

PART IV:
A Man's Guide to Women's Sexuality

CHAPTER 35:
Men and Women:
More Similar Than Different

WHEN NEGOTIATING SEXUAL relationships, as author John Gray, PhD, has opined, men and women often seem to hail from different planets—men from Mars, women from Venus. Yes, from initial infatuation to golden anniversaries, sexual relationships are huge challenges that require constant negotiation and endless mutual accommodation.

Yet, despite inevitable conflicts and the substantial risk of breakups, couples continue to fall in love and cavort between the sheets, many happily for decades. The gender chasm can be bridged. Despite their differences, people of all genders want pretty much the same attributes in lovers.

How Similar? How Different?
University of Wisconsin investigators analyzed more than 100 studies of what men and women desire in lovers. The upshot: the genders are considerably more similar than different.

- **Sexual satisfaction.** The analysis showed scant gender differences in overall sexual satisfaction.
- **Age at first intercourse.** Before 1970, most men lost their virginity a few years earlier than most women. But since the 1990s, the average age for everyone has been between sixteen and seventeen.
- **Frequency.** Dozens of studies show that men report more partner sex than women. But virtually every time a man does it, a woman does too, so what accounts for the difference? Men like to think of themselves as studs and tend to overestimate their frequency. Meanwhile, to avoid feeling slutty, women tend to underestimate frequency. In addition, as related in chapter 25, at some point in life, an estimated 15–20 percent of male Americans patronize sex workers, who number less than 1 percent of the adult female population. Many men's estimates include sex worker encounters. But sex workers often elude researchers, so their great frequency doesn't get tabulated. This raises men's average and reduces women's.

The Wisconsin review found gender differences in frequency significant—but only until age thirty. Then they largely vanish and the genders report fairly similar frequencies. Men report intercourse a little more often with slightly more partners (including sex workers), but given widespread belief in a huge gender gap, the actual differences are surprisingly small.

- **Oral sex.** From World War II through the 1960s, fellatio and cunnilingus (especially the latter) marked the sexual frontier. Today, oral is far from ubiquitous, with women still getting shortchanged on cunnilingus. But the substantial majority of lovers have given and received it, with shrinking gender differences.

- **Sexual regret.** In patriarchal cultures, women have always been more sexually constrained—and their violations of sexual norms more severely punished. So we would expect women to feel more sexual regret from lost opportunities and costly mistakes. In studies before 1960, this was the case. But since then, in the West, women have made major, though incomplete, strides toward social and sexual equality, and their sexual regret has decreased. Today, men and women report much smaller differences.
- **Extramarital sex.** The myth is that men have affairs and women don't. It's difficult to study stepping out. Even in anonymous surveys, many don't admit it. But the analysis showed a consensus—about 25 percent of men and 15 percent of women have had affairs, a smaller difference than the conventional wisdom suggests.
- **Masturbation.** Another subject that's difficult to research. Men yank the shank more than women butter the biscuit. But recent research shows converging rates of admitted self-pleasuring. The best current estimate is that during the past year, among those fourteen or older, 70 percent of men and 55 percent of women admit having masturbated, another difference that's smaller than the platitudes imply.

Are men really from Mars and women from Venus? It often feels that way, but surprisingly, the genders occupy largely common sexual ground between those two planets. Turns out men and women are both from Earth.

Sizzling Sex: Women Usually Know Best

Compared with most men, most women have a better intuitive understanding of high-quality sex, notably about the importance of whole-body loveplay.

Why do women usually know best? They're less influenced by testosterone and porn, and they place greater value on gentle loving touch.

As discussed in chapter 46, most men get much of their sex education from pornography or from friends heavily influenced by it. Porn is an efficient masturbation aid, but many men treat it as a sexual textbook. Actually, porn presents male sexual fantasies. It's a cartoon version of lovemaking as realistic as Superman flying. Way too many men consider porn a how-to manual and try to imitate it. Big mistake. Porn teaches sex all wrong.

Meanwhile, most women intuitively prefer lovemaking based on mutual massage of every square inch of the body. That's the type of lovemaking sexologists recommend, the sexual style that produces the greatest satisfaction. When men make love the way most women prefer, everyone is likelier to enjoy sizzling sex.

CHAPTER 36:
A Man's Guide to Women's Bodies

MEN KNOW WHAT goes where, but beyond that, many are in the dark about women's bodies and how men can enhance—or ruin—women's sexual pleasure.

Women's Deepest Sexual Insecurity

Data analyst Seth Stephens-Davidowitz, PhD, uses online searches to investigate America's greatest anxieties. He analyzed one month of Google sex searches and discovered that women search "vagina" almost as frequently as men search "penis size."

Women's biggest concern—odor. Women worry that what's down there smells like fish, vinegar, onions, ammonia, garlic, cheese, body odor, urine, or bleach. This worry sells tons of douches. Ladies, with regular bathing, your vaginas smell and taste fine. Gentlemen, I urge you to provide frequent reassurance: *You smell wonderful and taste delicious.*

After vaginal odor, women are most anxious about their physical appearance—and all the flaws they inevitably perceive. Turkish researchers surveyed 329 women, age nineteen to fifty-two, about their appearance and sexual functioning. As the number of features they considered unattractive increased—particularly weight, scars, and prominent bellies, thighs, and/or butts—their sexual function and satisfaction decreased. Gentlemen, you can never say this too often: *You are so desirable. I want you.*

Men's Breast Fascination—and Women's

Many men are obsessed with women's breasts:

- A huge vocabulary reflects men's interest: tits, titties, boobs, jugs, hooters, knockers, melons, cantaloupes, mounds, peaches, globes, knobs, headlights, mammaries, balloons, garbanzos, milkers, bazooms, ta-tas, chest toys, fun bags, the girls, the twins, and more.
- Many women complain that in conversations, men gaze at their breasts, not their faces. A New Zealand study that tracked men's eye movements supports this.
- Women bar and restaurant servers say revealing tops bring bigger tips.
- French researchers fitted women with various size padded bras and sent them to cafés where they sat alone. As bra size increased, so did the number of men who approached them.

Just as some women want men of a certain height, some men want women with a certain breast size—small, medium, or large. But when women shed their bras, most men love whatever emerges. That's what researchers at UCLA and Cal State Los Angeles found in an online survey of 52,227 heterosexual adults. Most of the men (56 percent) said they were "satisfied with their partners' breasts."

The Many Hazards of Douching

Ads for feminine hygiene products tout "that clean, fresh feeling." The implication is that the vagina is a foul, nasty organ. Actually, it's almost always fine.

Douching is unnecessary—and harmful. The healthy vagina contains various bacteria that coexist in complex relationships. Within ten minutes of douching, some get killed, upsetting the ecological balance. Vaginal flora usually revert to normal within a few days. But before that happens, bacteria no longer held in check by those that have been killed may multiply and cause problems:

- **Chlamydia.** It's the nation's top sexual infection. University of Washington researchers surveyed 1,692 women. Compared with those who never douched, those who did even once in the previous year had double the chlamydia risk. Douching weekly almost quadrupled risk.
- **Pelvic inflammatory disease (PID).** In women, chlamydia rarely causes symptoms. Unrecognized infections may move through the cervix into the uterus and fallopian tubes, possibly causing pelvic inflammatory disease (PID), a fertility- and life-threatening condition. Researchers at Mount Sinai School of Medicine in New York discovered that monthly douching doubles risk.
- **Bacterial vaginosis (BV).** Douching increases risk of BV, which causes a malodorous discharge. University of Pittsburgh researchers surveyed 1,200 women. Weekly douching doubled risk.
- **Trichomoniasis.** CDC researchers tested 3,754 women for this common vaginal infection. Regular douching increased risk.
- **Yeast infection.** Italian researchers surveyed 931 women. As douching increased, so did risk.
- **Cervical cancer.** US military researchers analyzed douching among 266 women with cervical cancer and 408 healthy controls. Weekly douchers had four times the risk.
- **Ectopic pregnancy.** This happens when the embryo implants not in the uterus but in a fallopian tube. Eventually, the growing fetus ruptures the tube, threatening the mother's life. As douching increases, so does risk.
- **Preterm delivery.** It raises risk of serious medical problems. CDC researchers surveyed 812 pregnant women. Regular douching almost doubled risk.

Cervical mucus and other natural secretions—including self-lubrication during lovemaking—keep the vagina clean. "It's a self-cleansing organ," says gynecologist David Eschenbach, MD, of the University of Washington. "With regular bathing, douching is completely unnecessary—and hazardous."

As the risks of douching have become more widely publicized, the practice has declined. In 2011, sales totaled $62 million, but by 2018, only $45 million, a 27 percent decrease. Ladies, if you still douche, please stop.

However, only 30 percent of the women felt satisfied with their own. "Younger, thinner women worried theirs were too small. Older, heavier women felt anxious about drooping." Self-conscious women swing into action:

- They choose fashions that direct attention elsewhere.
- Millions wear padded bras. In 1948, Frederick Mellinger, founder of Frederick's of Hollywood, introduced the push-up bra, which makes breasts appear larger. It's become a fashion staple. And in 1994, the cleavage-accenting Wonderbra became a sensation.
- Some women wear minimizing bras.
- Breast surgery is America's number one cosmetic procedure. The American Society of Plastic Surgery estimates 300,000 augmentations and 100,000 reductions annually. Augmentations typically involve an increase from A cups to B or C. Reductions usually trim one or two cup sizes.

Men's breast mania is clearly sexual. Women's breasts are among men's favorite sex toys. But what explains women's breast obsession? Men's opinions certainly play a role. In the study above, if 56 percent of men feel fine about their partners' breasts, then 44 percent don't. Many women who undergo augmentation say their men encouraged or pressured them.

Fashion also plays a role. From Jane Mansfield's 1950s torpedoes to the mostly smaller chests of today's top models, breast fashions evolve. But fashion is not destiny. While clothing designers generally favor petite chests, augmentations are three times more popular than reductions.

Finally, women's breast preoccupation reflects their mental health. Women sufficiently unhappy to have cosmetic surgery often feel depressed about other aspects of their lives. Several studies agree that women who seek augmentation are more likely to suffer depression.

So men and women are both breast-obsessed—but differently. Ladies, your man probably likes your girls better than you do. Gentlemen, if you like your gal's boobs, tell her. Often.

How to Caress Women's Breasts

Everyone is sexually unique. To discover how women like their breasts fondled, ask. In addition, some suggestions:

- As you begin to cuddle and kiss, don't immediately reach for her twins. Most women need time to warm up to breast play. Caress other areas first—her scalp, neck, shoulders, arms, back. As you move south, ask, *Is this okay?*
- Don't keep your hands clamped on her breasts throughout lovemaking. Caress every square inch of her.
- In porn, men often treat breasts and nipples roughly. When in doubt, always err on the side of gentleness, especially with nipples. In porn, men often pull, pinch, and twist them. Some BDSM submissives enjoy this, but most women do not. To learn women's limits, place your thumb and index finger on her nipple and ask her to press on your fingers until she reaches her comfort limit.
- Finally, most women enjoy men's mouths and tongues on their breasts and nipples, but not men's teeth. Ask for coaching.

High Heels: Why Women Torture Their Feet

High stiletto heels are also known as CFM shoes—*come fuck me*. With good reason.

High heels definitely excite men. French researchers placed young adult women posing as survey takers on sidewalks and in stores and cafés. They dressed identically, except for their heels—low, medium, or high. As heel height increased, men became more willing to take the survey.

Why? In high heels:

- Women's breasts look larger. Heels arch the back, pushing the chest forward. Breasts appear larger and more conspicuous.
- Women's buttocks look larger. High heels lift them, increasing their prominence. Several studies show that as women's butt size increases, so does men's interest.
- Walking in heels makes women's hips and butts sway more, which attracts men.
- High heels shorten women's gaits, increasing booty shaking. Most men like that.

But high heels substantially increase risk of foot pain, blisters, bunions, falls, ankle sprains, plantar fasciitis, ingrown toenails, knee and back pain, and foot and leg nerve damage.

Women complain about high heels, but most wear them. Apparently, many prefer desirability to comfort and health.

Women's Many Possible Sexual Response Cycles

During the 1960s, sex research pioneers William Masters, MD, and Virginia Johnson described a four-phase sexual response process—arousal, plateau, orgasm, and resolution—and called it universal. While almost all men and many women fit their framework, at the turn of the current century, Rosemary Basson, PhD, of the University of British Columbia discovered that many women feel differently:

- **Arousal.** Erection makes men's arousal hard to miss. But many women aren't so sure about theirs. Like men, women exposed to erotic media experience increased genital blood flow. But unlike men, many remain unaware of it. Most women must feel desired before they can experience arousal. And once aroused, many want emotional closeness as much as orgasm. Hence, the adage: *men become emotionally intimate to gain sex; women have sex to gain emotional intimacy.*
- **Plateau.** Masters and Johnson defined it as sustained arousal. The women in Basson's studies generally agreed.
- **Orgasm.** Masters and Johnson described it as a sharp spike, a climax. Some of Basson's women agreed, but many described their orgasms as mild and peakless, yet still satisfying. Others reported serial mini-orgasms. And some said they had satisfying sex without distinct orgasms.
- **Resolution**. After orgasm, men lose their erections and return to Earth. But postorgasm, many of Basson's women described continued arousal.

Masters and Johnson missed the breadth of women's possible sexual responses for two reasons. They believed men and women were not only equally sexual, but sexual *in the same way*. In addition, they studied only a subset of women: those willing to be observed and filmed during sex who were orgasmic during dildo play and intercourse—a small minority of women.

Masters and Johnson inadvertently ignored the more than 75 percent of women whose orgasms require direct clitoral stimulation. Consequently, they produced an incomplete view of women's sexuality.

One Breast Larger than the Other?

In around half of women, one side is noticeably larger than the other. This is normal.

Gentlemen, your lovers may not fit the Masters and Johnson model. That's fine. They're normal. Encourage all women partners to share how they experience their sexual response cycles.

More Than a Little Bump: The Clitoral System

What's the clitoris? Most consider it the visible little nub of erotically sensitive, orgasm-triggering tissue above the vaginal opening under the top junction of the vaginal lips. But as Rebecca Chalker explains in her compendium of the research, *The Clitoral Truth*, it's much more than that. Unfortunately, in the West for five hundred years, the clitoris has been misrepresented and misunderstood. Actually, it's as large and multifaceted as the penis, just arranged differently and mostly invisible.

Clitoris comes from the Greek *kleitoris*, meaning women's genitals—all of them, not just the button. The ancient Greek physician Galen said, "All parts men have, women also have. In men, they are outside, in women, inside." Modern anatomists have proved him correct—so correct, that we need a new term to describe the magical clit. Let's call it the *clitoral system*.

Just as the entire penis and surrounding tissue can become erotically aroused, the same goes for all parts of the clitoral system. Many men would feel shortchanged if lovers focused only on the head (glans) of their penises, ignoring the shaft, scrotum, anal area, and perineum, the skin between the scrotum and anus. Similarly, many women feel shortchanged when their lovers focus only on the little bump and ignore the rest of the clitoral system.

During fetal development, the penis and clitoral system develop from the same germ cells. At eight weeks, all genitals appear virtually identical. The little nub commonly called the clitoris develops from the cells that produce the head of the penis.

Beneath the clitoral nub lies another part of the clitoral system, the clitoral shaft, analogous to shaft of the penis, only much smaller. Like the penile shaft, it contains erectile tissue. When women feel aroused, extra blood swells the clitoral shaft. In many—but not all—women, this projects the little bump beyond the folds of the inner vaginal lips, making it more prominent and excitable.

As men's erections develop, they salute thanks to the suspensory ligament in the lower abdomen. Women also have suspensory ligaments, another part of the clitoral system. They tighten during arousal and retract the tissue that covers the little nub, the clitoral hood, analogous to the male foreskin. As penises become erect, uncircumcised foreskins retract, exposing the glans. Similarly, as women become aroused, their suspensory ligaments retract their clitoral hoods, making it more visible.

The inner vaginal lips are another element of the clitoral system. They develop from the embryonic cells that produce the penile shaft. Like the shaft, the inner lips contain touch-sensitive nerve endings. Some women say their inner lips feel as erotically charged as their clits. The inner lips also contain erectile tissue. As women become aroused, the inner lips swell and part a bit, making the vaginal opening more visible and accessible. Inner lips vary enormously—in color from pink to burgundy to gray, and in shape from thin and narrow to fluted or thick and fleshy. One side may be larger than the other. Some women feel self-conscious about theirs, thinking they don't look like they "should." Actually, inner lips—and vulvas—are like snowflakes, all unique, all beautiful.

Men's erectile tissue concentrates in the penile shaft. Women's pervades the clitoral system. Much of it occupies the area between the inner lips, particularly around the urethral opening, halfway between the bean and vagina. This tissue, the urethral sponge or root of the clitoris, wraps around the pubic bone and extends inside to the front wall of the vagina (the top when women lie supine). When this tissue becomes blood-engorged, it bulges slightly and becomes firmer. The urethral sponge forms a small mound an inch or two inside the vagina. This is another facet of the clitoral system, the G-spot (below).

South of the vaginal opening lies the perineum, the skin that separates the vagina and anus. It's very sensitive to erotic caresses, thanks in part to the pelvic floor muscles that surround the clitoral system. The best known is the pubococcygeus (pew-bow-coxy-GEE-us), or PC, the muscle that contracts when you squeeze out the last drops of urine. The PC also contracts during orgasm. It's the muscle strengthened by Kegel exercises, which increase the pleasure of orgasm. The pelvic floor muscles form a figure eight around the vagina and anus. Caressing them contributes to women's arousal. That's why some women enjoy gentle anal sphincter massage or fingering—some men, too.

Between the inner lips, around the urethral opening, lie the paraurethral glands. On orgasm, they may produce fluid similar to the prostatic fluid in semen. Not all women produce fluid, and among those who do, amounts vary from a drop to a tablespoon, sometimes more. This fluid is female ejaculate, similar to semen, but without sperm.

Finally, the outer vaginal lips develop from same embryonic tissue as the scrotum and are just as erotically excitable.

Ironically, one area between women's legs is *not* part of the clitoral system—the vagina. It's a key sex organ for men, but more of a reproductive organ for women. Most women enjoy loving vaginal intercourse. It creates a special intimacy. And many women delight in holding erections inside them. Nonetheless, the vagina is not part of the clitoral system. Intercourse may enable men to work up to orgasms, but at most only 25 percent of women are reliably

How to Caress the Clit

- **Allow women to warm up.** Many need at least twenty minutes of gentle, whole-body massage before they feel ready for genital play. Gentlemen, ask for coaching about this.
- **Be gentle.** The clitoris contains as many touch-sensitive nerve endings as the head of the penis, but they're packed into less space, making it, spot for spot, more sensitive than the penis. Many perfectly normal women feel discomfort, even pain, when men caress the little button in any way other than *very gently*. Many—but not all—women enjoy more intense clitoral play only as they approach orgasm.
- **Touch around it.** For some women, any direct clitoral caresses feel too intense. If so, touch and lick *around* it. Ask for coaching. Frequently.

Does Clitoral Size Matter?

Penis size rarely matters to men's sexual function. What about the size of the clitoris? The research is equivocal:

- One team of Cincinnati scientists used MRI to determine the size of thirty women's clitorises, ten of whom had trouble working up to orgasm. The latter had significantly smaller clits, suggesting that as size increases, so does sexual responsiveness.
- But another Cincinnati team surveyed twenty women's sexual function, then measured their clitoral size. Those with the greatest desire, easiest arousal and lubrication, and most reliable orgasms had the *smallest* clits.

Scientists don't know if clitoral size matters. Large ones are only slightly bigger than small ones. And no matter what their size, fingers, tongues, and toys can caress the large majority of women to orgasm.

orgasmic during intercourse—in part because only the vagina's outer third contains many touch-sensitive nerves. The inner two-thirds contains surprisingly few.

In the West, until around 1700, the penis and clitoral system were considered identical, except for their arrangement. After 1700, the concept of genital equivalence faded. Physicians and anatomists came to view women as less sexual than men and eventually denied the very existence of the clitoral system. By the nineteenth-century Victorian era, physicians considered women incapable of sexual arousal. The clitoris was reduced to the little nub the term connotes today. Sigmund Freud went so far as to tout the completely erroneous notion that only immature, neurotic women have orgasms triggered by clitoral play (clitoral orgasms). He claimed mature, mentally healthy women have them during intercourse (vaginal orgasms). Shame on Freud. Depending on the touch women receive, their orgasms may feel different, but physiologically, all orgasms are the same, triggered by caressing one or more parts of the clitoral system.

What explains Victorian denigration of women's sexuality? Feminists link it to the emergence of obstetrics and gynecology, when male physicians seized women's reproductive medicine from midwives. Historians contend that the change reflected the Industrial Revolution, the transition from men and women working side by side in agriculture as approximate equals to a division of labor—male breadwinners, female homemakers. Whatever the case, ancient appreciation of the clitoral system dwindled.

In the mid-twentieth century, Masters and Johnson refuted Freud's notion of the vaginal orgasm, restoring the clitoris to its rightful prominence. In the 1980s, sex researchers Alice Kahn Ladas, EdD, Beverly Whipple, PhD, and John Perry, PhD, documented the G-spot and female ejaculation, though both remain controversial (below). Today, most people consider the clitoris the little bump tucked beneath the top junction of women's vaginal lips. The full extent of the clitoral system has yet to become repopularized, with many men (and some women) still in the dark about its centrality to women's sexuality.

So where is the clitoris? It encompasses the entire vulva, from the clitoral hood to the anus, and has surprisingly little to do with the vagina. And why do so many women have difficulty with orgasms during partner lovemaking? Often because their lovers don't fully appreciate the majesty of the clitoral system.

There Is No "Typical" Vulva

Some women feel concerned that their external genitals look odd or abnormal. British researchers measured fifty healthy women's vulvas and found no "normal" and therefore no "abnormal":

- Width of the head (glans) of the clitoris: 3–10 millimeters (mm).
- Length of the clitoral shaft: 5–35 mm.
- Distance from the clitoris to the urethral opening: 16–45 mm.
- Length of the outer vaginal lips (labia majora): 7–12 mm.
- Length of the inner vaginal lips (labia minora): 20–100 mm.
- Length of the vaginal opening: 7–13 mm.
- Distance from the base of the vagina to the anus: 15–55 mm.
- Vulvar color compared with surrounding tissue: same, 18 percent; darker, 82 percent.
- Inner lips appearance: smooth skin, 28 percent; some fluting/wrinkling, 68 percent; very fluted/wrinkled, 4 percent.
- Pubic hair density and coverage: extremely variable, from sparse growth of silky hair over a small area above the clitoris to dense profusion of thick, coarse hair from the navel to anus.

The dimensions, appearance, and color of the women's vulvas had nothing to do with their age, race/ethnicity, sexual experience, number of children, or use of hormonal contraceptives.

Delivery of children stretches the vagina. Most mothers say it's temporary, that the vulva and vagina revert to baseline within several months to a year. But some women insist births cause permanent vaginal changes. In this study, "no difference was seen when comparing women with and without children."

Note that 82 percent of participants' vulvas were darker than their surrounding skin. Some women feel concerned about this. It's normal. The vulva is similar to the mouth. Compared with the rest of facial skin, lips are darker.

Women's external genitals are as unique as they are. As long as the tissue is healthy, all vulvas are normal.

The Controversial G-Spot

The G-spot excites great passion pro and con. One Italian researcher insists "the supposed G-spot does not exist." But reports from thousands of women and a dozen studies by researchers worldwide argue that the fabled spot is real and present in all women. Many women say G-spot stimulation enhances their lovemaking. It may not be a discrete spot, but a diffuse area of erotic sensitivity about one finger-length inside the vagina on its front (top) wall.

During the 1940s, two gynecologists, Ernst Grafenberg and Robert Dickinson, discovered "a zone of erogenous feeling" in the front wall of the vagina, an area known as the "urethral sponge." In a 1950 report, they asserted this zone contained erectile tissue that swelled when massaged, enhancing orgasm.

Their research faded into obscurity until the 1980s, when Ladas, Whipple, and Perry rediscovered that virtually all women have this area of erotic sensitivity. They unearthed the

Grafenberg/Dickinson research and decided to rename the urethral sponge the Grafenberg spot or G-spot.

In 1982, their book, *The G-Spot and Other Recent Discoveries about Human Sexuality*, became a bestseller and triggered a stampede of interest in the often-elusive spot. Millions of women and couples tried to find it, but only some succeeded. Consequently, the G-spot became controversial.

Other researchers dismissed the G-spot as a fantasy, citing reports that massage of the urethral sponge leaves many women feeling nothing erogenous. Ladas, Whipple, and Perry retorted that the G-spot lies not *on* the vaginal wall, but *deep inside* it, most easily found when women are highly aroused, when G-spot swelling makes it more palpable.

The most recent research suggests that the G-spot is part of the clitoral system. The clitoris includes two legs that extend around the pubic bone, producing the area of erotic sensitivity many women report in the front vaginal wall. US Army gynecologist Christine Vaccaro suggests that the G-spot should be renamed the "C-spot," in recognition of its connection to the clitoris.

Some women report mind-blowing orgasms from deep, sustained G-spot massage. Others call it a modest sexual enhancement. And some feel nothing or find G-spot stimulation uncomfortable. Whatever women experience is normal. Ask.

When they find the G-spot, some women feel a momentary urge to urinate. This usually passes. Women who feel concerned about this might urinate before sex so they know their bladders are empty.

How to Caress the G-Spot

The fabled spot is easiest to locate—and most sensitive to touch—when women feel highly aroused. Arousal engorges it with extra blood, causing bulging that men's fingers can usually feel.

- **G-spot toys.** It's not easy for women to touch their own G-spots, hence dismissals that it doesn't exist. Many women find the spot easiest to locate when lying supine using special G-spot sex toys, phallic vibrators, or dildos with curved tips. When women lie on their backs, they can insert G-spot toys a few inches with curved ends up and press them into the front/top wall. The most sensitive area may be off to one side.
- **Lovers can usually find it more easily than women themselves.** With women on their backs, insert a finger, hook it upward, and press gently. Ask for coaching.
- **G-spot intercourse.** The best position for G-spot stimulation during intercourse is rear entry (doggie style) with the woman on hands and knees and the man behind her. In this position, with deep insertion, the head of the penis presses the G-spot. This makes some evolutionary sense. All nonhuman mammals have intercourse only in this position. By pleasuring females, the G-spot evidently encouraged reproduction.

Female Ejaculation and "Squirting"

Tiny fluid-producing glands in the urethral sponge surround the urinary opening, the paraurethral glands ("para" means around). The first were discovered in the 1880s by Alexander Skene—Skene's glands. Since then, others have been identified, Bartholin's glands. Their secretions chemically resemble prostate fluid. Some anatomists call these glands the "female prostate." Recent research has strengthened the case that the paraurethral glands are analogous to the prostate. Ladas, Whipple, and Perry argued that when women feel highly aroused, G-spot play may trigger the paraurethral glands to release fluid on orgasm—"female ejaculation."

This observation explained some sexual history. Several ancient sources—Aristotle (350 BC), Galen (AD 150), the *Kama Sutra* (AD 300), and classical Japanese erotic works—agreed that many women release fluid on orgasm.

But the three founders of modern sex research—Kinsey and Masters and Johnson—all rejected female ejaculation, asserting that some women simply produced copious vaginal lubrication. However, lubrication does not emerge just during orgasm. Many women feel embarrassed about "urinating" when they come. Many women ejaculators have examined their fluid and determined by color and odor that it is not urine. The research confirms this. Female ejaculatory fluid is mainly paraurethral-gland secretions, possibly mixed with traces of urine.

How common is ejaculation in women? Depending on the survey, somewhere between 10 and 50 percent, with production varying from a drop or two to a tablespoon or more.

Female ejaculation is perfectly safe to produce and ingest. Lovers may need to change the sheets or make love on towels, but it causes no harm. One study even suggests that it protects women from bladder infections by expelling bacteria from the urethra.

It's also perfectly normal for women *not* to ejaculate. Many don't. If you don't but would like to, try extended loveplay with lots of deep G-spot massage.

Why do only some women ejaculate? No one knows. But it appears related to G-spot sensitivity. Women with erotically sensitive G-spots are most likely to release fluid. This makes physiological sense. The nerves surrounding the G-spot also excite the fluid-producing paraurethral glands.

Some couples love the juiciness female ejaculation adds to sex. Others feel put off, believing it's urine. Women who fear incontinence during sex should practice Kegel exercises to tighten their urinary sphincters.

Not: "I Can't Get Enough of Your Tits." Better: "I Can't Get Enough of You."

Gentlemen, how would you feel if women said, *I adore your thumbs.* You'd probably think, *Great . . . but I'm more than just my thumbs.*

Compared with men, women are more judged by their bodies—and often feel self-conscious. Don't just compliment body parts. Many women fear men don't see beyond their bits. Spotlight the whole woman.

Why Some Vaginas Feel "Tight"

Some women complain their vaginas are "too tight." Some men, too. Notions of vaginal tightness are fraught with mythology. Many believe that virgins' vaginas are extremely tight, first intercourse permanently loosens them, subsequent sex loosens them more, and childbirth causes permanent looseness. Possibly, but probably not.

Imagine a hand towel stuffed inside a sock held by two hands. The towel represents the folded muscle tissue inside the vagina. The sock is the vaginal wall. The hands are the pelvic floor muscles surrounding it.

The vagina's tightly folded muscle tissue is highly elastic. It expands considerably to allow watermelon-size babies to be born.

The vagina is like the mouth. Pull the corners of your mouth toward your ears, then let go. What happens? The mouth snaps back to its prestretched state. Pull on your lips repeatedly. The mouth quickly returns to normal and no one would ever suspect you'd stretched it. The same usually goes for the vagina—with a few exceptions (below).

Except during sexual arousal and childbirth, the vaginal muscles remain as tightly folded as a closed accordion. Anxiety makes this musculature clench tighter. That's why some adolescent girls initially have problems inserting tampons. Their vaginal muscle tissue is tightly folded to begin with, and many feel anxious about touching themselves and inserting anything, so those muscles contract more. Anxiety about first intercourse also explains many virgins' tightness. Painful tightness may also indicate vaginismus (below).

As women become sexually aroused, especially if they receive the caresses touted in chapter 5 and 8, vaginal muscle tissue relaxes somewhat. Sexologists call this "ballooning," but that's an overstatement. The vagina doesn't expand like a balloon. Instead its folded muscle tissue changes from resembling a tight fist to a fist loose enough to insert a finger or two. In evolutionary terms, this makes sense. Evolution is all about reproduction. A tight vagina would impede it, so women evolved to have sexual arousal relax vaginal tissue for easier erection insertion and greater chance of impregnation. If vaginas feel "too tight," in most cases, women are either not interested in sex or have not enjoyed enough warm-up time to allow their vaginal musculature to relax and become sufficiently lubricated for comfortable genital play.

Men who attempt fingering, intercourse, or toy insertion before women become fully aroused and lubricated are either sexually uninformed or boors. That's why extended, whole-body loveplay is so important. It allows women—and their vaginas—time to warm up to genital play.

Tightness may also result from medical conditions, for example, vaginismus, spasm of the vaginal muscles that may make fingering or intercourse painful or impossible. For suspected vaginismus, consult a gynecologist and/or a sexual medicine specialist. To find one of the latter near you, visit the Sexual Medicine Society of North America.

Other conditions that may cause unusual tightness include hysterectomy, vaginal trauma, pelvic radiation, and uterine prolapse, weakening of the connective tissue that holds the uterus in place. In prolapse, this tissue stretches. The uterus presses on the vagina. And women experience discomfort, possibly including tightness. Consult a gynecologist and/or sexual medicine specialist.

Despite extended loveplay and lots of lube, some normal, healthy women still feel tight. In older women, menopausal vaginal tissue thinning (atrophy) may exacerbate this. If so, transition your lovemaking away from intercourse to outercourse.

Why Some Vaginas Feel "Loose"

Loss of virginity and subsequent intercourse rarely cause permanent vaginal looseness. However, with age, vaginal muscle tissue loses some of its elasticity, possibly causing persistent looseness, especially after menopause.

In addition, any childbirth, especially multiple deliveries in rapid succession—three kids in six years—may cause long-term looseness. The vagina stretches a great deal during childbirth, like an accordion opened all the way. By the time the baby turns one, the organ usually returns to predelivery tightness. But not always.

Chinese obstetricians inserted pressure sensors into the vaginas of 165 women who'd recently delivered, eighty-eight vaginally, seventy-seven by cesarean. Pressure was greater, meaning tighter vaginas, in the cesarean group. However, the two groups reported the same sexual function and satisfaction. An Israeli study concurs, finding no difference in new mother's sexual functioning and satisfaction twenty-four weeks postpartum. Turkish investigators surveyed men after their wives delivered vaginally or by cesarean. Either way, the men reported the same sexual satisfaction.

To minimize looseness:

- Have intercourse in the man-on-top position. Once the man inserts, he lifts himself up and the woman closes her legs under him. Her thighs squeeze his penis and make her feel tighter.
- Do Kegel exercises daily. Kegels strengthen the muscles between the legs—so the hands holding the stuffed sock grip tighter. A few months of daily Kegels often make the vagina feel tighter.
- Women might also try ben-wa balls or vaginal cones. Sex toy marketers sell ben-wa balls in pairs. Women insert them, then walk around the house trying to keep them from falling out. With weak pelvic floor muscles, the balls drop quickly, but as the muscles grow stronger, women can hold the balls inside longer. Vaginal cones are similar but prescribed by physicians.
- Women's last resort is electrical vaginal muscle stimulation. A urologist or nurse inserts a probe similar to a tampon. It emits a mild electrical current that contracts the vaginal and pelvic musculature. Treatments take twenty to thirty minutes, usually twice a week for about eight weeks.

Finally, looseness is also possible if women go at it with several men in rapid succession. During extended group play, the vaginal muscles may not have time to revert to normal tightness.

Pubic Grooming: Farewell to Full Bushes
Until the 1980s, most American women retained all their pubic hair—"full bush." Today, the large majority (and many men) "groom" their pubes. Some women trim hair short. Others trim and shave the perimeter. Some shave the lips, leaving a small patch above the clitoris—a "welcome mat" or "landing strip." And some shave completely—"bald" or "Barbie doll."

The shift to grooming has occurred in little more than a generation. In 2016, a University of California, San Francisco, survey of 3,316 adult women showed full bushes, 16 percent, groomed pubes, 84 percent.

Grooming varies with age. It's most popular among young women, especially whites. As age increases, grooming decreases. Grooming also changes with education—more schooling, usually more grooming.

Some critics have castigated grooming, saying it makes women look like children and fuels male fantasies of pedophilia. But most American women shave their legs and underarms. Pubic grooming is simply an extension of that.

Many men have also jumped on the pubic grooming bandwagon. Another UCSF survey of 4,198 adult men showed that 51 percent groomed, particularly young adults.

For centuries, European and Asian artists have depicted female nudes both with and without pubic hair. Art historians continue to debate why. Some contend grooming became popular to control pubic lice. Others insist that medieval women retained their pubic hair and artists who painted it out indulged in artistic license. Early photography (1840s) shows the vast majority of models—but not all—with full bushes. The same goes for early motion-picture pornography (1890s).

America's major twentieth-century men's magazines, *Playboy* and *Penthouse*, didn't show models below the hips until 1970. From then until 2000, most had full bushes or modest trims. But after that, most showed little or no pubic hair.

Brazilian waxing, commercial removal of some or all pubic hair, was introduced by a New York spa in 1987. Since then, the term has become a part of the lexicon. But it's not clear how many women have had "Brazilians," let alone how many have them regularly.

Finally, there's Barbie. Since its 1959 introduction, Barbie dolls have been wildly popular with generations of girls. But Barbie's body is controversial. It's almost impossible, the equivalent of a five-foot, nine-inch-tall woman with a thirty-six-inch chest, eighteen-inch waist, and thirty-three-inch hips. Except for what's on her head, Barbie is completely hairless and may have contributed to popularizing grooming.

The practice's pioneers were women porn actors, who imbued it with naughtiness. Some critics charge that porn-addled men forced grooming on their lovers to imitate porn stars. But the Indiana survey just mentioned showed that male cajoling has little to do with women's decisions. Most women insisted they groomed for comfort and hygiene, believing it cleaner, safer, and healthier. In addition, women who groom believe it boosts the likelihood of cunnilingus, key to many women's orgasms.

Is grooming healthier? The main medical benefit is reduced risk of pubic lice. But downsides include the possibility of cuts that might become infected. And repeat shaving may irritate the hair follicles, causing folliculitis. One study suggested a possible increased risk of sexual infections (STIs), but a larger, better trial debunked that. No credible evidence shows that even going bald increases STIs risk.

For best grooming results:

- Beforehand, wash the area and your hands with soap and water to remove bacteria that may infect nicks.
- Washing also softens pubic hair, making it easier to trim or shave.
- Cover the area with soap or shaving cream. This reduces risk of nicks and cuts.
- Use razors with at least two blades. They shave closer than single-blade razors.
- Replace razors regularly. Blades dull.
- For hard-to-see areas, use a handheld mirror.

CHAPTER 37:
Women's Desire: Possibly Similar to Men's but Often Different

M EN LUST. WOMEN *yearn to feel desired.* Like all maxims, this isn't the whole story, but it contains some truth. Most men experience libido as a powerful drive that propels them to pursue sex, sometimes to their detriment, as illustrated by another adage: *men have two heads and the little one does the thinking.*

Meanwhile, few women feel a supercharged male-style sex drive. Instead, most yearn to feel wanted, to enchant men and capture their souls. Many women experience sexual urgency during the early, hot-and-heavy period of relationships. But for most couples, initial lustiness lasts only a year or so. After that, compared with men, most women want sex less.

Recognized, Then Dismissed

Ancient literature shows that many women had active libidos. Early Greeks invented the dildo and dramas of that era discuss women using them solo. But until recently, women's desire hardly mattered. In most ancient cultures, marriage implied wives' consent to sex on their husbands' terms. If wives refused, husbands were free to rape, divorce, and even kill them. Today, we remain closer to this barbarism than many imagine. In the US, marital rape wasn't outlawed by all fifty states until 1993. In many countries, it's still not a crime.

As the Middle Ages yielded to the so-called Enlightenment, men increasingly dismissed women's libidos. By the nineteenth-century Victorian era, physicians—virtually all men—considered women *incapable* of erotic desire.

During the mid-twentieth century, Masters and Johnson showed that women are just as sexual as men, sometimes more so. But the pioneering sex researchers erred in asserting that the genders experience their sexuality identically. The latest findings, largely by women sex researchers, show that while some women experience male-style lust, many, possibly most, experience desire differently, not as a drive but as enjoyable lovemaking's *result*.

The Challenging Lives of Highly Sexual Women

Today, in much of the world, men remain free to be horny goats constantly on the prowl for sex. Women rarely share this freedom. Men who bed many women are often the envy of their brethren, "studs." But women who act similarly are more likely to be castigated as "sluts," with friends raising questions about their mental health. Actually, some women are naturally very sexual. How many? No one knows. Few admit it and sex researchers have largely ignored this subject.

However, University of Chicago investigators asked a representative sample of 1,749 American women, eighteen to fifty-nine, if, during the previous year, they'd had partner sex four or more times a week. Among those age eighteen to twenty-nine, 11 percent said they had. Among older women the figure ranged from 7 percent for women in their thirties, down to 5 percent for those in their forties, and 2 percent for women over fifty. The all-age average suggests that around 6 percent of women are lusty ladies.

A Croatian study corroborates these findings. The researchers surveyed 2,599 Croatian women age eighteen to sixty. Those who were highly sexual—7 percent.

Highly sexual women aren't particularly numerous, but they're by no means rare—about one in twenty. This explains why many women have affairs, or become swingers, visit sex clubs, work in porn, enjoy gangbangs, and/or affirmatively choose sex work.

To my knowledge, only one researcher has explored the lives of highly sexual women, Michigan PhD candidate Eric Blumberg. In 2003, he advertised in Detroit's alternative weekly newspaper seeking to interview women who had six or more orgasms a week solo or partnered or who considered themselves highly sexual. Forty-four replied.

They ranged in age from twenty to eighty-two, in education from high school to graduate degrees, and in employment from entry level to CEOs. The newspaper's readers were over-whelmingly white. So were the respondents, with two Latinas and one African American. As a result, this study is hardly definitive, but it's still groundbreaking.

All respondents reported intense libidos that compelled them to have lots of sex, both solo and partnered. They all felt alienated from cultural expectations that women should be demure. And they'd all experienced distress about their sexual needs.

Growing up, they all realized they were different from other girls. More than half (57 percent) said they'd experienced "major conflicts" and "painful struggles" to accept themselves. All considered themselves "sluts," "nymphomaniacs," and "sex addicts." Most had been labeled as such by friends and lovers. All considered the name-calling cruel—but true.

Almost all eventually accepted their sexuality. For some (16 percent), this happened during their teens or twenties—thanks to sex-positive parents who accepted highly sexual daughters or to friends who reassured them that they were okay. But it took the rest (84 percent) well into adulthood to make peace with their powerful libidos. The process was gradual and fraught, often involving divorces from men incapable of accepting highly sexual wives.

All the women recalled innumerable flings and simultaneous relationships with two or more lovers. Twenty-three percent were married and 11 percent cohabiting, but two-thirds (66 percent) were single, having decided that they couldn't live with men's demands for monogamy. All said they were open to affairs, including those in committed relationships. Most described themselves as more comfortable with men than women. Many expressed pride that male friends considered them "one of the guys." Many complained that their women friends didn't understand them.

One-quarter reported histories of childhood sex abuse, well above the prevalence academic researchers have documented. Those who'd been sexually abused were unanimous in the opinion that their childhood experiences had little or nothing to do with their eventual sexuality. Almost all insisted they'd been born highly sexual.

Are highly sexual women "sex addicts"? The concept is controversial, but one hallmark involves feeling out of control. Blumberg decided that none of his interview subjects "were currently or ever had been sexually out of control. Some recalled occasional sexual impulsiveness, typically while drunk during their teens or twenties. But participants didn't fit typical depictions of compulsion or addiction, nor did they report the negative consequences typically associated with them." They just loved getting it on.

By the time they were interviewed, most had accepted themselves and enjoyed sex exuberantly. On balance, 80 percent said being highly sexual had enhanced their lives.

Little or No Desire: How Prevalent?

While around 5 percent of adult women are highly sexual, many more experience little or no desire. Sexologists call this "low libido" or "female hypoactive sexual desire disorder." Prevalence of low libido is unclear. Definitions differ and estimates vary substantially:

Studies	Proportion of women reporting low libido
Australia (2017), 2,020 women, forty to sixty-five	69%
US (2008), 1,550 women, fifty-seven to eighty-five	43%
Italy (2009), 427 women, twenty to seventy	40%
Iran (2012), 174 pre- and postmenopausal women	35%
US (2012), 806 women, forty or older	33%
US (1999), 1,749 women, eighteen to fifty-nine	29%
US (2006), 2,000 women, twenty to seventy	18%
US (2012), 701 women, over eighteen	7%
Average	35%

Worsley, R., et al. "Prevalence and Predictors of Low Sexual Desire, Sexually Related Personal Distress and Hypoactive Sexual Desire Dysfunction in a Community-Based Sample of Midlife Women." *Journal of Sexual Medicine* 14 (2017): 675.

Beigi, M., and F. Fahami. "A Comparative Study of Sexual Dysfunctions before and after Menopause." *Iran Journal of Nursing and Midwifery Research* 17, 2 suppl. 1 (2012): S72.

For additional citations, visit greatsexguidance.com/references-womens-desire.

Oddly, assuming an emotionally close relationship, these studies all agree that low-libido women can still become aroused and lubricated, enjoy sex, and call their lovemaking pleasurable—rather like those who rarely think about ice cream, but when it's offered, enjoy it.

Risk Factors for Low Desire

Why low libido? Two possibilities: something about the women or something about the sex. From the 1940s through the millennium, researchers focused almost exclusively on the women and identified many risk factors for lack of sexual interest:

- **Age.** Low libido increases with age, with desire often dropping sharply during early menopause.
- **Sudden menopause.** Menopause usually occurs gradually. But some women experience it suddenly after cancer treatment or ovary removal. Sudden menopause often causes a precipitous drop in libido that may be either temporary or persistent.
- **Body image.** Many heavy women (or "big beautiful women," BBWs) boast major libidos. But when women gain weight, body image and libido usually suffer.
- **Sedentary lifestyle.** Little or no exercise is associated with low desire.
- **Alcohol.** The first drink is disinhibiting and may lead to sex. But as drinking continues, alcohol becomes a central nervous system depressant—and may sabotage libido.
- **Relationship misery.** Couple unhappiness often kills libido.
- **Relationship duration.** After the initial hot-and-heavy period, desire almost always declines.
- **Hormonal contraception.** The Pill and other hormonal contraceptives may boost libido, have no impact, or reduce it. *Contraceptive Technology*, the bible of birth control,

estimates that 5 percent of users suffer libido suppression, but recent studies document declines in up to 37 percent of users, a big difference. My informal survey of sex therapists strongly suggests that birth control pills and other hormonal contraceptives are a leading cause of low desire in reproductive-age women.

- **Stress, anxiety, depression.** As emotional distress increases, libido typically declines.
- **Mood-altering medications.** Antidepressants, antianxiety drugs, and other mood-altering medications often reduce desire.
- **Illness.** Sexual desire tracks health. Acute illness and injury (colds, flu, sprains, etc.) typically depress libido for their duration. Chronic illnesses (asthma, diabetes, heart disease, etc.) may suppress it long term.
- **Vaginal dryness and pain during intercourse.** Chronic sexual discomfort depresses libido.
- **Sharp drop in income.** When income plummets, desire usually follows.
- **Partner sex less than monthly.** Over time, women who don't have much sex may stop wanting it.
- **History of sexual abuse or assault.** Sexual coercion usually reduces subsequent desire, usually temporarily, sometimes permanently.
- **Low androgens.** Androgens are the male sex hormones that govern women's desire. Unusually low levels torpedo libido.

Women's Desire and the Menstrual Cycle

In most female mammals, ovulation produces "heat," sexual enthusiasm, usually twice a year. Humans are different. Women ovulate year-round and don't experience heat. But many studies show that in reproductive-age women, libido is somewhat cyclical across the menstrual cycle, with peak interest around ovulation, midway between periods. It's evolution's way of spurring procreation:

- University of Virginia researchers surveyed the libidos of 115 reproductive-age women both premenstrually and midcycle around ovulation. At midcycle, they reported significantly more desire and sexual satisfaction.
- University of Rhode Island investigators asked ninety-six college women where they were in their cycles, then surveyed their reactions to various films: comedies, romances, action-adventure, and erotica. Around ovulation, they expressed increased interest in erotica.
- Arizona State University researchers asked 236 women to track their masturbation and basal body temperatures, which rise at ovulation. Masturbation peaked around ovulation.
- Finally, Spanish scientists reviewed the substantial literature on sex and the menstrual cycle: "At mid-cycle, women exhibit increased motivation."

Beyond the menstrual cycle, something else usually boosts women's libidos midcycle—being single. Compared with coupled women, single gals show a greater spike in desire.

However, two factors blunt the ovulatory libido surge:

- **The Pill.** Birth control pills alter the menstrual cycle. A few of the studies just mentioned sorted participants based on use of oral contraception. Women not using the Pill showed the expected monthly libido swings, but those taking birth control pills did not.

- **Work stress.** Chronic occupational stress depresses the midcycle libido spike. But on vacation, most job-stressed women return to increased desire at midcycle.

Gentlemen, if your partner is of reproductive age, consider tracking her menstrual cycles. Unless she uses hormonal contraception, she may feel the most desire around two weeks after her periods. Just remember, the menstrual cycle is *not* destiny. Risk factors for low libido may outweigh any increase around ovulation.

Women's Libido and the Seasons

Several studies show that interest in sex varies annually with peaks in summer and winter:

- Birth records consistently show more children conceived during summer and winter than spring and fall.
- Condom sales rise and fall seasonally, with spikes during summer and winter.
- Surveys of first intercourse consistently show two annual peaks, one in May and June, the other in December.
- Most sexually transmitted infections are diagnosed during summer and around Christmas.
- Finally, Rutgers and Villanova scientists compared millions of Google searches of sex-related and sexually neutral keywords. Searches for sex-neutral terms remained constant year-round, but searches for sex-related terms showed significant increases in summer and winter and dips during spring and fall.

Some researchers attribute twice-yearly libido increases to summer vacations and Christmas, the New Year, and Valentine's Day, when people are more likely to socialize—and do what comes naturally. Or perhaps sexual seasonality is an evolutionary echo of semiannual mammalian heat.

How Menopause Changes Women's Desire

During and after menopause, most women's libidos decline noticeably. So does their sexual frequency, in part because of reduced libido and in part because older women's partners are usually even older men with sex and/or health issues.

However, most studies of postmenopausal libido decline have surveyed women at one moment in time, for example, age fifty. Better information comes from tracking women for many years. But such studies are much more costly, so few get funded.

Fortunately, Australian researchers have conducted the world's longest-duration study of older women's sexuality, the Melbourne Women's Midlife Health Project (MWMHP). They interviewed 2,001 women age forty-five to fifty-five, then reinterviewed them repeatedly for at least eleven years. Over this long period, virtually all reported decreased sexual interest. However, the greatest declines occurred during early menopause, from age forty-five to fifty-five. After fifty-five, the rate of decline diminished—and in some women, libido rebounded.

Early menopausal changes distress many women—and the men who love them. But as women get used to postmenopausal living, most couples accommodate and some women's desire recovers.

The women showed the same pattern regarding sexual responsiveness. During early menopause, they reported a drop in sexual enjoyment. But as the years passed, it often improved. By their sixties, many reported almost as much pleasure as they'd enjoyed before menopause.

Reducing Risk Factors Boosts Desire

Some risk factors for low libido can't be changed—age and menopausal status. Others are more malleable:

- **Exercise.** Compared with couch sitters, physically active women usually report more desire.
- **Weight loss.** Dropping extra pounds means less weight to drag around, and more energy for other activities, including the bedroom dance.
- **Mood-altering drugs.** Women who reduce heavy drinking usually report increased libido. Ditto for those who stop other mood-altering medications. Some women experience increased desire after switching from the Pill to other contraceptives.
- **Physical health.** Healing of acute illnesses and injuries usually improves desire. Among women with chronic conditions, commitment to healthy lifestyle may boost libido: less meat, fewer high-fat and junk foods, more fruits and vegetables, regular exercise, and improved sleep.
- **Mental health.** Stress management often improves desire.

The Four-Part Program That Boosts Desire

University of British Columbia researchers tested a treatment for low desire that combined:

- Relationship counseling
- Instruction about risk factors for low libido
- Stress-reducing progressive muscle relaxation (PMR) exercises
- Mindfulness meditation, another stress reducer that focuses the mind on the present moment

The researchers enrolled twenty-six women with low libido and/or arousal difficulties in three ninety-minute counseling/education/mindfulness sessions two weeks apart. Between sessions, the women practiced mindfulness meditation daily at home. After six weeks, the program significantly increased participants' desire, arousal, lubrication, and satisfaction.

The same researchers tested a similar program on 117 low-desire women. Sixty-eight participated in the counseling/education/mindfulness program. Forty-nine were placed on a wait list. After six months, the treatment group reported significantly greater desire, arousal, and lubrication, easier orgasms, and greater satisfaction.

In a survey of 450 women, the same researchers also found that those who meditated regularly reported increased desire and enhanced sexual function as a result of "better overall mental health."

Investigators at Willamette University in Oregon analyzed eleven studies of mindfulness involving 449 women who complained of low libido and arousal and orgasm difficulties. "All aspects of sexual function and well-being exhibited significant improvement."

Why did the program work? The counseling element reduced relationship distress. The education component corrected sexual misconceptions. And the PMR and mindfulness pieces improved the women's ability to relax and savor erotic touch.

Self-Help That Enhances Women's Desire

Most women with desire issues feel exhausted by their jobs, marriages, families, and daily hassles. Their hectic lives often preclude the peace, quiet, deep relaxation, and erotic focus necessary to experience desire.

University of Florida researchers surveyed forty-five low-libido women who had been married for five to twenty-nine years. Some were placed on a waiting list. The rest read *A Tired Woman's Guide to Passionate Sex* by psychologist Laurie B. Mintz, PhD, which presents a self-help version of the programs just described.

The book discussed six subjects:

- **Thoughts.** Women with low desire often slip into negativity: *I'm overwhelmed; therefore, I can't be desirable.* The book promoted positive feelings about self and sexuality and mindfulness techniques to foster deep relaxation.
- **Talk.** Low desire often provokes relationship conflict. The book presented suggestions for constructive couple discussion of day-to-day irritants and the couple's love life, including mutual sexual coaching.
- **Time.** Low-libido women typically feel harried. The book promoted standard time-management strategies: setting goals, prioritizing them, dividing tasks into manageable chunks, and scheduling time to accomplish them.
- **Touch.** The book strongly advocated extended whole-body massage before genital play.
- **Novelty.** Sex ruts demolish desire. The book promoted making love at different times in new places in new ways.
- **Scheduling.** Many people believe sex "should" happen spontaneously when lovers feel "in the mood." That's true early in relationships, but after a year or so, sexologists almost universally recommend scheduling lovemaking in advance. The book advocated scheduling.

After six weeks, the participants who'd read the book reported significantly greater libido, arousal, and satisfaction.

University of Virginia investigators compared the self-help approaches just discussed with the two FDA-approved treatments for low libido in women, flibanserin (Addyi) and bremelanotide (Vyleesi). Self-help was as effective as the drugs.

Do Estrogen, Androgens, and Drugs Help?

After Viagra's 1998 approval, its maker, Pfizer, hoped the drug might also boost women's desire. The company funded many studies. A few hinted at benefit, but most showed none. After several years, Pfizer terminated all Viagra research on women. In a nutshell, that's the story of pharmaceuticals for low desire in women—intriguing possibilities but little compelling evidence of effectiveness.

Consider postmenopausal estrogen (hormone replacement therapy, HRT). Starting in the 1970s, many small studies suggested that HRT enhanced desire while reducing hot flashes and risk of heart disease, stroke, breast cancer, and dementia. But in 2014, the huge Women's Health Initiative, a fifteen-year study of 160,000 women, showed that while estrogen boosted desire—largely by eliminating hot flashes—it *increased* risk of heart disease, stroke, breast cancer, and dementia. Prescriptions plummeted. Today, few women take HRT.

Then came androgens. Some researchers theorized that low-desire women might benefit from supplements. However, androgen deficiency has never been well defined, so what's "low" is anybody's guess. Supplementation boosted women's desire, but also caused masculinizing side effects: male pattern baldness, voice deepening, acne, and uncomfortable clitoral enlargement. Women shunned androgens, and today, few physicians prescribe them.

Next doctors tried prescribing one androgen, dehydroepiandrosterone (DHEA). Some studies showed enhanced desire, but most have shown little or no benefit—and a risk of acne. Few women take DHEA.

Finally, researchers tried estrogen vaginal creams and transdermal androgen patches. Some studies suggested increased desire but most showed scant benefit and masculinizing side effects.

In 2015, the Food and Drug Administration approved the first nonhormonal treatment for low libido in women, flibanserin (Addyi, ADD-ee). Depending on the study, it boosts desire in 15–50 percent of users. It must be taken daily. When it helps, it's not particularly effective. An analysis of 5,914 users showed just one additional roll in the hay every eight weeks, six more a year. Meanwhile, flibanserin's possible side effects include dizziness, sedation, nausea, and low blood pressure, which may cause fainting, especially in women who use alcohol or the Pill. To prevent potentially fatal fainting while driving, women who take Addyi should not drink alcohol or take birth control pills. Few women use Addyi.

In 2019, the FDA approved a second desire drug, bremelanotide (Vyleesi). Women take it only before lovemaking, and it can be used safely with alcohol. However, it must be self-injected in the thigh or abdomen, off-putting for many women. In preapproval trials, 40 percent

Tribulus terrestris: Intriguing

Tribulus is a hairy-leafed, yellow-flowered annual that grows in temperate areas worldwide. Since ancient times, cultures from Eastern Europe to East Asia have considered it an aphrodisiac. Some research shows the plant increases synthesis of nitric oxide, a compound critical to sexual function.

Several studies show that *Tribulus* (750 mg/day) boosts women's libido:

- Brazilian researchers gave either a placebo or *Tribulus* to sixty postmenopausal women complaining of low desire. After ninety days, the *Tribulus* group reported significantly more desire, lubrication, and pleasure.
- Another Brazilian team gave thirty-six low-libido postmenopausal women a placebo or *Tribulus*. After four months, the plant group enjoyed significantly increased desire, arousal, lubrication, and satisfaction.
- Iranian scientists gave sixty-seven low-desire women a placebo or *Tribulus*. After four weeks, the *Tribulus* group reported significantly more desire, lubrication, and sexual satisfaction.

Side effects are unlikely but may include stomachache, cramping, diarrhea, nausea, vomiting, constipation, insomnia, and increased menstrual flow.

Studies to date haven't involved enough subjects to clearly establish *Tribulus* as beneficial. Questions also remain about how it works, best dosage, and long-term safety. However, findings so far have been intriguing. *Tribulus* is available over the counter at health food stores, supplement shops, and on the internet.

of users reported nausea, 21 percent experienced flushing, and 12 percent got headaches, all of which suppress libido. And Vyleesi should not be used by women with high blood pressure or cardiovascular disease.

Finally, libido-boosting drugs appear to have an unusually large placebo effect. Give people sugar pills for any complaint and around one-third report benefit. To be judged effective, new drugs must work significantly better than placebos. UCLA researchers analyzed drug treatments for low desire in twenty-four studies involving 3,959 women. Placebo treatment benefited two-thirds (68 percent), twice the benefit of most placebos. So it remains unclear if Addyi and Vylessi are as effective as their supporters claim or if their apparent effectiveness reflects this unusually large placebo effect.

Which Comes First—Desire? Or Good Sex?

As mentioned, low libido might involve something about the women, or something about the lovemaking. The studies discussed so far all focused on the women. But since the millennium, women sex researchers, notably Rosemary Basson, MD, of the University of British Columbia, have explored the sex. They've discovered that when women begin partner play, many feel erotically *neutral*. Then, as lovemaking unfolds, if they enjoy it, they eventually work up to feeling desire. In other words, for many women, good sex *precedes* desire—the opposite of the standard male model. Instead of desire compelling them to pursue sex, for many, possibly most women, desire isn't the *cause* of sex, but its *result*.

Now, most women experience pre-sex desire during the brief hot-and-heavy period of new relationships, and around 5 percent of women experience male-style lust for life. But if Basson is correct—and most sexologists agree with her—then many women's desire is fundamentally different from men's.

Basson's discovery that good sex produces desire explains why hormones and drugs haven't done much for women. These approaches assume that desire *precedes* sex, which puts the erotic cart before the horse.

Basson's perspective also explains why classes and self-help books work. They focus not only on the women, but also on how sex unfolds, promoting extended loveplay.

Finally, Basson's insight explains the consistent finding that women's low libido rarely precludes orgasm and sexual satisfaction. Women may initially feel erotically neutral, but if they enjoy the lovemaking, they work up to orgasm and emerge satisfied.

Ladies, if you don't feel aroused as kissing and cuddling begin, you're normal. If you're "slow" to become aroused, you're fine. If you like lots of whole-body massage before his fingers find your breasts or genitals, you're normal.

Gentlemen, women's sexual enjoyment usually has little if anything to do with your endowment, how long you last, or even if you can raise erections. The keys include deep relaxation, slow pace, whole-body massage, mutual coaching, lubricant, oral sex, novelty, and ongoing courtship that makes women feel desired. Don't imitate porn. Slow down—do everything at half speed. Kiss and cuddle more. Gently caress every square inch of women's bodies from head to toe for at least twenty minutes *before* you reach between their legs. Ask for coaching. Value sexual novelty. When erotic play progresses to the genitals, use lubricant. And offer extended cunnilingus every time.

According to Basson and a good deal of other sex researchers' recent studies, the question is *not* What provokes women's desire? The real question is What kind of lovemaking allows women to feel sufficiently desired, relaxed, caressed, and loved to enjoy sex so they can eventually feel desire?

CHAPTER 38:
Why So Many Women Have Trouble with Orgasm

THE GOAL OF sex is not orgasm but mutual pleasure. Satisfying lovemaking is quite possible without climaxing. Sex without orgasm doesn't necessarily reflect badly on you, your lover, or your relationship. And even cataclysmic orgasms can't redeem sex that's boring or fraught. But just as banquets don't feel quite finished without dessert, many lovers feel that lovemaking is incomplete unless they come.

The Great Orgasm Divide

During the 1920s, two decades before Indiana University's Alfred Kinsey officially launched sex research, New York gynecologist Robert Dickinson, MD, quietly surveyed one thousand married women about their sexuality. Their main complaint—no orgasms during partner sex. Almost all were orgasmic solo, but with their husbands, even those in loving marriages often found climax maddeningly elusive.

Kinsey's much larger studies in the 1940s confirmed that during partner lovemaking, considerably fewer women than men have orgasms. And since Kinsey, the orgasm gender divide has been consistently reconfirmed in dozens of studies. With partners, men report orgasms around 95 percent of the time, but depending on the study, the figure for women is only 50–70 percent. Why? Like low libido in women, there are two possibilities—something about the women or something about the sex.

For decades, the conventional wisdom has favored the former explanation. Many people believe women are the more emotionally complicated gender, and that even minor emotional upsets might derail their orgasms.

Many women concur, believing that orgasm difficulties are a reflection on them. Investigators at Valparaiso University in Indiana asked 452 women why they had trouble coming. Their list: anxiety, pain, little self-lubrication, and body image upsets.

In many studies, researchers have documented four elements that make modest differences in women's rate of partner sex orgasms:

- **Demographics.** As women's age, education, and income rise, their likelihood of orgasm increases a bit.
- **Beliefs.** Compared with women who embrace religious fundamentalism (sex only for procreation) and traditional gender roles (male breadwinners, female homemakers), women who embrace more liberal views are a little more likely to have orgasms.
- **Relationships.** As relationship happiness increases, women's likelihood of climaxing increases modestly.

- **Sexual trauma.** Compared with survivors of child sexual abuse and/or sexual assault, women free from sexual trauma are somewhat more likely to come.

However, add up all these impacts and they don't come anywhere near explaining the magnitude of the orgasm gap.

Since the millennium, several sexologists have turned away from female psychology and have focused on the nitty-gritty of lovemaking. They've discovered that, compared with the factors above, what lovers do—or don't do—in bed makes a much greater difference and largely explains the orgasm gap. Women's ability to have orgasms has less to do with their emotional complexity than with the erotic caresses they receive.

Not the Women, the Sex

Australian researchers surveyed 5,118 men and women age sixteen to fifty-nine about the four factors discussed above, then asked them to describe the genital touch they'd received during their most recent partner play—and if they'd come. As usual, 95 percent of the men reported climaxing, but among the women just 69 percent. The women's demographics, beliefs, relationships, and trauma histories made only a small difference.

During their most recent erotic tangos, participants reported three types of genital play: vaginal intercourse (95 percent), massage or fingering (80 percent), and oral sex (25 percent). Among the men, orgasm likelihood varied only slightly based on genital play:

- **Just intercourse:** Men reporting orgasms—96 percent
- **Hand job and intercourse:** 95 percent
- **Hand job, intercourse, and fellatio:** 98 percent

But for the women, orgasm varied considerably based on genital caresses:
- **Just intercourse:** Women reporting orgasms—50 percent
- **Vulvar massage, fingering, and intercourse:** 71 percent
- **Vulvar massage, fingering, intercourse, and cunnilingus:** 86 percent

For reproduction, sex is all about intercourse. But for women's orgasms, it's mostly about men providing *all three kinds of genital touch.*

Other studies corroborate this:

- Compared with partner lovemaking, women consistently come faster and more reliably from self-sexing, which involves direct clitoral caresses.
- Indiana University researchers surveyed 1,055 women age fourteen to ninety-four. Fewer than one in five (18 percent) reported orgasms solely from intercourse. Most said they needed direct clitoral touch. And many of those who could come during intercourse said their orgasms felt better with direct clitoral caresses.
- Scientists from several universities surveyed 407 lesbians and 370 heterosexual women. The two groups were demographically comparable, but the lesbians reported significantly more orgasms. They received more clitoral massage and cunnilingus.
- Researchers at Chapman University in Southern California analyzed orgasms among 52,588 American adults. Lesbian women reported coming in 86 percent of encounters, heterosexual women only 65 percent. The lesbians kissed more, shared more mutual whole-body massage, and received more vulvar massage, fingering, and cunnilingus.

- One of the world's largest porn sites, PornHub, tracks searches by gender. Compared with men, women are three times more likely to search "cunnilingus" and "pussy eating."

Clitoral? Vaginal? G-Spot?

All women's (and men's) orgasms involve involuntary, rapid, serial, wavelike contractions of the pelvic floor muscles that run between the legs.

But early in the twentieth century, Sigmund Freud, founder of psychoanalysis, postulated two kinds of female climaxes—"immature" clitoral and "mature" vaginal orgasms. He made this up. Sexologists have never produced any evidence of vaginal orgasms, and there's nothing immature about those triggered by clitoral stimulation.

Starting in the 1980s, some women said they experienced a third type, G-spot orgasms, produced by pressing on the front vaginal wall.

Orgasms may *feel* very different based on women's (or men's) mood, relationships, arousal, fantasies, drug use, type of stimulation, and other factors. But physiologically all orgasms are the same. They all involve rapid, involuntary contractions of the pelvic floor muscles.

Gentlemen, Unless She Requests Otherwise, Eat Her Every Time

The head of the penis contains the largest concentration of orgasm-triggering nerves. Intercourse rocks these nerves, which explains why, among men whose partner sex involves only intercourse, 95 percent have orgasms.

But women's orgasm nerves don't reside inside the vagina. They're concentrated in the clitoris an inch or two north of the vaginal opening under the upper junction of the vaginal lips. Intercourse provides sufficient stimulation to bring some women to orgasm, but for many women, intercourse alone falls short.

What fraction of women consistently work up to orgasm during intercourse? Elisabeth Lloyd, author of *The Case of the Female Orgasm*, analyzed thirty-three studies:

- At most, only 25 percent of women are consistently orgasmic during intercourse.
- Around 50 percent come from shagging sometimes.
- About 20 percent seldom have orgasms during intercourse.
- And 5 percent rarely, if ever, climax from the old in-out.

Gentlemen, this bears repeating: Only one-quarter of women are reliably orgasmic during intercourse—no matter how large your penis, how long you last, or how the woman feels about you.

Unfortunately, many men believe women "should" have orgasms during intercourse. In countless books, movies, and TV shows, both lovers climax simultaneously during intercourse. Actually, this is rare. Meanwhile, during porn intercourse, the women thrash and moan, looking like they come. Actually, they don't. I've interviewed several women porn actors. None ever came on camera. Porn sex, largely fellatio and intercourse, didn't turn them on. But all were orgasmic at home with their partners—thanks to direct, gentle, extended clitoral caresses from vibrators, lovers' hands, and especially their tongues.

Compared with intercourse, hand jobs, fingering, and cunnilingus are considerably more likely to excite the clitoris. That's why, in the Australian study discussed earlier, lovemaking that included them made such a difference in women's rate of orgasm.

Most women's need for clitoral kisses also explains the demographics of women's orgasms:

- As age and education increase, so do women's rates of orgasm. Older, better educated women are more likely to ask for direct clitoral touch and more likely to be involved with older, better educated men willing to provide it.
- As women move from fundamentalism toward religious liberalism and from home-making into the labor force, their rates of orgasm also increase. They're less likely to feel cowed by tradition and more likely to assert their need for clitoral touch and be involved with men willing to provide it.

I'm not dismissing the pleasure of intercourse for women. Many love its special closeness, saying they cherish holding lovers inside them. But as far as women's orgasms are concerned, intercourse usually proves inadequate. Gentlemen, if you want her to come, review part I, especially the discussion of oral sex, and provide gentle, extended clitoral caresses and cunnilingus every time. Or as many men would say, *eat more pussy*. Go down and feast for a nice long time every time.

"Did You Come?" How to Recognize Women's Orgasms

Some women accuse men of not caring if they come. University of Michigan scientists surveyed 810 men. The vast majority cared deeply about their partners' orgasms. It was crucial to the men's sexual self-esteem.

But many men, especially teens and young adults, can't tell if their lovers have climaxed. Gentlemen, if you feel the need to ask, *Did you come?* chances are she didn't, especially if you make love drunk, rush into intercourse, and don't provide gentle, extended clitoral massage and cunnilingus.

What Proportion of Women Fake Orgasm? Why?

Depending on the study, one-third to two-thirds of women say they've faked orgasm at least once:
- University of Kansas researchers surveyed 101 women college students. Those admitting faking—67 percent.
- Finnish scientists surveyed 1,421 adult Finnish women. Those who'd pretended at least once—34 percent.

Women fake orgasms to:
- Boost partners' egos
- Avoid hurting partners' feelings
- Avoid interrogations, accusations of inadequacy, and shame
- End the sex

Faking is age-related. As women mature, many become better able to ask for the caresses that trigger their orgasms and many men gain insights into the moves that help their lovers come.

Actually, if you know what to look for, orgasms are pretty hard to miss. Women's resemble men's. Think about your own and you should be able to identify women's. Most begin with a quickening of breathing often accompanied by gasps or moans followed by several seconds of rapid, involuntary contractions of the muscles around the vulva and anus, usually with convulsive movements of the hips and often the whole body. Orgasms conclude with release into relaxation and dreamy contentment. In addition, if you eat women to O's, your lips and tongue are likely to feel her vaginal muscles contract. If you'd like to see what women's orgasms look like, watch the video *Orgasmic Women: 13 Self-Loving Divas.*

How to Boost Women's Likelihood of Orgasm during Intercourse

Three-quarters of women are *not* consistently orgasmic during intercourse. But many couples would like women to come that way. Three intercourse positions allow men to provide direct clitoral massage quite easily and a slight variation on the man-on-top (missionary) position may also help.

- **Woman-on-top.** The man lies on his back, legs together. The woman straddles his hips and sits on his erection. She can reach down and caress her clit by hand or vibrator. Or he can make a fist and place it at the junction of their pelvises. She can lean forward and press her clitoris into it.
- **Rear entry (doggie).** She's on hands or elbows and knees. He kneels or stands behind her. He can reach around and caress her clit. Or she can reach between her legs or use a vibrator.

  Note: Rear entry allows deep insertion that may hurt women. Except for consensual BDSM, sex should *never* hurt. Gentlemen, during doggie intercourse, remain still and allow women to specify their comfort limits. Ask for coaching.
- **Spooning.** With her back to his chest, his hands are free to massage her clitoris. Or she can caress herself by hand or vibrator.
- **Pelvic motion.** During man-on-top intercourse, many women remain fairly still while the man pumps. But women are more likely to come if they move. Swiss researchers surveyed 1,239 women, age eighteen to seventy-five. As their pelvic movements during intercourse increased, so did their likelihood of orgasm. The women's movements increased clitoral stimulation.
- **The coital alignment technique (CAT).** During conventional man-on-top intercourse, erections move almost horizontally. In 1988, New York sex researcher Edward Eichel announced the CAT, a minor adjustment that shifts the man forward and to one side, his chest over one of her shoulders. With this change, erections move more up and down, and the pubic bone at the base of the penis makes more direct contact with the clitoris. Eichel asked eighty-six couples how often the women had orgasms during intercourse, then taught them the CAT. The women quickly became significantly better able to climax during intercourse, and with continued CAT practice, their rates of orgasm rose further.

  By the mid-1990s, the CAT was largely forgotten. Then in 2000, studies by Texas investigators reconfirmed its effectiveness. The researchers worked with thirty-six women unable to have missionary-position orgasms. They and their lovers enrolled in an eight-week sexual-enrichment course that emphasized mutual whole-body massage. In addition, half learned the coital alignment technique. With the course, women's missionary-position orgasms increased 27 percent, but with the CAT, 56 percent, twice as much.

Coital alignment is no substitute for gentle, extended clitoral caresses by hand, mouth, or vibrator, nor does it guarantee orgasm during missionary intercourse. Many women just don't come that way—and that's fine. But the CAT improves women's ability to come with lovers on top of them.

- **Have a ball.** During man-on-top intercourse or the CAT, a small soft ball—Nerf, hacky sack, and so forth—can be placed between the woman's clitoris and the man's pelvis. As he presses on the ball, she receives more clitoral stimulation and is more likely to come.
- **Mock intercourse.** Instead of inserting, he positions his erection so it presses against the sensitive groove between her inner vaginal lips. His glans caresses her clit.

Help for Women with Orgasm Difficulties

University of Chicago researchers surveyed a representative 1,749 women age eighteen to fifty-nine and another 1,550 women fifty-seven to eighty-five. In every age group, one-quarter to one-third of the women reported difficulty working up to orgasm.

Fortunately, the overwhelming majority of women can learn to have orgasms. In the words of sexologist Erwin J. Haeberle, "Orgasm is learned. The teacher is masturbation." Review chapters 1–10 and 36. In addition:

- **Buy a vibrator.** Today, half of adult American women own at least one. Vibrators produce more intense sensation than hands and tongues can provide. Many women who can't have orgasms without vibrators can come with them.
- **Read *Becoming Orgasmic: A Sexual and Personal Growth Program for Women.*** First published in 1976, this classic self-help book by sexologists Julia Heiman, PhD, and Joseph LoPiccolo, PhD, guides women through a step-by-step process of self-discovery focusing on barriers to pleasure, self-touch, vibrators, and coaching lovers. A companion DVD is also available.
- **Coaching.** Ladies, does your man kiss and cuddle playfully? Does he provide at least twenty minutes of gentle hand jobs and oral? If not, speak up. Ask for what you need. If you don't, nothing changes.
- **Sex coaching or therapy.** If you can't speak up, a sex coach or therapist can help you find your voice.

Why Do Women Have Orgasms?

If only 25 percent of women are reliably orgasmic during intercourse, women don't need orgasms to have children. And if evolution doesn't require female orgasms for procreation, why do women have them?

Scientists once believed that women have orgasms because men do. Traits biologically necessary for one gender often develop in the other—if there's no evolutionary pressure *against* them. Consider nipples. Women need them to nurse infants. Men don't need nipples, but there's no evolutionary pressure against them, so men retain them. It's possible that women have orgasms simply because men do.

However, evolution is remarkably energy efficient. Over thousands of generations, traits that consume energy but produce no survival advantage usually disappear. It takes no energy for men to have nipples, but orgasms consume energy—women's more than men's. Men's orgasms last around ten seconds, women's often longer. In addition, more women than men are multiorgasmic, able to have successive orgasms in fairly rapid succession.

A growing body of evidence suggests that orgasms help women send their genes into the next generation:

- Women's rates of orgasm during intercourse fluctuate with the menstrual cycle. They're mostly likely around ovulation.
- Women's orgasms during intercourse often trigger men's, sending sperm toward eggs.
- Orgasms release the hormone oxytocin, which stimulates rhythmic contractions of the uterus. These contractions help suck semen from the vagina into the womb.
- When women come during intercourse, sperm entering the uterus are less likely to spill out, so more swim toward eggs.
- And women's orgasms release the hormone prolactin, which energizes sperm to swim faster and farther.

Meanwhile, women can raise children alone, but a man helps. Which man? Some evidence suggests that orgasm plays a role in women's mate selection:

- In both men and women, orgasm releases the hormone oxytocin, which fosters attachment.
- Women who have orgasms with men are also likely to want more sex with them, which helps them retain mates.

But if orgasm helps women conceive and retain mates, why are only 25 percent consistently orgasmic during intercourse? That's still a mystery.

CHAPTER 39:
A Man's Guide to Women's Sexual Pain

RESEARCHERS AT SEVERAL US universities—Columbia, Purdue, and Indiana—reviewed data from the 2018 nationally representative US National Survey of Sexual Health and Behavior. They identified 382 adult women who'd reported at least one painful sexual experience during the previous year, and asked them three questions:

- How painful was it?
- Did you tell your partner?
- And if not, why not?

Of those reporting pain, only half (51 percent) told their partners. The women were most likely to speak up if pain felt severe, but 82 percent said theirs was "only" mild to moderate, not sufficiently agonizing to warrant discussion. However, even mild pain significantly interfered with the women's erotic pleasure and satisfaction. Their silence cost them, but many grew up believing that sex *should* hurt and that their erotic pleasure should be subordinate to their men's.

Gentleman, women's sexual pain is more prevalent than you probably imagine. Many women suffer pain of the external genitals (vulvodynia, vestibulodynia). Others experience discomfort or pain during intercourse (dyspareunia). And some endure chronic pelvic pain independent of lovemaking but aggravated by it.

Some men dismiss women's sexual pain, accusing them of feigning it to avoid sex. A few even believe sex *should* hurt women—some popular songs say sex "hurts so good." And until the 1980s, some (mostly male) doctors dismissed women's genital pain as "neurotic," leaving them doubly wounded—in pain and feeling ridiculed.

Except for intense sensation during carefully choreographed consensual BDSM, sex should *never* hurt. If she says it does and you dismiss her complaints, you're at best a jerk. In addition, she's unlikely to become aroused, which means you *both* have lousy sex. Fortunately, most women's sexual pain can be relieved—and men's support helps.

How Many Women Suffer Sexual Pain?

University of Chicago researchers surveyed a representative 3,299 women age eighteen to eighty-five. Depending on the age group, 8–21 percent complained of sex-related pain, and across all age groups, an average of 15 percent reported it. Other studies have estimated pain prevalence at up to 30 percent.

Sexual pain is most likely among young women, who may not be sufficiently informed or experienced to minimize it with assertive partner coaching. But as they mature, most young women become more willing to speak up. The likelihood of pain declines with age until menopause, when vaginal dryness and tissue thinning (atrophy) increase it.

Pain is a body-mind experience with both physical and emotional components. Physically, noxious events trigger the body's pain nerves. Emotionally, anxiety, depression, and relationship woes may aggravate pain. It's important to explore both physical and psychological components. Each responds to different treatments. If physical pain can't be eliminated, psychological interventions—including lovers' support—may still reduce it.

Start with a Checkup

Ladies: if you have sexual pain, consult your primary care physician or gynecologist. If they can't cure you, consider a sexual medicine specialist. To find one near you, visit the North America Society of Sexual Medicine (SexHealthMatters.org/resources/find-a-provider). Or try a sex therapist. Many work with physicians trained in sexual medicine. Helpful organizations include the International Pelvic Pain Society (pelvicpain.org), the National Vulvodynia Association (nva.org), or the Vulvar Pain Foundation (vulvarpainfoundation.org).

Doctors should investigate these possibilities:

- **Relationship turmoil.** One possible consequence is sexual pain.
- **Imperforate hymen.** At birth, the hymen covers part of girls' vaginal openings. The membrane often wears away during childhood and causes no discomfort on tampon insertion, fingering, or intercourse. In others, residual hymen tissue may cause sexual discomfort or pain.
- **Menopause.** After forty, vaginal dryness and atrophy become increasingly prevalent. Intercourse may become uncomfortable or painful.
- **Vaginismus.** Affecting around 10 percent of women, vaginismus causes muscle spasms that constrict the vaginal opening or clamp it shut, making any insertions painful or impossible. My informal survey of sex therapists suggests it's a leading cause, if not the number one cause, of women's sexual pain.
- **Sexual infections.** Chlamydia, genital warts, and pelvic inflammatory disease may cause pain on intercourse.
- **Other vaginal infections.** Vaginal yeast infection or bacterial infection (vaginosis) may cause sexual pain.
- **Vulvar skin conditions.** Many women's external genitals become irritated from sunburn, pubic shaving, latex allergy from barrier contraceptives, or contact dermatitis from perfumed soaps, bubble baths, douches, or underwear made from synthetic fabrics.
- **Vulvar vestibulitis (VV).** This condition involves inflammation of the tiny vestibular glands just inside the vagina. Q-tip pressure causes sharp pain.
- **Oxalate irritation.** Women sensitive to the oxalates in some foods may develop urethral irritation and sexual pain.
- **Other medical conditions.** Uterine prolapse, endometriosis, interstitial cystitis, irritable bowel syndrome, gynecological cancers, and other conditions may cause pelvic pain.
- **Birth control pills.** Andrew Goldstein, MD, editor of *Female Sexual Pain Disorders*, says birth control pills are "a leading causes of women's sexual pain." The Pill increases release of sex hormone-binding globulin that attaches to vulvar cells, triggering biochemical changes that may cause pain.

- **Sexual trauma.** Childhood sexual abuse and/or sexual assault may cause chronic sexual pain.

Effective Treatments
These approaches often help:

Abuse recovery. Professional therapy is usually necessary.

Relationship issues. Consult a couples counselor or sex therapist.

Lifestyle changes. Stop douching. Use unscented soaps. Don't use bubble baths. Wear cotton underwear. Switch from barrier contraceptives or birth control pills to another method. Pill-related sexual pain usually resolves within six months.

Low-oxalate diet. Try avoiding high-oxalate foods: celery, coffee, chocolate, rhubarb, spinach, and strawberries. The Vulvar Pain Foundation publishes a larger list. It can take three to six months on a low-oxalate diet to experience improvement. Calcium citrate supplementation (Citracal) may also help.

Coaching. In three trials, Canadian researchers surveyed 87, 107, and 179 couples struggling with the women's sexual pain. In every study, as the women coached the men more assertively, their pain decreased.

Cognitive therapy. *Cognitive* means thinking. Cognitive therapy involves changing how you think about your life. If sex hurts, women might think, *This is unbearable. I'm dying.* That's often an overreaction psychologists call "catastrophizing." When people catastrophize, they tense up and pain hurts more. But with cognitive therapy, women might face the same physiological pain and think, *This hurts, but I can do something about it.* Then the pain is less likely to feel debilitating:

- Swedish scientists surveyed 133 women's sexual pain and how they felt about it. As catastrophizing increased, so did their pain.
- Canadian researchers assessed seventy-eight women's sexual pain, then assigned them to vestibulectomy (below), biofeedback (below), or cognitive therapy. All three significantly reduced their pain.
- The Canadian team surveyed the sexual pain of 97 women, then taught them cognitive therapy or asked them to use an inflammation-reducing topical steroid cream. After six months, both groups reported less pain, but the cognitive therapy group reported greater relief.

Relaxation regimens. Emotional stress aggravates pain. Relaxation therapies reduce stress and help relieve it:

- Researchers at the University of California, San Francisco, asked sixteen women to rate their pelvic pain. Then they took an hour-long yoga class twice a week and practiced yoga regularly at home. After six weeks, their pain decreased significantly.

- Swedish investigators gave forty-six women with vulvar vestibulitis either a relaxation therapy (biofeedback) or a topical anesthetic. A year later, both treatments were equally effective.
- Canadian scientists surveyed pain in eight women with vulvar vestibulitis, then treated them with a relaxation therapy (hypnosis). After six months, they reported significant relief.

Acupuncture. University of Illinois researchers used acupuncture on thirty-six women with genital pain. It significantly reduced their pain.

Intrarosa (prasterone, dehydroepiandosterone, DHEA). Approved in 2016, Intrarosa is a vaginal suppository that may relieve pain in postmenopausal women with vaginal dryness and atrophy. Canadian researchers gave 696 postmenopausal women suffering sexual pain either a placebo or Intrarosa. After three months, the drug reduced pain 50 percent. In another trial, men involved with women taking Intrarosa said it significantly enhanced their partner lovemaking. Intrarosa's most common side effects include vaginal discharge and abnormal Pap tests.

Vaginismus treatment. Therapies include muscle relaxants, Kegel exercises, biofeedback, other relaxation regimens, and insertion of graduated dilator rods that gradually coax the vagina back open. An Italian analysis of forty-three studies found this combination of therapies effective for 82 percent of women. For best results, assemble a physician-sex therapist team.

Vulvar vestibulitis treatment. Some VV clears up with time and increased lubrication. Other treatments include Kegel exercises, biofeedback, cognitive therapy, a low-oxalate diet, a support group, and removal of the glands (vestibulectomy).

Pelvic floor physiotherapy. This branch of physiotherapy focuses on the muscles, joints, connective tissue, and nerves of the pelvis, low back, and hips.

Adjust Your Lovemaking

Women's pain may also result from how couples make love—with porn-style sex often the culprit.

Rushed intercourse. In porn, boy meets girl and moments later, he's hiding the salami. In fantasy, that's fine, but in real life, rushed intercourse often hurts women.

Before women can enjoy intercourse comfortably, most need at least twenty minutes of nongenital loveplay, which spurs vaginal relaxation, making the organ more receptive to fingers, erections, and toys.

Gentlemen: never imitate the rushed intercourse of porn. Inserting can wait. Give women all the time they need to relax and become receptive. Ask for coaching about your lovers' preferences. Occasionally, quickies can be fun. But sex coaches and therapists almost universally recommend leisurely, playful, extended, nongenital loveplay and oral before attempting any insertions—especially if women suffer sexual pain.

Lack of lubrication. Even with extended loveplay, poorly lubricated intercourse is a major cause of women's sexual pain. Many perfectly normal women don't produce much natural lubrication. After forty, as women become menopausal, lubrication issues increase. That's one reason why many older couples switch from intercourse to outercourse. For sizzling sex, intercourse is *not necessary*. Mutual pleasure and fabulous orgasms are quite possible without it.

Gentlemen: never insert anything into vaginas that feel dry. Saliva is often an effective lubricant. Provide generous, gentle, extended cunnilingus every time. Or use a commercial lube. Apply it to both the vagina and anything you insert.

Porn-style pounding. Even if women are well lubricated and highly aroused, they may experience pain if men "pound" them, imitating the furious fucking in porn.

Gentlemen: the vagina is not a hollow space. It's packed with tightly folded muscle tissue that relaxes and yields to insertions most comfortably when well-lubricated fingers, erections, and toys enter *slowly*. To learn how slowly women prefer, ask, and/or use the woman-on-top position and notice how slowly she sits on your erection.

Inserting too deeply. If you're the rare guy with an unusually long banana, your length may hurt women in any position. But rear-entry (doggie style) intercourse is most problematic. The penis may bang into the cervix and cause pain.

Gentlemen: to enjoy pain-free doggie intercourse, remain still and invite your lover to back onto your erection to a depth that feels comfortable to her. Notice her comfort limit and never push in deeper.

Uninformed anal play. The anus is the least receptive erotic opening. Unschooled anal play often hurts recipients. However, with patience, a very slow pace, and copious lubrication, it's quite possible to enjoy pain-free anal eroticism.

Bottom line: most women's sexual pain can be reduced or eliminated. Women appreciate men who take their pain seriously, provide emotional support, and are willing to make erotic adjustments for women's comfort.

Some Men Also Suffer Sexual Pain

Indiana University researchers surveyed 1,738 adults and discovered that 7 percent of the men reported pain during intercourse. Causes include anxiety, depression, chafing, prostatitis, herpes, other infections, unusually persistent erections (priapism), a tight foreskin (phimosis), and an unusually curved erection (Peyronie's disease). Men with sexual pain should consult their doctors or urologists, or a sexual medicine specialist.

PART V:
Other Ways to Play

CHAPTER 40:
A Consumer's Guide to Vibrators

L ISTEN CAREFULLY. THAT faint buzzing you hear just might be the woman—or couple—next door enjoying a vibrator. Today, more than half of adult American women own
at least one, and vibes are becoming increasingly popular in couple lovemaking. In the 1980s,
vibrators were mostly sold by small catalogs. Today, one of the largest marketers is Walmart.

Vibrator Myths versus Truth

MYTH: Vibrators are for loners and losers.
TRUTH: Actually, an Indiana University study shows that single women are *less* likely to use
them than married women—29 percent versus 50 percent. Compared with singles, most married women think about sex more and are more likely to reach for vibes. Compared with
women who never used vibrators, those who did reported more interest in sex, more self-
lubrication, easier arousal and orgasms, and greater sexual satisfaction.

MYTH: If women need vibrators to come, something is wrong with them.
TRUTH: Not at all. Some women just need more intense stimulation than fingers, penises, and
tongues can provide.

MYTH: If women need vibrators to have orgasms, their men are lousy lovers.
TRUTH: Possibly—but not necessarily. Gentlemen: review chapters 4–10 and 35–39. Even
when men provide the whole-body lovemaking most women prefer, some perfectly normal
women need intense vibrator stimulation to climax.

MYTH: If women use vibrators, men are replaced by machines.
TRUTH: Absolutely not. The best carpenters use power tools. Vibrators provide only one thing,
intense stimulation. They don't smile, converse, kiss, embrace, warm the bed, tell jokes, say
I love you, or share women's joys and heartaches. Vibrators don't replace men any more than
power tools replace carpenters.

MYTH: Vibrators are unnatural.
TRUTH: They're as natural as other erotic enhancements: lingerie, perfume, music, candlelight,
lubricants, champagne, clean sheets, or massage lotion.

MYTH: Vibrators ruin women for sex without them.
TRUTH: Does driving ruin you for walking? No, it just gets you there faster. The same goes for
vibes. Using vibrators—even frequently—doesn't change the body's ability to respond to other
sexual caresses.

MYTH: Vibrators are addictive.
TRUTH: Many people use the term "addiction" too loosely. Some women become *very fond* of vibrators. But unlike addictions, vibrators don't cause tolerance. In fact, over time as vibes teach women about the full range of their erotic responsiveness, many find it takes *less* vibrator stimulation to get the job done. And unlike addicts who organize their lives around their addictions, it's virtually unheard of for vibe users to do that. I've answered more than twelve thousand sex questions. Here are two I've never received: *Should I be worried about how often I use my vibrator?* And: *Why does my girlfriend/wife use her vibe so much?*

MYTH: Vibrators numb the genitals.
TRUTH: Sometimes, but not often. In the Indiana survey, 11 percent of users reported occasional numbness and 3 percent experienced it frequently. For numbness or tingling, use lubricant and press less. Or try a lower-power vibe. Or vibe less.

MYTH: Vibrators cause urinary tract infections.
TRUTH: No. Vibrators don't cause UTIs, but using them carelessly might. UTIs are caused by digestive-tract bacteria that leave the body during defecation. Residual bacteria may contaminate the anal area. If vibrators (or fingers) touch them, then contact the vulva, the bacteria may travel up the urine tube (urethra) and infect the bladder. If you enjoy anal play, always wash thoroughly beforehand. Keep track of what vibrators touch. Or cover them with condoms for anal play and remove them for vulva/vaginal play.

Increasingly Popular among Women

When the nation's first woman-friendly erotic boutiques opened—Eve's Garden in New York City (1974) and Good Vibrations in San Francisco (1977)—few women owned vibrators. Fast-forward to 2009, when Indiana University researchers surveyed a representative 3,800 adult American women and found that more than half (53 percent) owned at least one. They said that using vibrators:

- Is a healthy part of women's sexuality—Agree: 77%. Disagree: 23%.
- Adds excitement to partner sex—Agree: 75%. Disagree: 25%.
- Enhances partner sex—Agree: 74%. Disagree: 26%.
- Makes it easier to have orgasms—Agree: 73%. Disagree: 27%.
- Reduces pressure on partners to bring users to orgasm—Agree: 68%. Disagree: 32%.
- Increases women's sexual independence—Agree: 66%. Disagree: 34%.
- Is only for single women—Agree: 13%. Disagree: 87%.
- Is embarrassing—Agree: 28%. Disagree: 72%.
- Makes women too dependent on them—Agree: 35%. Disagree: 65%.
- Intimidates men—Agree: 37%. Disagree: 63%.

Herbenick, D., et al. "Prevalence and Characteristics of Vibrator Use by Women in the United States: Results from a Nationally Representative Study." *Journal of Sexual Medicine* 6 (2009): 1857.

Herbenick, D., et al. "Women's Vibrator Use in Sexual Partnerships: Results from a Nationally Representative Survey in the U.S." *Journal of Sex and Marital Therapy* 36 (2010): 49.

Herbenick, D., et al. "Beliefs about Women's Vibrator Use: Results from a Nationally Representative Probability Survey in the United States." *Journal of Sex and Marital Therapy* 37 (2011): 329.

Increasingly Popular among Men

Until the millennium, women asked me only one question about men and vibes: *How can I persuade him to include one in our lovemaking?* I still get that, but less frequently.

Indiana University investigators interviewed 1,047 adult men. Forty-five percent said they'd been involved in partner vibrator play at least once, 10 percent frequently. Men who included vibrators regularly in partner lovemaking reported more desire, firmer erections, better orgasms, happier lovers, and greater satisfaction. It remains unclear if vibrators, per se, improve sex for men or if men who have sizzling sex are more apt to use them. My guess: some of both.

The Indiana survey of attitudes about vibes included more than one thousand men. They said that using vibrators:

- Is a healthy part of many women's sexuality—Agree: 80%. Disagree: 20%.
- Adds excitement to partner sex—Agree: 81%. Disagree: 19%.
- Enhances partner sex—Agree: 82%. Disagree: 18%.
- Makes it easier for women to have orgasms—Agree: 81%. Disagree: 19%.
- Reduces pressure on men to bring users to orgasm—Agree: 68%. Disagree: 32%.
- Increases women's sexual independence—Agree: 61%. Disagree: 39%.
- Is only for single women—Agree: 15%. Disagree: 85%.
- Is embarrassing—Agree: 23%. Disagree: 77%.
- Makes women too dependent on them—Agree: 35%. Disagree: 65%.
- Intimidates men—Agree: 30%. Disagree: 70%.

Still, many men hesitate to incorporate vibrators into partner play. To change that, ladies, I suggest you and your man watch *The OH in Ohio*, a comedy starring Parker Posey, Paul Rudd, Danny DeVito, and Liza Minnelli. Posey plays a Cleveland advertising executive who has never had an OH. Her husband (Rudd) considers the marriage a failure because she can't come. A friend sends Posey to a sexuality workshop led by Minnelli, who introduces her to vibrators. It's love at first buzz. And when our heroine sets her phone on vibrate and slips it into her underwear before a business meeting, hilarity ensues. Meanwhile, her husband fears he's being replaced by a machine. A friend persuades him that vibrators rock partner sex.

Many men wonder how best to use vibrators on women. Ask for coaching. The main problem is overstimulation from pressing vibes into the vulva too forcefully. When in doubt, hold the device motionless and invite your lover to dance her vulva on it.

The Astonishing History of Vibrators

Who invented vibrators? Nineteenth-century male doctors who didn't care about women's pleasure. What they wanted was a labor-saving device to prevent the fatigue they suffered providing clitoral massage to a steady stream of well-to-do ladies who suffered "hysteria," then a vaguely defined ailment involving anxiety, insomnia, irritability, nervousness, erotic fantasies, and wetness between the legs, easily recognizable today as sexual frustration.

Physicians first described hysteria, from the Greek for uterus, during the thirteenth century. The quick, effective treatment was masturbation to orgasm, which most women discovered on their own or learned of from friends. But by the nineteenth century, Victorian physicians, all men, and the arbiters of decency, including many upper-class women, had demonized solo sex as "self-abuse."

Lower-class women continued to self-sex as they always had and didn't suffer hysteria. But many upper-class women embraced the notion that "ladies" had no sexual inclinations and put up with getting down entirely to retain husbands and have children.

Fortunately, doctors discovered a reliable, socially acceptable treatment—reaching under women's skirts and massaging their genitals, especially the clitoris. Fairly quickly, most hysterical women had orgasms and experienced relief. But doctors didn't call women's climaxes "orgasms." Everyone knew women didn't have them. The clinical term was *paroxysm*.

As physician-assisted paroxysms became popular among well-to-do European and American women, doctors reaped a financial and public-relations bonanza. During the nineteenth century, medicine was primitive and the public had little faith in it. But doctors could treat hysteria successfully, and a steady stream of paying customers returned regularly for treatment.

But frequent hysteria treatment had a downside for doctors—achy, cramped hands. In nineteenth-century medical journals, doctors lamented that treating hysterics taxed their endurance, and prevented some from continuing treatment long enough to produce relief.

Physicians experimented with mechanical replacements for their hands. They tried all sorts of genital massage contraptions, among them steam-driven dildos and water-driven gadgets, the forerunners of today's shower massagers. But the machines were costly, cumbersome, unreliable, and sometimes dangerous.

During the late nineteenth century, the first electric appliances appeared: fans, toasters, and sewing machines. In 1880, an enterprising English physician, Dr. Joseph Mortimer Granville, patented the electromechanical vibrator. Doctors loved it. Granville's device produced paroxysm quickly, safely, reliably, and as often as women desired.

Vibrators quickly became home appliances. They were advertised in popular women's magazines and the *Sears and Roebuck Catalog*, that era's Amazon.com. One 1903 Sears advertisement touted a popular model as "a delightful companion . . . pleasure will throb within you. . . ."

However, to make vibrators socially acceptable, their real purpose had to be disguised. Ads called them "personal massagers" (still the case in some catalogs). But discerning women understood their real purpose.

During the 1920s, vibrators showed up in porn, stripping their veil and quickly rendering them taboo. Vibrator ads disappeared from the consumer media, and until the late 1960s, they were largely unavailable (as substitutes, some women leaned into washing machines and dryers, or lay supine in bathtubs with the water at full blast hitting their genitals).

In 1968, as rising feminism spotlighted women's sexuality, Hitachi introduced its Magic Wand, currently the world's most popular vibrator. Today, more than half of American women own vibrators. And to think we owe them to physicians' finger fatigue.

Which Vibe Is Best?

Most users own one or two vibrators, but many own several. Among the dozens of models, what's "best" depends on individual women's inclinations, their circumstances, and the kind(s) of buzz they enjoy.

All vibes contain motors that produce vibration. Beyond that, they vary tremendously:

- Some resemble realistic erections, others impossibly huge ones, and some are more abstract cylinders, possibly with curved tips for solo G-spot play.
- Some are wands capped by plum-size vibrating balls, among them Hitachi's Magic Wand.

- Bullets are minivibrators—good for travel. A wire connects a thumb-size vibrator to a unit that houses the battery and controls.
- Dual-action vibrators have small protrusions extending from their shafts. With the main shaft nestled inside the vagina, the appendage stimulates the clitoris.
- Tongues are cylindrical vibes whose tips flatten into a tongue shape that wags back and forth, approximating cunnilingus.
- Butterfly vibes are pancake shaped. They cup the vulva and often include thigh straps to hold them in place.
- Materials include hard or soft plastic, jelly (like gummy-bear candies), or materials that feel like skin.
- Vibrators use disposable or rechargeable batteries or wall current. Battery vibes are lighter than plug-in models, useful where wall current is unavailable. But batteries must be changed or recharged and may lose power when you want it most. Plug-in vibrators are heavier but have more powerful motors and deliver more intense sensations.
- Some vibes have only one speed, others several, allowing a range of sensation.
- Most vibrators are *not* waterproof. Don't use them around water. However, there are many models of waterproof vibes, whose electrical components sealed inside their housings for fun in tubs, showers, and swimming pools.
- "Kits" include basic cylindrical vibes and attachments that alter their look and the sensations they produce.
- Plug-in models are usually more durable. Battery-powered vibes use lighter-weight motors that break more easily.
- Multispeed vibrators are among the most versatile—and popular. Sometimes you want a gentle buzz, other times intensity. But multispeed models require controls that may break.
- Use affects longevity. Frequent users usually employ plug-ins or switch among models depending on the setting.
- Most battery-powered vibes are not designed to operate continuously for more than twenty minutes at low speeds and ten minutes at high speeds. Plug-in models can be used longer. If you enjoy extended play with battery-powered vibrators, alternate among several.
- For whole-body massage, lovers can use vibrators on each other. For genital play, many women insist on handling them themselves—the clitoris can be *very* sensitive to touch, especially the intense sensations vibrators provide. But as women handle their vibes, many appreciate being held, kissed, caressed, and encouraged by their lovers.
- For greatest enjoyment, lubricate vibrators and whatever they touch.
- There is no "best" vibrator for everyone. Preferences and circumstances differ. That's why sex toy marketers offer such large selections.

Caring for Vibrators

- Many battery-powered vibrators have rechargeable batteries, so there's nothing to change. If not, change batteries frequently. Motors operate best at full power. As batteries age, they produce less juice—and pleasure.
- Remove batteries after each use. This increases vibrator longevity by keeping contacts clean. It also prevents damage in case of battery leakage.
- Before using waterproof vibrators, check for cracks that may allow water intrusion, which increases risk of shock and short-circuiting. If you find cracks, buy a new vibe.

- If you need an extension cord for your plug-in, use a heavy-duty cord, not one designed for lamps.
- Wash vibes with soap and water. Keep water away from batteries and motor compartments. Soap may leave a residue. Sex toy marketers offer "adult-toy cleansers," mild detergents they claim clean better than soap and leave no residue. You might also try diluting dish detergent.
- After washing, allow vibes to dry, then dust them with cornstarch for storing.
- Water-based lubes are usually best with vibrators. They wash off easily. Silicone lube should not be used with silicone vibrators. They degrade the vibrator surface. And Crisco and Vaseline may leave vibes feeling greasy.
- Vibrators have become so popular that many are cheap knockoffs that don't hold up. Look for brand names you recognize: Hitachi, Panasonic, and so forth.

CHAPTER 41:
Other Sex Enhancements

BRITISH RESEARCHERS ANALYZED one million purchases from Lovehoney, a leading UK sex toy marketer. The top ten accounted for 83 percent of sales:

- Lubricants, 22 percent of sales
- Vibrators, 18 percent
- Lingerie, 12 percent
- Anal toys, 7 percent
- Cock rings, 6 percent
- Penis sleeves, 5 percent
- Ben-wa balls, 4 percent
- Dildos, 3 percent
- BDSM toys, 3 percent
- Novelties (penis-shaped lollipops, etc.), 3 percent

Lubricants are discussed in chapter 7, vibrators in chapter 44. This chapter deals with other sex toys.

The Man's Guide to Buying Lingerie for Women

Lingerie adds novelty and ignites fantasies that enhance pleasure. Many men dream of seeing their partners "undressed up." But few men have any idea how to buy lingerie for women.

The conventional wisdom says women wear lingerie to excite men. That may be true for the minority of couples with high-libido women and lower-desire men. But few men need to see their lovers in lingerie to feel turned on. Gentlemen, she's more likely to enjoy wearing lingerie if you consider lingerie a tool to arouse *women*. You want lovers in lingerie to look in the mirror and feel *flattered and desirable*. Then tell them how desirable they look.

There are two ways to buy lingerie for women—with them or as a gift. Ask which she prefers.

If you shop together, she can try things on. When she asks your opinion, remember: the issue is *not* how hot she looks to *you*, but how *desirable* she feels. Shopping together also simmers incipient arousal so you can't wait to get home.

Meanwhile, many men want to surprise women with gifts of lingerie. If so, try to abide by these pointers.

For most women, forget skimpy. Porn often features women who appear thrilled to flaunt their assets, and in the real world, some—usually young—women feel that way. But most women feel self-conscious about their bodies and with age, discomfort grows. The best research suggests that only about 2 percent of women are exhibitionists. If *she* wants to surprise *you* with a fishnet body suit, fine. But if you're shopping for her, skimpy is risky. You're better off with greater coverage.

Forget bras, panties, thongs, and G-strings. To look flattering, these items must fit like gloves, which means knowing her size. Do you? Probably not. So you peek into her underwear drawer. But unlike the sizing of men's clothing—small, medium, large—women's sizes are a minefield: misses, petites, juniors, woman's, and more, each with a raft of sizes that are by no means standard.

For male shoppers, bras are particularly tricky. Professional corset fitters often chide women for buying bras that don't fit, so even if her bras say 36C, there's no guarantee that size will flatter her. If you buy a bra that's too large, she might conclude you think she's a whale. But if you select one that's too small, she may believe you want her to lose weight. My advice: avoid bras and panties.

Silky. You want her to feel special. Fabric should feel soft and sensual. Discuss this with salespeople. When in doubt, go with silk.

Full coverage. You may adore her boobs or butt, but she may feel differently. You want her to feel comfortable and self-confident so she can forget her insecurities and focus on playing with you.

Your best bet is loose-fitting, full-coverage outfits: robes, baby dolls, and negligees. Lingerie robes resemble bathrobes, but they're lighter weight and often semisheer. Baby-doll nighties are short nightgowns, usually thigh-high and sleeveless. Negligees are longer, calf- or ankle-length, and may have sleeves. Some include lace, ruffles, spaghetti straps, or slits up the sides. "Many women like lingerie that disguises what they consider flaws," says Joan Price, author of *Naked at Our Age*, a sex guide for older lovers. "Shop for full-coverage items. That way she decides what to reveal and what remains hidden."

Another advantage of full coverage—warmth. Warmth helps many women feel hot. Even with the thermostat cranked up, skimpy lingerie may leave women shivering. Warmth is another advantage of silk.

Buy several and invite her to model them. If you buy a few baby dolls, negligees, and/or robes in different colors and styles, imagine the fun you both can have at your own intimate fashion show. As she models each outfit, tell her why you selected it: "You look so hot in red." "That semisheer bodice drives me wild." "Those straps show off your shoulders so beautifully." Then decide together which one(s) she'll keep. Return the rest. Most lingerie shops and catalogs prohibit returns of panties, thongs, and G-strings, but accept returned baby dolls, negligees, and robes. Ask.

Butt Plugs, Anal Beads

Few lovers engage in penis-anus intercourse, but many play with sphincter massage, anilingus, and insertion of fingers or toys—butt plugs, anal beads, and/or anal dildos.

Unlike the vagina, the anus does not self-lubricate. Be sure to use lube for anal play. Lubricate the receiving anus and everything you insert. Watery lubes may not prove sufficient. Consider thicker gel lubricants or Crisco.

Never force anything into the anus. In partner anal-toy play, the inserter should hold the toy still with its tip just touching the receiving anus. The recipient should move back onto it, controlling the speed and depth of insertion. Good positions for this include hands and knees or standing bent at the waist.

Butt plugs come in several sizes—thin to thick, short to long. They have flared bases that keep them from getting lost inside. They can be enjoyed as part of loveplay or used beforehand to prepare the recipient for other insertions.

Anal beads enable serial opening and closing of the sphincters, which some find pleasurable.

Rings

Also called cock rings, these donut-shaped devices or belt-like straps slip over the erect penis. They may help maintain erections, but don't expect miracles. The arteries that deliver blood to the penis run through the central shaft, but the veins that carry blood out lie close to the surface. Rings compress these veins, somewhat reducing outflow, which helps maintain erection. Rings also help some men relax, which opens the arteries, increasing inflow for possibly firmer erections.

Rings may be made from jelly, plastic, or leather. Some are adjustable. Some include built-in bullet vibrators that nestle against the clitoris during intercourse. And some include butt plug attachments.

Use lubricant to increase pleasure of rings, and to prevent bruising.

Penis Sleeves

These male masturbation toys approximate the feel of fellatio or intercourse. The most popular is Fleshlight. It looks like a flashlight, but unscrewing the cap reveals a realistic-looking mouth or vulva rendered in latex or another soft plastic. A man or his lover can guide his erection inside and work the device to stroke him. Use a water-based lubricant.

Ben-Wa Balls

About the size of golf balls, they come in pairs. Women slip them inside the vagina and try to hold them inside while standing or walking. At first, they usually fall out. But over time, women learn to hold them in. Like Kegel exercises, ben-wa balls help tone the pelvic floor muscles, the ones that contract during orgasm. When used over time, the balls help intensify orgasms.

Dildos

Dildos are cylindrical or penis-shaped objects inserted into erotic openings.

Some are realistic penis surrogates made from latex, jelly, or silicone. Others are plastic wands tapered at one end. Some are two headed, for two-opening insertion or simultaneous use by two people. Some have curved ends for G-spot stimulation. Others have two shafts, one for the vagina, the other for the anus or clitoris. For lovers who enjoy playing with size, some dildos are much larger than the vast majority of penises. Use lubricant.

Strap-On Dildos

In some porn featuring two women, one wears a strap-on and penetrates the other. Many lesbians enjoy strap-on play, but any couple can enjoy them.

Strap-ons include a dildo that fits into a harness worn around the waist or hips. Strap-ons give women artificial penises right where they should hang, or they give men an extra penis that may be firmer and more cooperative than their own.

Why not just use a regular dildo? Strap-ons offer a different experience. They:

- Free the hands for other caressing.
- Allow men to play with having more between their legs.
- Compensate for erectile dysfunction, allowing intercourse for couples who might not otherwise be able to accomplish it.
- Invite gender-bending. Women can play with male-style hip thrusting.
- Deepen intimacy. Strap-ons expand erotic possibilities, encouraging discussions that enhance emotional connections.

Unfortunately, two myths may interfere with strap-on play:

MYTH: Men who enjoy being on the receiving end are gay.
TRUTH: Not at all. Sexual orientation is all about the gender you play with, not how you play. Many 100 percent straight men enjoy receptive anal play, including strap-ons.

MYTH: Women who wear strap-ons secretly want to be men.
TRUTH: Possibly. But the vast majority of women who wear them feel fine about being women. For most, strap-ons carry no gender-bending implications, just new erotic possibilities.

Strap-ons come in two basic styles: thongs and jocks. Both have straps that circle the waist. In addition, thongs have a strap that runs between the legs, while jocks have two straps that circle the thighs. How to choose?

- Some find one style more comfortable than the other.
- Thong harnesses require fewer adjustments.
- Thong straps between the legs provide stimulation some enjoy.
- With jocks, the extra strap provides additional support for the dildo.
- Jock harness straps don't touch the genitals and anus, which some prefer.

Straps may be leather, nylon, or elastic. Each has a different feel. Nylon and elastic can be popped into washing machines. Leather requires more care. Front pieces' materials also vary: leather, velvet, neoprene, or rubber. Harnesses typically come in kits, including dildos that fit them. Tips for enjoyment:

- Be patient with initial strap adjustments.
- Use lubricant on dildos and receiving openings.
- At first, inserters should remain still. Recipient should do the moving.
- Women may have little experience with male-style hip thrusting. Offer coaching.
- Strap-ons free the hands so users can caress each other all over.
- If men with firm erections wear the harness, they may alternate inserting one then the other, or play with simultaneous vaginal and anal intercourse.
- If women wear the harness, the dildo holder typically covers the clitoris. Some women enjoy the clitoral stimulation that results when the holder presses against it.

Finally, for women who'd like a strap-on without the straps, there's InJoyUs. Instead of a harness, InJoyUs offers a base that fits inside the vagina with a dildo that attaches (newlovecreations.com).

BDSM Toys: Paddles, Canes, Riding Crops, Restraints, Whips, Floggers, and Nipple Clamps

Light BDSM involves obedience play, spanking, and blindfolds. Heavier play adds other accoutrements.

According to an Indiana University study, 30 percent of American adults have tried erotic spanking: with the palms, hand in oven mitts, or with spatulas, ping pong paddles, riding crops, or canes.

Restraint is also popular—20 percent of American adults have tried it. Restraint ranges from commands (*Clasp your hands behind your back and don't release until I say so*) to binding with thread, ribbon, Velcro, scarves, rope, leather, handcuffs, and contraptions like stocks. Start with commands and, if you like, progress to thread, which confers much of the excitement while allowing the submissive to break free at any time. Then consider double- or triple-thread restraints before progressing to other devices.

Unless players negotiate other arrangements, during restraint play, doms should always remain in close physical proximity to bound subs and provide reassurance that subs are safe and in control of the scene.

Whips and floggers have been used by 13 percent of American adults. Whips have one long tail. Floggers have several short tails (cat-o'-nine-tails). Whips are more difficult to control. The longer the whip, the sharper the snap. As a result, whips might exceed subs' sensation limits. If you're new to BDSM, use floggers.

Finally, many sex toy catalogs feature large arrays of nipple clamps: alligator clothespins and many adjustable pinchers. Some look like jewelry. Others vibrate. And some look like torture devices. Negotiate the type, tightness, and duration of any clamping.

CHAPTER 42:
Anal Sex — without Pain

WHAT EXACTLY IS anal sex? To many, it means penis-anus intercourse. Ironically, this is the *least* popular variation. Most backdoor eroticism involves noninsertive sphincter massage, shallow fingering, insertion of small toys (butt plugs), or oral-anal play (rimming, anilingus).

Many lovers consider any anal sex, particularly rimming, dirty, disgusting, and hazardous, and have zero interest in it. If that's how you feel, you have every right to decline anal invitations. But with clear consent and careful hygiene, anal sex is clean, safe, and free from fecal contact.

For many lovers, anal play is a major turn-on. The anal area is richly endowed with touch-sensitive nerves. Many lovers revel in rear-end caresses and gentle probing. For some, rimming adds spice to oral sex. The novelty of anal play can be erotically exciting. It fuels fantasies, hence its frequent depiction in porn. And it often deepens intimacy.

Compared with heterosexuals, a larger proportion of gay men enjoy anal play. But heterosexuals substantially outnumber gays. Consequently, hetero couples account for the majority of anal sex.

Unfortunately, many women—and some men—have had bad experiences on the receiving end of anal insertions. The anus is much less receptive than the mouth or vagina. Inexperienced anal recipients may experience sharp pain and decide *never again*. But with information, negotiation, planning, and plenty of lubricant, anal play can feel comfortable and enjoyable—and, for some lovers, marvelous.

How Popular?

Ancient Greek pottery (ca. 500 BC) shows men engaged in homosexual penis-anus intercourse (PAI). The oldest known representations of hetero anal appear on Peruvian pottery (AD 300). Chinese and Japanese woodblock prints (sixteenth to nineteenth centuries) also feature hetero anal intercourse. And since the invention of photography (1840) and motion pictures (1890), pornography has presented every imaginable type of heterosexual anal play.

Today, anal sex is a staple of both commercial and amateur porn: sphincter massage, licking, fingering, butt plugs, intercourse, enemas, and pegging (women doing men with dildos). Why? In part, because many people who don't actually play that way fantasize about it and gravitate to material that shows it. And in part because anal sex is more popular than many believe.

Indiana University researchers surveyed 5,865 Americans age fourteen to ninety-four (2,936 men, 2,929 women). Forty percent admitted having tried PAI, with peak prevalence in the broad age range of twenty-five to thirty-nine.

But day-to-day, anal remains a minority pleasure. During the year before being surveyed, anal intercourse ranged in popularity:

- 5 percent (ages fourteen to nineteen)
- 10 percent (twenty to twenty-four)
- 25 percent (twenty-five to thirty-nine)
- 12 percent (forty to forty-nine)
- 10 percent (fifty to fifty-nine)
- 5 percent (over sixty)

Anal Sex and AIDS

Receptive PAI is a major risk factor for contracting HIV. The reason is not anal sex per se, but rather that anal intercourse is more likely than oral or vaginal intercourse to cause bleeding. It may rupture anal capillaries and allow semen-blood contact. Anal intercourse with condoms is just as HIV-safe as any other safe sex.

Among the youngest and oldest lovers, PAI is not rare, but it's not prevalent. However, from twenty to thirty-nine, it's fairly popular.

Other studies corroborate these findings. The National Survey of Family Growth (2011–13) asked 9,175 Americans, and found that 42 percent of the men and 36 percent of the women said they'd tried anal intercourse.

Anal experimentation appears to be increasing. In 1992, the CDC asked 2,500 Americans if they'd ever tried it. Saying yes: 26 percent of the men, 20 percent of the women. Fifteen years later (2006), it was 38 and 33 percent respectively—significant increases.

Despite increasing experimentation, anal play, particularly intercourse, remains an occasional minority pleasure. Australian researchers asked 5,118 adults what they'd done during their most recent partner sex. Only 1 percent mentioned PAI.

All these studies tracked penis insertion, but nonintercourse anal play is more popular. A 2010 Indiana University study of 1,478 heterosexual men showed that during the previous month:

- 24 percent had performed anilingus.
- 15 percent had received it.
- 53 percent had anally fingered a woman.
- And 24 percent had received anal fingering.

If we include all types of partner anal eroticism, it appears that more than half of heterosexual American couples have indulged at least once.

Initial anal play is often unplanned. A tongue, finger, toy, or erection on its way into the vagina finds the anus instead. Some recoil, but others become intrigued.

What's the allure?

- **Novelty.** Anal is different. Novelty enhances sex.
- **Forbidden fruit.** Many lovers consider anal play taboo, therefore exciting.
- **Experimentation.** Some try it accidentally or on a whim, like it, and continue.
- **Intimacy.** To some, anal feels uniquely self-revealing. It's a way for recipients to say: *I'm all yours.* And for inserters to reply: *No part of you turns me off. Every square inch of you turns me on.*
- **BDSM.** Anal play fits easily into consensual BDSM.
- **A special gift.** Some recipients said they reserve anal intercourse as a treat for special partners.

- **Pleasure.** In a Czech survey of women who engaged in regular PAI, more than half (58 percent) called it "very arousing and pleasurable."

Researchers at California State University, Long Beach, asked focus groups of women why they engaged in receptive PAI. The main reasons were their own pleasure and to please lovers. They also considered it a unique gift for special partners. Their main problems: pain and disgust.

Anal Anatomy Surprises

One reason anal play may hurt is that few lovers understand the fine points of backdoor anatomy. The visible pucker is only half the story. The body has two anal sphincters—one visible, the other an inch or so inside. The external sphincter is fairly easy to relax, the internal one more difficult. Different nerves control the two. But over time, most people can learn to relax their inner sphincters.

Moving internally from the inner sphincter, the narrow, muscular anal canal extends an inch or two. The sphincters and anal canal are richly supplied with touch-sensitive nerves, the reason many people find anal play erotic. In addition, the anus borders the pelvic floor muscles that contract during orgasm. Anal stimulation can excite these muscles and intensify orgasm.

The anal canal widens into the rectum, a five-inch tube of soft tissue. The rectum is not a straight cylinder. It has curves that vary from person to person. Anything inserted must negotiate these turns—always proceed *very slowly*, with lots of lubrication and the recipient in control of the speed and depth.

The rectum and anal canal don't contain much stool. Most fecal material is stored above the rectum in the descending colon. When you feel "the urge," stool moves into the rectum and fairly quickly passes out of the body. However, residual stool in the anal canal and rectum may leave traces on anything inserted.

Unlike the vagina, the anus and rectum are not self-lubricating. For comfortable anal sex, use plenty of lubricant. Even with lots of lube, anal insertions and/or vigorous movement may abrade anal tissue, possibly causing minor bleeding, especially if the recipient is among the ten million Americans who have hemorrhoids.

Minor bleeding, pink streaks on toilet paper, is usually no cause for concern—unless the object inserted is an erection and the inserter is infected with HIV. If HIV-laden semen contacts the recipient's blood, infection is possible. Unless you're confident your lover is

Anal and Hemorrhoids

Hemorrhoids make anal play uncomfortable or impossible. Hemorrhoids are swollen (varicose) veins in or around the anus. Symptoms include itching, bleeding, and/or pain. The cause is pressure on the anal veins, usually from the weight of a fetus or from straining to defecate, largely the result of chronic constipation.

To eliminate hemorrhoids, cure constipation. Eat a high-fiber diet: more fruits, vegetables, beans, and whole grains, and a bran cereal at breakfast. Limit consumption of constipating foods (bananas, rice) and supplements (iron). Drink plenty of nonalcoholic fluids—coffee often helps. Get daily, moderate exercise. Never ignore the urge. And if you use laxatives, the safest contain bulk-forming psyllium (Metamucil). If home care doesn't resolve things, consult a physician.

HIV-negative and free of other sexually transmitted infections, condoms should be used during anal intercourse.

Hygiene: How Dirty Is It?

"Our culture considers the anus dirty and disgusting," the late sex therapist Jack Morin explains in *Anal Pleasure and Health*. "Intellectually, people might like to explore anal pleasure, but emotionally, they can't handle it. The anal taboo can be overcome, but it takes time. Take all the time you need. Otherwise, anal sex is no fun and might become coercive."

Cleanliness is crucial. Wash, bathe, or shower beforehand. Some people insert soapy fingers, but soap works best on skin and not on the mucous membrane of the anal canal, where it may cause irritation. A finger without soap is usually sufficient. Slowly insert a finger one knuckle or two. This cleans the area and helps locate your inner sphincter, which begins the process of relaxing it.

Some people also rinse with enemas. Disposables (Fleet) are available over the counter at pharmacies. Occasional enemas—once or twice a month—rarely cause problems, but if used more frequently, enemas may cause irritation.

If you're new to enemas:

- Use the prepared solution or fill the plastic container with warm water.
- Lubricate your outer sphincter and the nozzle.
- Bend over or position yourself on elbows and knees.
- Insert the nozzle an inch or two, gently squeeze the bottle, wait a minute or two, then discharge into the toilet.

Rinsing not only cleans the area, but also helps both lovers relax about anal play. If the receiving partner washes well beforehand and uses an enema, then anal play—including rimming—is hygienic.

I consulted several people very experienced with receptive anal play. Their consensus opinion: it's best not to go overboard with enemas and soap. Regular bathing and an unsoaped wet finger or two are usually sufficient.

However, despite washing, fecal bacteria may remain in the vicinity. Nothing that touches the anal area should be introduced into the vagina. Anal bacteria may cause urinary tract infections.

Anus-to-mouth moves, often depicted in porn, should be avoided. It may spread digestive bacteria.

Recipients, Start Solo

Researchers at California State University, Long Beach, asked women why they tried anal sex. The majority said, *It just happened*. Their anal play was unplanned, not discussed, and happened when most were drunk. That's a recipe for pain and regret.

Lovers interested in anal play should negotiate it beforehand. If you decide to proceed, partner anal should wait until receiving partners have practiced by themselves, feel comfortable, and are clear about their limits. Recipients should be free of hemorrhoids and begin with solo sphincter massage, then proceed to self-fingering:

- Use plenty of lube. Saliva and water-based products may be your choice for vaginal sex but may not work as well for back door play. Consider the thicker water-based lube,

Slippery Stuff. Some anal players use vegetable oils, Vaseline, or Crisco, but they can be problematic. They may damage latex and should not be used with condoms. Also, their effect on the anal mucosa has not been well researched, so safety questions remain.

- Massage around the external sphincter.
- Using one lubricated finger, enter slowly.
- Where you encounter resistance, that's your inner sphincter. Breathe deeply. Probe gently. If the sphincter yields and your finger slips through comfortably, you're on your way to enjoyable anal. If you feel any discomfort, back off, perhaps returning to gentle probing another time. Or limit yourself to shallow insertions that don't cross the internal sphincter.
- Some anal aspirants numb the area with topical anesthetics or dull their sensibilities with alcohol or other drugs. Bad idea. Deadening sensation teaches nothing, reduces pleasure, and may lead to injury.
- Try different positions: bent at the waist, on hands or elbows and knees, or on your back with legs raised or knees on your chest.
- If you feel inclined, proceed to experimenting with two fingers or a small, well-lubricated butt plug. Plugs have flared bases that prevent losing them inside. They come in many sizes. Once inserted, they're designed to stay in place, leaving your hands free for other erotic play. Or try anal beads. Designed to serially open and close the sphincters, they trigger sensations some find erotic.
- The receiving lover should become comfortable solo before attempting partner anal play. Remember, few anal aficionados ever attempt penis-anus intercourse. They limit things to sphincter massage, anilingus, fingering, and plugs (many women in porn refuse to participate in anal scenes).

Rimming (Anilingus): The Curious Lovers' Guide to Oral-Anal Eroticism

Heterosexuals typically stumble on anilingus accidentally during cunnilingus. The man's tongue slips further south than intended and both realize they've crossed a line.

Anilingus is a minority pleasure, but with good hygiene, it's neither abnormal nor harmful. If you reflexively condemn it, remember, until 1961, oral sex was considered a perversion and largely outlawed in the US.

Anilingus feels erotic for the same reasons that anal play in general is arousing (above). Of course, rimming also involves a big fear, oral-fecal contact. Not to worry. Washing beforehand with soap removes any traces from the external sphincter and the area around it and leaves the external back door clean enough to lick.

Millions of digestive bacteria pass through the anus, notably *E. coli*, and despite washing, some may remain around the opening. If they come in contact with women's urethras, urinary tract infection is possible. Rimming may also transmit *Shigella*, *Salmonella*, and *Giardia*. Discuss these risks and don't rim anyone who has any of these infections. But among healthy, monogamous lovers who practice good anal hygiene, anilingus is unlikely to transmit infection.

It Should Never Hurt

If anal play hurts, four causes are possible:

- Hemorrhoids (above).
- The recipient is tense.
- The receiving anus and the object being inserted are not sufficiently lubricated.
- The inserter is uninformed and insensitive or pushy.

Pain and fear of pain are major reasons why recipients nix backdoor play. "Women's biggest complaint about anal," New York sex educator Betty Dodson explains, "is that men push in too quickly. That can really hurt. In my twenties, my first attempt at receptive anal intercourse was a disaster. We were both young and inexperienced. I wasn't relaxed. We didn't even know enough to use lube. He pushed in and I felt a hot, burning sensation. I cried out in pain, but my boyfriend mistook my screaming for arousal and pushed in deeper. I pulled away, furious. It was twenty years before I tried anal again."

Dodson is typical. Croatian researchers surveyed 2,002 women age eighteen to thirty. Pain compelled half (49 percent) to abort their first attempted PAI. And an Indiana University survey of 1,738 adults showed that 72 percent of the women experienced moderate to severe pain during anal intercourse—but rarely told their lovers.

Recipients: if it hurts, say so immediately. No one can read your mind. Except in carefully negotiated consensual BDSM, sex should *never* hurt. If you feel pain and say nothing, you suffer and your lover remains in the dark. That's unfair to both of you.

Recipients Should *Always* Be in Control

Enjoyable anal play requires deeply relaxed recipients. Tension contributes to clenching of the sphincters—and pain when anything pushes against them.

Begin deep relaxation by taking a hot bath or shower, solo or together. Wash the external sphincter with soap and water and slip a finger into one sphincter or both to begin the process of accommodating insertions.

Next enjoy at least twenty minutes of kissing, cuddling, and whole-body mutual massage. It's relaxing and arousing, and anal sex is usually most enjoyable when both lovers feel deeply relaxed and highly aroused. Then proceed to well-lubricated partner massage of the external sphincter.

If you're interested in fingering, recipients should *always* be the ones in control, the ones who move. Inserters should position a finger on the external sphincter and then remain still. Recipients should back onto it, controlling the speed and depth of insertion. Once recipients feel comfortable, inserters can move a bit. If you'd like to try a small butt plug, use the same procedure. That's as far as most couples go.

If you're inclined toward penis-anus intercourse—or strap-on dildo play—it's even more important for recipients to be in control. Inserters should position the head of the penis or toy on the external sphincter and stay still. Recipients should back onto it, controlling speed and depth. Good positions include recipients standing bent at the waist or on hands or elbows and knees. Inserters should not move until recipients invite it, then slowly and gently.

How deep can inserters go? That varies. With practice, some recipients can hold much of the penis. But unlike what's depicted in anal porn, most cannot. Many feel uncomfortable accepting anything but the head of the penis, if that. Some recipients feel more receptive if they wear a butt plug for about thirty minutes before attempting to accommodate an erection. Don't rush things. Deep insertion often takes months of practice and most recipients never feel comfortable with it. This bears repeating: most anal play involves only sphincter massage, fingering, small plugs, and rimming—not intercourse.

Adding anal play to more conventional lovemaking can lead to particularly intense orgasms. Some recipients love having a finger or plug inserted as they or their lovers bring them to orgasm by hand, mouth, or vibrator.

Many anal inserters dream of coming inside recipients. But many recipients prohibit this. Orgasm causes involuntary hip movements and during anal, they may cause pain. Discuss this. It's the recipient's call.

If One Wants It and the Other Doesn't

Frequently, one lover is eager to explore anal play, but the other is reluctant or adamantly opposed.

Attention, eager lovers: never force it, and don't nag. In a calm, loving manner, explore your partner's reluctance. *What exactly is so off-putting?* Listen carefully and try to address your lover's concerns. Ask if there is *any way* your partner might feel comfortable exploring this variation. Do only what's mutually agreed. If your partner says stop, do so immediately. Learn your partner's limits and always respect them.

Attention, reluctant lovers: you're under no obligation to be sexual in ways that turn you off. Your lover should respect your limits. But try not to dismiss anal play automatically. Many couples play that way enjoyably and hygienically. Tell your partner specifically what you object to. The anal taboo? Previous painful experiences? By discussing your issues, the two of you learn more about each other—and that sharing enhances intimacy even if you *never* engage in anal play.

During insertions, recipients may feel the urge to defecate. It may be real or a false alarm, the reaction of a rectum not yet used to anal sex. If this is a concern, use an enema beforehand so you know you're empty.

Many potential recipients worry that sphincters stretched during anal play may never return to normal, and lead to soiled underwear. Unlikely. Your anal sphincters have opened and closed your entire life. They can't tell if material is exiting or entering. Assuming your sphincters close normally after defecation, they should do the same after anal play.

If a Man Enjoys Receiving, Is He Gay?

On my Q&A site, GreatSexGuidance.com, many have asked:

- Does a man's interest in receptive anal suggest he's gay?
- Does a man's desire to enter a woman's back door mean he wants to hurt, dominate, or humiliate her?
- If a woman uses a strap-on dildo on a man, is she "too dominant"?

Sexuality exists in cultural contexts. In the US, anal sex is most associated with gay men, so it's not surprising some would link it to homosexuality. But gay men also hold hands, hug, cuddle, kiss, and enjoy oral sex. Is kissing "gay"? Sexual orientation is all about who you play with—not how you play with them.

Anal rape occurs with abominable frequency in men's prisons. It's usually less about pleasure than domination and humiliation. Outside prison, it's certainly possible for men to use anal sex to dominate and humiliate women. It's equally possible for women wearing strap-ons to do the same to men. But most free-world anal play is loving. Usually, it means nothing beyond mutual pleasure and intimacy.

Compared with oral or vaginal play, anal sex requires more negotiation. That extra communication can deepen intimacy and bring couples closer. Anal play is just another sexual variation that some lovers enjoy.

If any aspect of anal play causes chronic relationship conflict, consult a sex coach or therapist.

CHAPTER 43:

Hall Passes, Threesomes, Swinging, Sex Clubs, and Polyamory: The Curious Couple's Guide to Consensual Nonmonogamy

THE VAST MAJORITY of American couples profess monogamy—while, in secret, many men and women have affairs and many men patronize sex workers. Meanwhile, some couples temper demands for absolute monogamy with negotiated arrangements that allow each to play on the side. This isn't cheating. It's based on mutual consent, full disclosure, and diligent safe sex, though one spouse may be more into it than the other.

Consensual nonmonogamy doesn't mean daily orgies or long-term ménages à trois. For most it's an occasional break from sexual exclusivity. Nonmonogamists say it enhances libido, prevents boredom, adds spice to the primary relationship's lovemaking, and deepens spouses' intimacy, love, and devotion.

Orgies through the Ages

In the Bible, men were free to be polygamous, assuming they could support more than one wife. However, for the past 1,500 years, most Western cultures have embraced monogamy—with exceptions.

After long winters came spring and "spring fever." As the days lengthened and crops were planted, many cultures developed religious rituals to petition their deities for bountiful harvests and livestock fecundity. Many included relaxation of sexual restraints, and some involved raucous, drunken, public group sex.

Spring-fever sex parties had rough edges. They included alcohol, which led to sexual assaults of both women and men. But there's every reason to believe that back then, like today, around 5 percent of women were highly sexual and that other women, especially teens coming of age, were also up for erotic excitement. Historians agree that in spring-fever group-sex rituals, women were often enthusiastic participants.

The earliest known springtime public-sex parties took place in ancient Egypt. Early Egyptian mythology includes a tale similar to the story of Noah. The sun god, Ra, recoiled from humanity's wickedness and killed almost everyone along the Nile. Then he relented and flooded the fields with beer. The few survivors got drunk and beseeched Ra for bountiful harvests. They also engaged in public free-for-all sex that repopulated Egypt. In commemoration, every spring as the Nile flooded, the Egyptians held fertility festivals involving public drunkenness, dancing, and group sex. It's not clear what proportion of the population participated, but apparently, many did.

Egypt's fertility festival influenced ancient Greece, where Dionysus was the god of wine, pleasure, fertility, and religious ecstasy. In ancient art, Dionysus rides a chariot pulled by wild beasts, followed by dancers—the women naked, the men with huge erections. The god's acolytes weren't particularly numerous, but they celebrated him during festivals called *orgia*. Participants were required to abstain from sex for nine days before these orgies, so they were eager to party.

In early Rome, the fertility god was Liber. Springtime parades honoring him featured huge carved wooden phalluses that were carted around the city and through the fields. Liber's springtime festivals culminated in a sacred ritual involving a married noblewoman and a priest doing the deed in public with the community watching.

Around 200 BC, the Romans adopted Dionysus, changing his name to Bacchus. The Roman historian Livy reported that early celebrations in the god's honor, Bacchanalia, were held three times a year and restricted to women who abstained from sex for ten days beforehand. But eventually, Bacchanalia included men and for years took place monthly featuring public drunkenness and communal lasciviousness. Bacchanalia became scandalous, not for their wild, public sex, but because the action crossed class lines, low-born men doing it with aristocratic women (aristocratic men were always free to debauch their women servants).

Ultimately, Bacchanalia devolved into mass rapes of both women and men, with murmurs of rebellion against the state. The Roman Senate had no objections to public intoxication or humping but could not abide any hint of sedition. In 186 BC, when the population of Rome and its environs was estimated at almost one million, Livy reported the arrest of seven thousand Bacchanalians (0.7 percent of the populace), most of whom were executed.

Despite this slaughter, around the Roman Mediterranean, springtime fertility rituals continued. In some, priests petitioned the gods for good harvests during ceremonial public sex with temple prostitutes. In others, celebrants repaired to newly planted fields for drunken orgies.

As Christianity supplanted paganism, its solemn springtime holiday, Easter, followed forty days of quiet reflection beginning on Ash Wednesday. But the day before was a big party, Fat Tuesday—in French, *Mardi Gras*, in Spanish, *Carnival*. Ever since, Mardi Gras and Carnival have been celebrated with oceans of alcohol and relaxation of sexual constraints.

Several Renaissance popes celebrated Carnival year-round. In 1501, the Italian nobleman and Catholic cardinal Cesare Borgia, Duke of Valentinois, organized a party at the Papal Palace featuring the pope, high-ranking clergy, and fifty courtesans, who dined together, then stripped and played.

Renaissance Italian nobility enjoyed masked balls, masquerades. Many of the masks featured exaggerated noses resembling erections. With participants' faces and identities obscured, masquerades often included communal sex that sometimes devolved into rape and even murder.

In medieval England, the springtime fertility ritual, Beltane, took place in late April, eventually settling on May 1, May Day. Participants danced around a huge phallic symbol, the May Pole, then repaired to the fields where they drank and played. In 1644, the Puritans banned May Day partying as immoral.

In seventeenth-century England and Europe, brothels were commonplace and stratified by social class. Upper-class men also joined fraternal organizations, gentlemen's clubs. Many clubs regularly contracted with madams to send dozens of sex workers to country estates for group romps.

This tradition continued into the twentieth century. In 1961 at a pool party at an English country estate, Secretary of War John Profumo cavorted with sex worker Christine Keeler, who was simultaneously involved with a Russian naval attaché and suspected spy. The ensuing scandal almost brought down the government.

American colonists were surprised that many Native American tribes had no qualms about masturbation, homosexuality, nonmonogamy, public nudity, cross-dressing, and childhood sex play. The Europeans were particularly nonplussed by nonmonogamy, which clouded paternity. The Native Americans replied, "You love only your own children. We love all our children."

From the American Revolution through the late nineteenth century, a small minority of Americans joined frontier utopian communities, each with its own relationship rules. The Shakers insisted on celibacy. The Mormons embraced polygamy. And in 1848 in Oneida, New York, John Humphrey Noyes established a "communist" community. All property was held by the group and traditional marriage was abolished in favor of "complex marriage." Men could invite member women to bed. Women could accept or decline, but the community opposed exclusivity and encouraged multiple partners. Most Oneidans maintained several simultaneous relationships. At its height, the Oneida commune numbered three hundred. It lasted thirty-one years, until 1879.

During the 1870s in New York, Victoria Woodhull was a sex worker who became the nation's first woman stockbroker. She gained notoriety for promoting "free love"—not unconstrained promiscuity, but arrangements we'd call swinging. Woodhull condemned traditional marriage for enslaving women. She encouraged women to pursue their attractions by choosing as many lovers as they wanted, even if the men were married.

Modern American swinging developed at World War II air bases. American fighter pilots suffered substantial casualties. Pilots and their wives understood that many flyers would not return. Before the men flew off, pilot couples intermingled sexually—then called "wife swapping"—in a tribal bonding ritual that cemented a tacit commitment by surviving flyers and their wives to look after the widows. The couples held "key parties." The men tossed their house keys into a hat. The women picked keys and spent the night with the man whose door they opened. After the war, swapping spread throughout the military, then to surrounding communities.

Today the North American Swing Club Association (NASCA) includes more than 350 clubs around the US and Canada. Its conventions draw thousands of couples. Travel agents who specialize in swing destinations book couples on swinger cruises and into swing resorts worldwide. Meanwhile, most swinging is organized on a smaller scale at private homes with two or more couples and occasionally some singles. Thousands of informal swing groups play in all fifty states.

Do Men Coerce Women into Nonmonogamy?

Many critics view nonmonogamy as inherently abusive, a way for horny men to get off at the expense of prim women who would rather not. That's possible, but quite often, couples become and remain nonmonogamous at the *women's* initiative. A *New York Times Magazine* writer interviewed swinger couples. Who pushed to play? In some, the men, but in quite a few, the women. Among long-term nonmonogamous couples, the women are usually equally sexually active and enthusiastic, if not more so. The most comprehensive book on the subject, *The Lifestyle: A Look at the Erotic Rites of Swingers* by Terry Gould, quotes many women insisting that the spouse in the driver's seat of swinging is usually the woman.

How Many North Americans Are Nonmonogamous?

No one knows, but many dream about it. One of the most popular erotic fantasies involves rolling around with someone new. That's why so much porn depicts threesomes, swapping, gangbangs, and orgies.

Sexologists estimate that 3–5 percent of married couples have tried swinging, with 1–2 percent regularly playing that way. These estimates may be low. Among a representative 2,003 Canadian adults, 4 percent said they were in open relationships, and 12 percent said it was their relationship ideal. A Temple University survey of 2,270 US adults also found that 4 percent reported ongoing consensual nonmonogamy.

Around 5 percent of American women are highly sexual, complemented by at least twice that proportion of men. NASCA suggests that 15 percent of American couples have swapped at least once. An Indiana University study of 2,021 adults agrees, finding that 10 percent of women and 18 percent of men have participated in at least one threesome. Finally, based on census samples of 8,718 single American adults, Indiana University researchers found that 21 percent—one in five—reported at least one experience of consensual nonmonogamy.

For argument's sake, let's accept the conservative estimate that only 3 percent of couples enjoy occasional unconventional pairings, with another few percent sufficiently curious to experiment, a total of, say, 6 percent of couples. US census figures estimate 78 million couples—60 million married, 18 million cohabiting. If 6 percent are occasionally nonmonogamous, that's 4.7 million couples, enough to support sex and swing clubs in almost every metropolitan area and many rural locales—which is the case. Just search "sex clubs" or "swing clubs" and any US or Canadian locale—urban, suburban, or rural. Or try AdultFriendFinder. com, a Boca Raton, Florida–based swinging-oriented social network launched in 1996. It claims more than 40 million members. If you're interested in nonmonogamy, potentially like-minded singles and couples are rarely far away.

The Wide World of Nonmonogamy

Consensual nonmonogamy takes many forms:

- **Sex clubs.** These commercial establishments are generally open to both couples and singles. Admission is low for couples and single women, much higher for single men. Once patrons enter, partner sex is available at no additional charge, but it's by no means guaranteed, and often not desired. Some couples prefer to watch, then once aroused, return home for the prone boogie. At most clubs, a small number of exhibitionist or swing couples get down and dirty, watched by a larger number of single men, who openly masturbate. Clubs insist on safe sex and provide free condoms and lubricant.
- **Swinging.** Swingers engage in threesomes, swapping, or group sex, usually in private homes. Players find each other through personal networks or swing-oriented websites. Some swingers play at clubs that typically admit couples and single women but exclude single men. Several states have no clubs, but according to NASCA, Michigan and Illinois boast seventeen, Texas twenty-three, New York thirty, Florida thirty-two, and California forty-one. Swing clubs insist on safe sex and provide free condoms and lubricant. Some club operators interview prospective couples in advance to make sure both spouses are into playing.
- **Open relationships.** This is a catch-all term for nonmonogamy. It usually implies mutual consent, but some invoke it when pursuing affairs without their mate's knowledge.

- **Polyamory.** Literally "loving many," polyamorists aspire not only to sex with others, but also to spousal emotional commitments in multiple sexual relationships. This takes a tremendous amount of time, commitment, negotiation, and patience. Polyamorists joke that being "poly" is much less about sex than conversation.
- **BDSM clubs.** Many completely monogamous couples enjoy bondage, discipline, and sadomasochism. BDSM clubs don't encourage nonmonogamy, but are open to it.

Are Swingers Psychologically Healthy or Mentally Ill?

Many people believe that nonmonogamists must be at least emotionally troubled if not deranged. On the contrary, several studies show that swingers are the people next door—with a few intriguing differences. Compared with monogamous couples, swingers usually:

- Express more nonsexual affection with their spouses
- Consider their lives more exciting, and their sex more satisfying
- Report more marital sex
- Enjoy more marital communication
- Praise their primary partners more
- Report greater marital happiness
- Express less jealousy
- Enjoy greater overall relationship satisfaction
- Are about as likely to say that swinging strengthened their marriages (27 percent) as that it contributed to their divorces (24 percent)
- Are no more likely than the general population to suffer anxiety, depression, and other mental health problems
- In some studies are a bit less likely to divorce, in others, somewhat more likely
- In some studies are more likely to make love sober, in others, less likely
- Have more friendships and more active social lives, but often feel more distant from relatives
- Are more likely to have had psychological counseling, usually before they began swinging
- On standard psychological tests, usually fall within the normal range

The consensus among researchers is that nonmonogamists are demographically, socioeconomically, and politically a snapshot of mainstream America—and psychologically healthy.

How to Explore Consensual Nonmonogamy — Happily

Like virginity loss, first swing experiences often happen by accident while drunk. However, you're most likely to feel happy with nonmonogamy if you discuss it extensively and plan it carefully before anyone disrobes.

The first issue is mutual consent. Ideally, both partners should be equally into it. If not, couples typically try it once or twice, then the less interested spouse says *never again*.

For More on Consensual Nonmonogamy

I recommend *The Ethical Slut: A Practical Guide to Polyamory, Open Relationships, and Other Adventures* (3rd edition) by Janet W. Hardy.

Attention, more eager partners: don't badger your partner. No one should ever feel pressured to be sexual in ways they'd rather not.

Attention, less interested partners: at sex and swing clubs, there's never any coercion to get it on. You're free to just watch or play exclusively with your partner.

Assuming you're both interested, ground rules are key. What exactly interests you? What can you tolerate your spouse doing? Are you more into clubs or private get-togethers? How do you feel about threesomes? Couple swapping? Group play? Other races and ethnicities? Or play partners who are considerably older or younger? What about incidental same-sex contact? Bisexual liaisons? People whose bodies look better than yours? And how would you feel if your partner has hotter sex with strangers than with you?

Before experimenting, couples happiest with nonmonogamy take lots of time to discuss their "what-ifs." Sex with strangers accounts for only part of nonmonogamy's allure. Equally compelling are the what-if discussions that deepen partners' emotional intimacy. Be as specific as possible. For example, "I'm okay with you kissing strangers, getting naked, touching, and hand jobs. But not oral or intercourse." Or "I don't mind us playing with others at clubs, but no dating or sleepovers with anyone else."

Another issue is spousal presence. Many nonmonogamous couples insist on same-room play to keep an eye on each other. Others feel comfortable with separate rooms, hall passes, or mutual permission to date and arrange overnights. Discuss this. Remember, the goal of nonmonogamy is to draw primary partners closer, not drive them apart.

However, despite extensive negotiations, when one spouse sees the other cavorting naked with strangers, freak-outs are always possible. Occasional nonmonogamy usually works best when, like those into BDSM, players have "safe words" that signal discomfort, for example, *yellow light* and *red light*. The former means, *I need a brief break to make sure both of us are okay with what's happening.* The latter means, *I need to stop everything right now.* When one utters a safe word, both should immediately disengage from their play. The couple regroups and spends as much time as necessary deciding to either continue playing or go home. Couples should abide by their safe words absolutely.

If you've discussed nonmonogamy but have never indulged, you might consider visiting a sex or swing club and watching others play while touching only your partner. Most clubs work hard to make newcomers feel comfortable and never pressure anyone to be sexual. Rules are clearly posted, typically: always be polite. "No" means no. And condoms are required for insertion.

Some clubs allow alcohol. Others do not. Most provide free condoms and lube. Some have monitors who circulate and enforce the rules. Some newbies watch during initial club visits, and subsequently become more adventurous. Or not. It's up to you. A slow, step-by-step approach usually works best, complemented by plenty of what-if discussions.

Learn the lingo. Swingers may or may not use that term. Many say they're "in the lifestyle." At swing gatherings, "hard or full swaps" mean intercourse. "Soft swaps" involve everything-but or any limits players declare.

Practice safe sex. More partners means greater risk of STIs. A Belgian study of 392 swingers showed that 26 percent had experienced a sexual infection. Use condoms.

At clubs, new connections may develop quickly. But many nonmonogamists feel happiest when they get to know prospective partners before anyone undresses. Meeting beforehand allows all parties to state their hopes, concerns, play preferences, and limits.

Unless you and your new friends have affirmatively opted for quickies, the best nonmonogamous sex resembles sizzling sex in general. Review chapters 5–10. Forget porn-style wham-bam. Instead, savor extended loveplay.

What Kind of Women Enjoy Groups of Men?

Some porn depicts one woman with a series of men (tag team, pulling a train) or several men simultaneously (gangbangs). In real life, this is rare—but far from unheard of. Some women enjoy being the center of sexual attention for groups of men. San Diego researchers found 132 ads in swing publications placed by women seeking consensual gangbangs and sent them questionnaires. Thirty-seven (28 percent) responded. That's not many, but this is the only published study, and its results are intriguing:

- The women lived in all regions of the United States: cities, suburbs, small towns, and rural areas.
- Ages ranged from twenty to fifty-seven and averaged thirty-seven.
- Those in committed relationships, 92 percent, with 76 percent saying their mates were always present and usually participating.
- About half had children.
- Two-thirds had some college education. Nineteen percent had graduate degrees.
- Frequency of the women's play with multiple men ranged from once a year to twice a week and averaged once a month.
- Their preferred number of men: three to ten.
- All excluded some men, most frequently smokers, heavy drinkers, drug users, obese men, and those who wouldn't send photos. Many preferred or excluded men based on race and ethnicity.
- Fourteen percent said they'd had sexually transmitted infections.
- Their biggest problems: finding likeable men and dealing with men who misrepresented themselves, had erection problems or poor hygiene, or who played too rough.
- Most said their first multipartner experiences had occurred at swing clubs with the support of their partners. They'd enjoyed them and continued.
- Why multiple partners? Eighty-six percent said they provided unique pleasure that could not be duplicated any other way.
- Their advice to women considering this: have a supportive partner who helps select the men, is present during the play, and is quick to intervene if things seem headed out of control.

Before, during, shortly after, and the morning after partying, check in with your partner. *Are you okay? Any second thoughts? Regrets? Want to play again? Anything you'd do differently?* Always remember, nonmonogamy has twin goals—novelty and deepening primary relationships.

Many couples interested in nonmonogamy don't pursue it for fear they might run into people they know. To prevent this, they play only at clubs far from home. Ironically, your friends probably feel similarly, meaning you might be *more* likely to bump into acquaintances far away than close to home. If you see people you know, why feel embarrassed? You've both opted to experiment with unconventional sexuality, so you have something new in common. Who knows? Chance encounters might turn into new erotic friendships.

Beginning nonmonogamists often gravitate toward threesomes, believing it's easier to deal with one stranger than two or more. But threesomes have disadvantages. When two of the three play, the third might feel ignored. In addition, it's much easier to find single men than women, who are so rare, they're called "unicorns." Foursomes are often preferable. While it's more challenging to get along with two others, there's someone for everyone. No one feels abandoned. And it's less difficult to find women.

It's rare for both spouses to feel equally into nonmonogamy. If one is much more into it than the other, conflicts may arise. If you can't resolve differences on your own, consider sex therapy.

CHAPTER 44:
BDSM: A Loving Introduction to Bondage, Discipline, and Sadomasochism

IN THE CHILDREN'S playground game Trust Me, one youngster stands behind another. The one in front willingly falls backward. The other promises to catch the one falling before that person hits the ground. Trust Me combines danger and faith. If those who fall don't get caught, they get hurt. But when the catch happens as planned, both players share a closeness and exhilaration that's difficult to duplicate in other ways.

BDSM is similar. The myth is that it's perverted and abusive—*whips and chains!* Actually it's about trust. When trust prevails over possible harm, the result can feel so intense, intimate, and ecstatic that people who play this way often call BDSM thrilling and fulfilling "beyond sex." A good deal of BDSM doesn't even include genital sexuality. It's role-playing, scripted theater involving mutual power play that may or not include genital play.

BDSM versus Kink

The two terms are not synonymous. *BDSM* refers to erotic bondage, discipline, and sadomasochism. *Kink* is a more general term for sex that's unconventional, for example, consensual nonmonogamy. All BDSM is kinky, but not all kink involves BDSM.

Varieties of BDSM
BDSM involves many possibilities:

- **Domination-submission (D/s, obedience training, role play, power play, or power exchange).** One person, the submissive (sub, bottom), grants nominal control to the other, the dominant (dom, top). Men and woman may play either role, though more men play doms, more women subs. Some enjoy both roles (switches).
- **Sadomasochism (SM).** This involves what's usually called pain: spanking, flogging, hair-pulling, nipple clamps, and so forth. But in BDSM parlance, it's not pain but "intense sensation."
- **Bondage and discipline (BD).** Subs get physically restrained with ropes, scarves, neckties, handcuffs, or other devices.

In nonconsensual contexts, all of the above are abusive. But erotic BDSM is completely consensual. It's also ironic. Bottoms play at submissiveness, but *always retain total control.*

Aficionados call BDSM the most loving, nurturing, and intimate form of human relations. Many people have sex without negotiating the particulars, without any intimate, that is, deeply self-revealing, emotional connection. But in loving BDSM, the players *always* negotiate the action in detail in advance, including what-ifs and mutual nurturance that creates special bonds often absent from conventional ("vanilla") lovemaking.

The Marquis de Sade and Leopold von Sacher-Masoch

No one knows when humanity discovered BDSM, but ancient Greek art depicts it. The classic Indian sex guide, the *Kama Sutra* (ca. AD 300), promotes erotic spanking with accompanying shrieks and is particularly enamored of biting and scratching: "There are no keener means of increasing passion than acts inflicted by tooth and nail."

European BDSM flowered during the eighteenth century, when some brothels began specializing in restraint, flagellation, and other "punishments" administered by women sex workers who topped willingly submissive men.

The first detailed discussions of SM appeared in two novels, *The 120 Days of Sodom* (1785) and *Justine* (1791), by Donatien Alphonse Francoise, comte de Sade, better known as the Marquis de Sade (1740–1814). His name gave us the word *sadism*. De Sade's controversial writings appalled many but also popularized BDSM and the gear it often involves: floggers, restraints, riding crops, nipple clamps, and so forth.

De Sade was imprisoned as criminally insane. Contemporary BDSMers revile him for nonconsensual abuse of women and for failure to embrace safe words (below).

In 1870, Austrian writer Leopold von Sacher-Masoch (1836–95) published the novel *Venus in Furs* about his ecstatic sexual submission to his mistress, Baroness Fanny Pistor. In 1886, Austrian psychiatrist Richard Freiherr von Krafft-Ebing published the influential medical text *Psychopathia Sexualis* (*Sexual Pathology*). He nodded to Sacher-Masoch by coining the term *masochism*.

In 1905, Sigmund Freud declared that "sadomasochism" signaled severe neurosis. For more than a century, mental health professionals agreed. The first edition of the American Psychiatric Association's bible of mental illness, the *Diagnostic and Statistical Manual of Mental Disorders* (DSM-I, 1952), pathologized sadism. DSM-II (1968) added masochism. And DSM-IV (1994) listed BDSM as a psychiatric disorder.

But DSM-5 (2013) redefined mental disorders as "characterized by clinically significant disturbance in cognition, emotion regulation, or behavior." Consensual BDSM does not meet these criteria. Its main result is mutual pleasure—see "Is BDSM Mentally Healthy?" page 341—so it was deleted as a mental disorder. BDSM is just another way for psychologically normal, healthy people to play.

How Popular in Fantasy? In Real Life?

In erotic fantasies, BDSM is remarkably popular:

- In Kinsey's mid-twentieth-century surveys, 24 percent of men and 12 percent of women admitted arousal from BDSM stories (some wouldn't admit it, so actual proportions were undoubtedly higher).
- In a 2009 survey of Canadian college students, 62 percent confessed fantasies of tying up lovers, with 65 percent saying they'd daydreamed of being restrained.
- In 2017, scientists surveyed a representative 1,027 Belgians. Those admitting BDSM fantasies—69 percent.

- Also in 2017, Canadian researchers surveyed 1,040 Quebecois, age eighteen to six-ty-four. Among the women, 28 percent reported fantasies of sexual submission, and 5 percent fantasized domination. Among the men, 19 percent admitted sub daydreams and 10 percent dom fantasies.
- Pornography is a window into men's sexual fantasies. A good deal of porn depicts BDSM.
- Some think kinky fantasies are most common among sex offenders. On the con-trary, University of Tulsa scientists surveyed 302 male sex offenders, along with 124 men incarcerated for nonsex crimes and 135 male college students. The sex offenders reported the *fewest* BDSM fantasies.
- Most astonishing is the BDSM romance novel trilogy, *Fifty Shades of Grey*, which fol-lows a brash young dom billionaire and his naive lover as she becomes his sub, at first hesitantly, then willingly, and finally enthusiastically. First published in 2011 on an obscure Australian website, by 2019, it had sold 150 million copies worldwide in fifty languages, the only book to ever to sell that many copies so quickly. The *Fifty Shades* film series has grossed more than $1 billion.

Clearly, many people's erotic imaginations include BDSM. And after considering it—for an average of six years, according to a Portuguese study—quite a few lovers incorporate some BDSM into partner lovemaking:

- In a 1971 University of Miami study, 8 percent of men and 5 percent of women admit-ted engaging in sexual spanking. A book of that era, *Sexual Behavior in the 1970s* (1974), suggested similar interest in BDSM—3 percent of men and 5 percent of women.
- In 2015, Indiana University researchers surveyed a representative 2,021 American adults. Many had tried some BDSM: spanking (30 percent), D/s role-playing (22 per-cent), restraint (20 percent), and flogging (13 percent).
- In the Belgian survey (above), 47 percent said they'd experimented with BDSM. Thirteen percent said they played that way "regularly." Eight percent said they were "committed" to BDSM.
- Shortly after *Fifty Shades of Grey* became a bestseller, BDSM sex toy sales surged. Target introduced a "Fifty Shades" line of lubricants and blindfolds. And hardware stores reported an unusual spike in sales of rope.
- A survey of 30,000 people by condom maker Durex shows that 36 percent of American adults have used blindfolds and/or bondage gear during lovemaking.

If you believe no one you know is into BDSM, think again. The National Coalition for Sexual Freedom, a Baltimore-based civil rights organization, surveyed 3,058 players nationwide. Almost half (43 percent) said they never mentioned their kinky play to anyone outside BDSM circles. Those who discussed it kept their involvement secret from coworkers and family (60 percent) and non-BDSM friends (41 percent). Their top reason for secrecy was fear—of fam-ily condemnation (68 percent), getting fired (58 percent), friends' disapproval (54 percent), harassment (38 percent), and loss of child custody (11 percent).

Most BDSM takes place in players' homes, but BDSM clubs operate in every US met-ropolitan area and many rural communities. Search "BDSM" and any locale. Or search "munches," informal restaurant gatherings where prospective players meet, socialize, and con-sider new partners.

Is BDSM Mentally Healthy?

DSM-5's recognition that it's sane reflected substantial research showing that, compared with the general public, BDSM players are no more likely to suffer psychiatric problems and have no psychological disorders unique to their kinky proclivities:

- A Los Angeles investigator administered standard psychological tests to several hundred BDSM aficionados and concluded they were mentally healthy.
- Dutch researchers gave standard personality tests to 902 BDSM players and 434 controls. The same proportion of both groups tested psychologically healthy, but the kinksters were "less neurotic, more conscientious, more extraverted, more open to new experiences, less sensitive to rejection, and showed greater subjective well-being." Those who scored most mentally healthy were the doms, followed by the subs, and in last place, the vanilla controls.
- Australian researchers surveyed 19,370 Aussies age sixteen to fifty-nine. Among the 2.2 percent of men and 1.3 percent of women who called themselves "committed to BDSM," all tested psychologically healthy and reported no disproportionate history of childhood sex abuse or sexual trauma.
- University of Illinois scientists took before and after saliva samples from 58 BDSM players, measuring their levels of the stress hormone cortisol. After BDSM scenes, cortisol decreased, showing that they found BDSM play relaxing.
- Finally, researchers at Idaho State University asked 935 players what BDSM meant to them: personal freedom (90 percent), adventure (91 percent), self-expression (91 percent), stress relief (91 percent), positive emotions (97 percent), and, above all, pleasure (99 percent).

Those into BDSM are a cross-section of the population, mentally healthy, and typical in every respect—except that they find vanilla sex unfulfilling and want something more exciting, intense, and intimate.

Domination, Submission, and the Human Condition

So BDSM is mentally healthy. Still, what kind of person becomes sexually aroused by imposing or surrendering control, or by inflicting or receiving intense sensation? Actually, dominance and submission are fundamental to social organization among mammals, including us.

From elk to chimps, dominant alpha males fight to subdue other males. The winners' reward? Exclusive sexual access to harems of submissive females. For millennia, humans have made war to dominate others. Capitalism assumes a dog-eat-dog world where succeeding means domination of resources and markets.

Consider sports. Players strive to dominate opponents. When they perform well, teammates often grab, slap, or punch them. It looks violent, but recipients accept this "abuse" gratefully as signs of appreciation.

Consider a long hike up to a mountain peak. Insects bite. Thorns scratch. The sun is brutal. Approaching the summit, you're tired, aching, and feeling punished. Yet at the peak, you feel exhilarated.

Former Secretary of State Henry Kissinger once called power "the ultimate aphrodisiac." For some, it is. In *Fifty Shades of Grey*, Christian Grey revels in playing the top. But exercising power can also be a burden—so much responsibility. To those desiring brief breaks from executive decision-making, playing the sub may feel therapeutic. Researchers at New York Medical College interviewed dozens of high-end sex workers and were astonished at the number who reported playing the demanding dominatrix ("pro-dom") during sessions with wealthy, powerful men—judges, government officials, captains of industry—who enjoyed playing the sub.

Sadly, the media often portray BDSM as violent and abusive. However, in actual violence, victims have no control over the force used against them and recoil from it. In BDSM, subs retain total control (below) while actively seeking "punishment."

Fundamentally, BDSM is theater. Encounters are called "scenes." In the theater, staged fights may look savage, but they're acting. No one gets harmed. BDSM is similar. When orchestrated by ethical doms, it's *never* abusive.

"BDSM is always consensual," says Jay Wiseman, author of *SM 101*. "Abuse is not. In loving hands, gags, whips, and other equipment heighten sensual excitement and allow both players to enjoy scenes as good, clean, erotic fun."

When BDSM inflicts intense sensation, it's always carefully choreographed beforehand with subs clearly specifying their limits. Most subs are very particular about the sensations that bring them pleasure.

"Within their limits, subs may enjoy being spanked," Wiseman explains, "but they experience dog bites, bee stings, and street assaults exactly like everyone else, and dislike them just as much."

The Magic of "Safe" Words

Like theater, BDSM players script their scenes in advance. Participants agree on safe words, stop signals that subs may invoke at any time. If subs are gagged, players arrange nonverbal safe signals—a series of grunts or the sub might hold a device that makes noise.

Many players arrange two levels of safe terms, for example, *yellow light* and *red light*. The former means *I'm uncomfortable. Without terminating our scene, we need to discuss things.* The latter means *Stop right now.* Safe terms immediately suspend scenes—until players discuss subs' concerns and mutually agree to resume play.

Some words should *not* be used as safe signals: "stop," "no," or "don't." Many players enjoy it when subs "beg" doms to stop, secure in the knowledge that they won't.

What happens if doms don't honor safe words? Like athletes who break the rules, word gets around and no one plays with them. Tops who fail to honor safe words face ostracism from the BDSM community.

BDSM Might Help Deter Sexual Assault

Some rape-prevention efforts promote affirmative consent—yes means yes—which requires sexual initiators to obtain explicit permission for every erotic escalation. Northern Illinois University researchers assessed college men's support for affirmative consent, comparing the attitudes of men who engaged in only vanilla sex with those into BDSM. Compared with the vanilla group, the kinky men evinced greater support for affirmative consent, greater willingness to negotiate lovemaking, and less acceptance of the myth that women who get raped "ask for it."

The Irony of BDSM: Subs Are in Charge

Although bottoms feign subservience, the irony of BDSM is that the subs are always in charge. They can invoke safe words whenever they wish, and if they do, tops suspend play immediately.

Tops act dominant, even sadistic, but must always be caring and nurturing, taking bottoms to their pre-agreed limits, but no further. In this way, BDSM provides an opportunity for everyone to experiment with taking and surrendering power, while always feeling safe and protected.

It's easier to play sub than dom. After specifying their limits and safe words, all subs do is surrender to whatever doms orchestrate. Playing dom is more complex. Within subs' limits, doms must choreograph fresh, imaginative, exciting scenes, which takes imagination and effort.

Learning the Ropes

Before experimenting with BDSM, get oriented. Good books include *SM 101* by Jay Wiseman, *Fifty Shades of Kink* by Tristan Taormino, and *Screw the Roses, Send Me the Thorns* by Philip Miller and Molly Devon. Some BDSM clubs and groups offer classes. Or visit BDSM sites.

Before scenes commence, Wiseman urges players to negotiate clear agreements covering:

- **People.** Who will participate? Will anyone watch? Will photography or video recording be permitted?
- **Roles.** Who's the top? The bottom? What kind of scene will be played out? Will players remain in their initial roles? Or switch? Will the submissive obey immediately? Or "resist" for a while?
- **Place.** Where? How private is it? How will privacy needs be honored?
- **Time.** When will the scene begin and end?
- **Safe signals.** What are they? If subs invoke safe signals, do both parties agree to discuss the reason constructively?
- **Health.** Does either party have medical conditions that might affect the scene?
- **Sex.** Will there be any? If so, what? What about contraception and sexual infection prevention?
- **Intoxicants.** Which, if any, will be permitted? How much?
- **Bondage.** Will the submissive allow restraint? If so, what? Will unassisted escape be possible?
- **Intense sensation.** Will the sub allow it? If so, how intense? Only inflicted by hand? Or with instruments? Which?
- **Marks.** Will the sub allow evidence of scratching, biting, and so forth? If so, what? Where? Temporary or permanent?
- **Verbal humiliation.** May the dom call the sub names? If so, which?
- **Follow up.** Will you see each other afterward?
- **More.** Does either player need to discuss anything else?

In addition, beginners should:

- **Stay sober.** Intoxication impairs judgment and may compromise commitment to safe words.
- **Start without equipment.** Before playing with blindfolds, try this command: "Keep your eyes shut until I tell you to open them." Before trying gagging: "Keep your mouth shut." Before restraint: "Clasp your hands behind your head."

- **Start softly.** If you're interested in erotic spanking, begin with something soft, for example, the top's hand in an oven mitt. If the sub wants greater intensity, move to a bare hand. More? Discuss paddles, riding crops, and other equipment.
- **Be particularly cautious about restraint.** Before you try handcuffs, ropes, stockings, or neckties, first experiment with thread, so the bottom can break free at any time.
- **Doms must always treat subs lovingly.** Don't jump right into hair-pulling or spanking. Instead, lead up to them with hair combing, or touch with a feather, massage mitt, or fingertips.
- **Stay present.** If you restrain anyone, don't leave the room.
- **Marks.** Be extra careful with anything that can burn or leave marks, for example, whips and hot candle wax.
- **Bottom line.** Safe words and every detail of scenes should be negotiated in advance with explicit mutual consent—ideally, written contracts.

What Is Intimacy?

Relationship authorities define intimacy as clear, frank, self-revealing emotional conversation. Many people equate *intimacy* and *sex*. But it's quite possible to have enjoyable sex with lovers you hardly know—"perfect strangers."

Most couples hardly discuss their lovemaking, which diminishes its intimacy. But BDSM *requires* detailed negotiations. Players must plan every aspect of scenes beforehand and evaluate them after. Many BDSM aficionados consider these discussions as intimate, erotic, and relationship enhancing as the scenes themselves.

Couples who enjoy occasional BDSM often remark that it enhances their vanilla sex. Negotiating scenes helps them discuss their other lovemaking. The communication skills required for BDSM enhance relationships and lovemaking—no matter how you play.

Curious about BDSM? Consider Blindfolds

Blindfolds are a fun, nonthreatening portal into BDSM. Blindfold play incorporates the dominant-submissive element of role-playing without the intense sensations of heavier BDSM. Blindfolds also provide an opportunity for tops to be nurturing. Blindfolded subs are vulnerable. Loving doms can practice keeping them safe from harm.

Sight deprivation may feel especially powerful when women wear blindfolds. Sexologists agree that most men become most aroused visually. It's no coincidence that women wear the vast majority of lingerie. Men love *seeing* women in it. When women wear the blindfolds, men see them in all their submissive glory.

Of course, some men enjoy being blindfolded, and some women don't care for it.

Sexologists also agree that most women become most aroused by sensual touch: massage, hot baths, spa treatments, the feel of silk, and extended kissing, cuddling, and whole-body caresses. When women don blindfolds, they can focus more deeply on being touched.

Blindfolds are also discreet. If anyone stumbles upon yours, just say, *I sleep better that way.* It's more difficult explaining handcuffs. Blindfolds also travel easily, enabling sexy spice wherever you go.

Blindfolds are available from drug stores and sex toy catalogs.

Many BDSM enthusiasts pity those who engage only in vanilla sex. They contend that conventional lovemaking cannot approach the intimacy and thrills of BDSM.

How Kinky Women Play

A San Francisco State University researcher used BDSM websites to survey how 1,580 women devotees, age nineteen to seventy-two, played. Eighty percent were Americans living in forty-nine of the fifty states. The remaining 20 percent hailed from two dozen other countries. About half described themselves as partnered: married, cohabitating, or polyamorous. They enjoyed an enormous range of erotic fun from conventional sex to extreme BDSM.

The figures below represent percentages of the total sample who participated in any way—dom, sub, or voyeur. Activities that attracted at least two-thirds of respondents included:

Vanilla sex:

99.62%	Touching (caressing, cuddling, massage, tickling)
99.56%	Kissing
98.76%	Masturbation solo
90.26%	Mutual masturbation with partner
97.06%	Cunnilingus
93.83%	Hand job
91.89%	Fellatio
91.39%	Anal insertions (fingers or penis)
89.74%	Penis-vagina intercourse
88.95%	Vaginal sex toy (vibrators, etc.)
79.12%	Swallowing semen
71.88%	Phone sex
78.19%	Anal sex toys (vibrators, butt plugs, etc.)
76.69%	Mammary intercourse (rubbing penis between breasts)
70.30%	Anilingus (rimming)

BDSM:

95.70%	Spanking
93.16%	Hair-pulling
92.03%	Biting
90.06%	Scratching, leaving marks
87.53%	Use of bondage gear (rope, cuffs, gags, etc.)
86.39%	Moderate bondage (can move but can't escape unassisted)
85.13%	Light bondage (can escape unassisted)
84.24%	Paddling
83.16%	Breast torment (slapping, pinching, clothespins, etc.)
81.90%	Flogging
80.38%	Genital torment (slapping, kicking, pinching, clothespins, etc.)
80.06%	Ice play (ice cubes on the nipples, genitals)
79.62%	Hickeys
78.61%	Hot candle wax play
77.53%	Physical humiliation (face-slapping, forced begging, crawling)
75.70%	Whipping
68.67%	Caning
66.77%	Verbal humiliation (yelling, name-calling, etc.)

Role play:

83.53%	Master-slave play
69.56%	Obedience training
69.44%	Occupation play (boss-employee)

Exhibitionism:

87.83%	Model for erotic photos, video	Rehor, J. E. "Sensual, Erotic,
78.56%	Share erotic images of yourself with others	and Sexual Behaviors of Women from the 'Kink'
75.92%	Model erotic clothing (lingerie, corsets, etc.)	Community." *Archives of Sexual*
71.36%	Breast flashing in public	*Behavior* 44 (2015): 825.

Many believe that BDSM is a realm unto itself, that those into it don't engage in conventional sex and vice versa. Actually, most BDSM aficionados combine it with vanilla sex. Many are primarily vanilla and use BDSM for occasional spice.

In this study, the most popular form of kinky play was spanking (95.7% of respondents). But among BDSMers, several conventional sexual moves were more popular: caressing (99.62), kissing (99.56), masturbation (98.76), and cunnilingus (97.06).

Cunnilingus was the kinky women's favorite genital play (97.06), ahead of hand jobs (93.83), fellatio (91.89), and vaginal intercourse (89.74).

Some people characterize BDSM as "whips and chains." Those activities are popular: paddling (84.24), flogging (81.90), and whipping (75.70). But noninstrumental BDSM is more popular: hair-pulling (93.16), biting (92.03), and scratching (90.06).

With the exception of master-slave play (83.53), other forms of role-playing were not particularly popular—obedience training (69.56) and boss-employee scenarios (69.44).

The study's author concluded, "Respondents willingly engaged in BDSM behaviors for their own enjoyment. Their willingness to disclose such personal details indicate ardent participation in kink eroticism."

What *Fifty Shades* Got Wrong—and Right

Fifty Shades of Grey got one aspect of BDSM horribly wrong: it depicts dom Christian Grey as the product of horrendous child abuse and implies it propelled him into kink. Actually, BDSM players are no more likely than anyone else to have suffered child abuse or sexual trauma.

Otherwise, author E. L. James depicted BDSM quite realistically:

- **Communication.** Before Grey lays a hand on Anastasia Steele, they discuss their play in great detail.
- **Contracts.** Grey hands Steele an extensive contract proposal and they discuss it point by point. Steele agrees to some clauses, modifies others, and nixes a few. Not all BDSM players use written contracts, but many do.
- **Limits.** Grey quizzes Steele on the hard boundaries she can't conceive of crossing and the soft limits she might cross under the right circumstances. Both players declare their limits and pledge to honor the other's.
- **Safe word.** Grey tells Steele she is always free to invoke their safe word. No matter how anything looks or feels, she always retains total control over their play.
- **Intimacy.** Steele is astonished by the depth of self-revelation involved in BDSM, and how emotionally close it brings her to Grey.

CHAPTER 45:
Minority Sexual Orientations, Minority Gender Identities:
Lesbian, Gay, Bisexual, Transgender, Queer, Nonbinary, Intersex, and Asexual

CONVENTIONAL SEXUALITY IS hetero. But since the dawn of literature, some people have been depicted as homosexual, bisexual, transgender (dressing or living as the other gender), or intersex (ambiguous gender). Asexuality (never feeling sexual attractions) probably also has ancient roots, but sexologists did not recognize it until the 1970s. And since the millennium, another gender option has emerged, nonbinary, identifying as neither male nor female.

This book focuses on heterosexual (straight) sexuality. But both sexual preference and gender identity can be remarkably fluid, a flexibility no umbrella term captures. I propose *curved*. Many self-identified straights enjoy curved lovemaking—some in the past, others currently but occasionally, and some regularly throughout life. Adolescents and young adults are the demographic most likely to experiment with curved sexuality, but many older, ostensibly heterosexual adults also explore gay/lesbian/bi relationships and gender-bending.

On the surface, the various sexual and gender options appear quite distinct. But considerable research shows that straight and curved relationships are much more similar than different and that sexual preference and gender identity play only minor roles in most couples' happiness.

How Many People Are Not Exclusively Heterosexual?
The conventional wisdom says 10 percent of the population is homosexual. We owe this estimate to Alfred Kinsey. His post–World War II surveys showed that many people identify as gay/lesbian/bi and that many self-identified straights have enjoyed curved sex.

Kinsey suggested a sexual preference continuum, a six-point scale still used today—one signifying exclusively hetero, six exclusively homo, and two through five varying degrees of bisexuality. Kinsey himself was bisexual, married to a woman and predominantly straight, but with many gay experiences.

Kinsey concluded that 4 percent of men were exclusively gay, with 13 percent predominantly homosexual. His figures for women were 2 and 15 percent respectively. During the 1970s, the emerging gay-rights movement justified its slogan (*We Are Everywhere!*) by averaging Kinsey's findings and proclaiming that 10 percent of the population is lesbian/gay.

However, Kinsey committed a sampling error. His team interviewed anyone who would talk to them, including patrons of many gay bars. Kinsey's sample was not representative. Critics accused him of overestimating the curved population.

More recent surveys based on representative samples of up to tens of thousands of Americans have produced these findings:

Survey	Exclusively heterosexual	Exclusively lesbian/gay	Bisexual	Identify hetero with curved experiences
US National Survey of Men (1991)	96.6%	1.1%	2.3%	No data
The National Survey of Family Growth (2006–8)	96.3%	1.4%	2.3%	8.8%
General Social Survey (2008)	97.2%	1.7%	1.1%	7.5%
California Health Interview Survey (2009)	96.8%	1.8%	1.4%	No data
National Survey of Sexual Health & Behavior (2009)	94.4%	2.5%	3.1%	11%
National Survey of Sexual Attitudes & Lifestyles (2010)	95.1%	2.5%	2.4%	No data
UCLA (2011)	96.5%	1.7%	1.8%	No data
National Center for Health Statistics (2013)	96.6%	1.6%	0.7%	No data
Average	**96.2%**	**1.8%**	**1.9%**	**9.1%**

Copen, C. E., et al. "Sexual Behavior, Sexual Attraction, and Sexual Orientation among Adults Aged 18–44 in the United States: Data from the 2011–2013 National Survey of Family Growth." *National Health Statistics Report* 7 (2016): 1.

Gates, G. J. *How Many People Are Lesbian, Gay, Bisexual, and Transgender?* Los Angeles: Williams Institute, UCLA School of Law, 2011.

Spiegelhalter, D. "Is 10% of the Population Really Gay?" *Guardian.* April 5, 2015.

Ward, B. W., et al. "Sexual Orientation and Health among U.S. Adults: National Health Interview Survey, 2013." *National Health Statistics Report*, no. 77 (July 15, 2014).

Depending on one's perspective, Kinsey was either way off the mark or fairly close to it. Only a small proportion of the population admits being exclusively lesbian/gay—1.8 percent. But 11 percent are not entirely heterosexual—the 1.9 percent who identify as bisexual and the 9.1 percent of self-identified straights who report curved sex. Kinsey's seventy-year-old estimate has held up pretty well.

Straight versus Gay/Lesbian: Any Differences in Sexual Satisfaction?

The genders don't always see eye to eye. Some assume that same-gender couples understand each other better and consequently have better sex. Actually, no.

Canadian psychologists surveyed 423 people age eighteen to fifty-eight, all coupled, 322 women, 101 men, 253 heterosexuals, 170 gays/lesbians. They found "far more" sexual similarities than differences.

- **Libido.** Most men are hornier than most women, so in decreasing order, we would expect men in gay couples to feel the most desire, followed by heterosexual men, and then the women. But sexual desire was fairly close for all respondents, with gay men expressing slightly more than heterosexuals and lesbians.
- **Communication.** Similarity breeds comfort, so compared with heteros, we would expect lesbian and gay couples to feel happier with their erotic negotiations. But sexual communication was "virtually identical" for all groups.
- **Activities.** "All groups displayed very similar sexual repertoires." The main differences: men prefer more genital play, women more whole-body caressing. Gay men engage in more anal play. And lesbians don't have penis-vagina intercourse, but most insert fingers and dildos.
- **Orgasm.** All groups reported the same fulfillment from orgasm.
- **Satisfaction.** All groups reported very similar sexual pleasure and satisfaction.

Other studies have reported almost identical findings. Straight and gay/lesbian couples largely share feelings about affection, decision-making, conflict resolution, reasons for getting it on or abstaining, and relationship quality and satisfaction. The most prominent differences: gay men have sex a little more often than straight couples, who do it a bit more than lesbians. But lesbian couples are the most emotionally intimate.

Straight and curved relationships are different, but across all orientations, lovers report similar happiness.

Bisexuality: Controversial

Bisexual individuals enjoy fantasizing and possibly playing with people of all genders. They might be involved in heterosexual or same-gender relationships, but still fantasize about sex across the gender spectrum. They "swing both ways," or are "AC/DC."

Bisexuality has been depicted in literature since the Bible's David fell in love with King Saul's son, Jonathan. The biblical Book of Samuel is a bit coy about their relationship, but the clear scholarly consensus is that they were lovers. They also had wives, meaning they were bisexual.

Kinsey called bisexuality fairly prevalent. However, it's long been controversial:

- Some have argued it doesn't exist, that people are straight, lesbian/gay, or *lying*—with the liars often gays/lesbians who feign straight attraction to avoid stigmatization as homosexual.
- Others have dismissed it as youthful experimentation before people embrace their "real" orientations, straight or gay/lesbian.
- Some have said bisexuals are heterosexuals in single-gender institutions (prisons, monasteries) who reluctantly make do.

These dismissals linger today. College women involved with women are sometimes called LUGs, lesbians until graduation, after which they presumably embrace AC or DC. Meanwhile, some lesbians and gays view bisexuality as a cowardly refuge for homosexuals who lack the courage to come out.

Heterosexuals began celebrating sex for pleasure during the 1960s. Lesbian/gay sexuality emerged from the closet beginning in 1969 when a group of drag queens fought police who'd raided the Stonewall Inn in Greenwich Village, New York City. Soon after, the media spotlighted bisexuality. A 1974 *Newsweek* article was titled "Bisexual Chic: Anyone Goes." Around that time on both coasts, bi activists founded the first bisexual organizations: in Boston, a discussion group, the Bivocals, and in San Francisco, the Bisexual Center. But research into bisexuality lagged. The *Journal of Bisexuality* didn't launch until 2001, and books about lesbian/gay issues vastly outnumber those dealing with bisexuality.

Starting in the 1980s, AIDS transformed our understanding of bisexuality. A surprising number of apparently straight, often married men developed the disease. It soon became clear that sexual identification often differed from behavior. Men could identify as hetero, live straight lives, and enjoy happy marriages with women, yet have periodic, even regular, curved experiences—not just experimentally, but for decades.

Then in 2005, Northwestern University researchers made headlines by declaring that bisexuality did not exist. They asked 101 young men—straight, gay, and self-identified bisexual—to watch erotic videos with their genitals wired to detect arousal. The straight men were aroused only by heterosexual videos and the gays only by male-male action. Among the self-identified bisexuals, three-quarters were aroused by the gay porn and one-quarter by the straight videos, with *none* aroused by both—in other words, straight, gay, or lying.

Bisexual groups cried foul. The researchers had recruited participants by advertising only in gay media. Six years later in 2011, the same researchers repeated the study, only this time they recruited through bi websites. They found that almost all self-identified bisexuals became aroused by *both* straight and gay/lesbian porn.

Bisexuality is real and, for many, lifelong. Around 2 percent of the population identifies as bisexual, some six million Americans.

Continuing Prejudice against Bisexuals

In the US, homophobia is becoming culturally unacceptable, but "bi-phobia" is alive and well. During the mid-1990s, college students were asked how they felt about curved sexuality. Fewer than half disapproved of homosexuality, but more than half objected to bisexuality. A 2013 University of Pittsburgh study showed that many straights and gays/lesbians expressed prejudice against bisexuality, with 15 percent of the straight men insisting it doesn't exist. In other studies, many people call bisexuals promiscuous, unfaithful, unable to make long-term commitments, and more likely than straights or gays/lesbians to transmit STIs.

Bisexuality: Myths versus Truth

One myth is that most bisexuals are involved with men and women simultaneously. This is possible, but the research shows that only a minority maintain concurrent relationships with lovers of more than one gender. Most switch back and forth. In one report, self-identified bisexuals were asked if they'd played with both men and women during the past twelve months. Two-thirds said yes (66 percent of the men, 70 percent of the women). However, only one-third said they'd been involved with men and women simultaneously.

About promiscuity: bisexuals are potentially attracted to more people and may jump into bed more often. The research is scant, but one study of 105 bisexual men, age nineteen to sixty-two, showed a lifetime average of twenty-three male sex partners and twenty-three female lovers. That's considerably more than most heterosexuals, but fewer than many gay men (I found no studies of women bisexuals' lifetime number of partners).

"Coming Out Twice"

Many bisexuals use this phrase. When they first realize same-gender attractions, they come out as gay/lesbian. Later, when they acknowledge continuing other-gender attractions, they come out a second time as bisexual (or, alternatively, assuming themselves straight for many years, then later realizing they're also attracted to the same gender). This process is more complex than simply declaring one is lesbian/gay, and it typically takes longer. Most gays/lesbians realize they're homosexual during their teens or early twenties. But most bisexuals don't acknowledge being AC/DC until their late twenties or after.

Coming out as bisexual can feel socially isolating. Gays and lesbians are much more visible, with robust cultures that includes publications, websites, organizations, community centers, and neighborhoods in several cities. Bisexuality is comparatively invisible. Fortunately, the internet has fostered bisexual community. A search of "bisexual" produced forty-two million hits.

If you're bisexual or think you might be, you're in good company. In addition to Kinsey, a partial list of notable bisexuals includes singers Lady Gaga, Debbie Harry, Janis Joplin, Amy Winehouse, Billie Holiday, and Bessie Smith; actors Marilyn Monroe, Anthony Perkins, Greta Garbo, James Dean, Drew Barrymore, Montgomery Clift, Anne Heche, Laurence Olivier, Lindsay Lohan, and Sal Mineo; dancers Isadora Duncan and Alvin Ailey; musician/conductor Leonard Bernstein; and artist Frida Kahlo.

For more about bisexuality, visit Bisexual.org or the American Institute of Bisexuality (americaninstituteofbisexuality.org).

New Insights into Relationships Thanks to Transgender Men and Women

Mention "raging hormones" and most people think of horny teens. Eventually, most people's hormones stop raging, but the transgender community has shown that they never stop *arranging* us.

Ever since paleolithic humans began telling stories, some have dealt with men and women who lived as the other gender. But anatomical gender-switching dates from 1931, when German surgeons performed the first male-to-female reassignment surgery.

Being transgender had little cultural impact until the 1990s, when increasing acceptance of homosexuality led to growing appreciation that some people suffer "gender dysphoria," deep discomfort with the gender assigned at their birth ("cis" gender) and strong yearnings to transition.

What proportion of the population is transgender?

- A 1993 Dutch survey of 8,064 people showed that 1.1 percent of the men and 0.8 percent of the women identified more strongly with their nonbirth gender.
- A 2013 survey of 2,730 San Francisco middle-schoolers revealed that 1.3 percent identified as transgender.
- That same year, the National Center for Health Statistics interviewed a representative 34,557 Americans. Those who identified as other than straight, lesbian/gay, or bi—1.1 percent.

It appears that around 1 percent of the population is inclined toward gender-switching—some three million Americans—though only some take hormones and fewer have surgery.

Many people wonder about transgender folks' mental health. The research shows that the vast majority score in the normal range on standard psychological tests.

Transitioning has significant sexual impact. The most consistent findings are that trans men express increased interest in sex, masturbate more, and have more partner sex. Trans women report reduced libido and less sex, both solo and partnered.

Postsurgically, when trans men and women get it on, they generally report good sexual function—reasonable erections in the men, vaginal lubrication in the women, and satisfying orgasms. But orgasms often change. Trans men typically report shorter but more powerful climaxes, trans women longer but less jolting release.

One element of gender change is unpredictable—posttransition sexual preference. Some maintain their cisgender preference and appear lesbian/gay. Others switch preference, appearing straight. And some realize they're bisexual.

Nothing Personal, It's Just Hormones

Transitioning involves another change that's rarely discussed and hardly researched: trans folks' relationship to intimate, that is, self-revealing conversation. I'm acquainted with a few trans women. In addition to the changes just discussed, they've all reported increased interest in talking about their emotional lives and their relationships with others. Meanwhile, trans men typically become somewhat quieter.

Not all men badger women for sex, but in common parlance, the word that follows "horny" is *guy*. Many women don't understand how men can want so much sex. As transsexuality demonstrates, libido is largely hormonal. Trans women take estrogen and quickly feel less sexual urgency. Trans men take testosterone and suddenly want to get laid. If they don't, they masturbate. That's the power of hormones.

In addition, many women complain that men have trouble controlling their tempers. This, too, is hormonal. Italian researchers assessed anger in fifty trans men as they took testosterone during their transitions. During the seven-month trial, their anger significantly increased.

Meanwhile, some men complain that women talk too much, and many women fret that their men are "the silent type" and don't listen. Like all stereotypes, this isn't the whole story. Some woman are reserved, and some men can't shut up. But in common parlance, the word that follows "chatty" is *Cathy*.

Many men love to discuss sports, politics, and business, but don't understand women's fascination with intimate conversation. Transgender people show that enthusiasm for self-revealing exchanges is also largely hormonal. Trans women take estrogen, talk more about their emotions, and criticize men's silence. Trans men take testosterone, retreat from intimate conversation, and tend to feel annoyed by women's preference for it.

No doubt women will continue to complain that men are insatiable horndogs and men will continue to complain that women can't stop talking about their feelings. But transgender people show us that neither gender is out to drive the other crazy. It's nothing personal, just hormones.

Nonbinary, Gender Neutral, Queer

Traditionally, people were either male or female—the gender assigned at birth. But in the twenty-first century, a third option has gained traction: nonbinary, gender neutral, or queer (which used to mean gay). Instead of he, she, his, and hers, nonbinary individuals usually use "they" and "their." Instead of Mr., Miss, Mrs., or Ms., they often use "Mx."

At this writing, ten countries allow nonbinary identification on passports, drivers licenses, and other documents: Australia, Bangladesh, Canada, Denmark, Germany, India, Malta, Nepal, New Zealand, and Pakistan. Currently in the United States, California, New Jersey, New York City, Oregon, and Washington allow nonbinary birth certificates. A few others allow gender-neutral driver's licenses but not birth certificates, and a few prohibit any alteration of birth certificate gender. The issue is emotionally charged and evolving.

Official forms often equate sex and gender. They say, *Sex: Male. Female.* Actually, it should be "gender." Gender-neutral individuals may claim any sexuality: heterosexual, lesbian, gay, bisexual, or asexual.

Intersex: Neither Conventionally Male nor Female

Intersex means being born with genitals or sex chromosomes that don't fit standard male-female parameters. Genitals may appear ambiguous or, instead of male or female chromosomes (XY or XX), there may be something else, for example, XXY (Kleinfelter syndrome).

Intersex folks used to be called hermaphrodites. *Intersex* was coined in 1917 and has largely replaced it.

It's not clear how many people are intersex. Estimates vary from one in one thousand to one in ten thousand. Intersex includes Kleinfelter, Turner syndrome (female but missing an X chromosome), and ovotestis (having both ovaries and testicles).

Until recently, when infants were found to be intersex, doctors and psychologists pressed parents to approve surgery and hormone treatments to make them more clearly male or female. Today the situation is in flux. In some locales, surgery and hormones continue to be the norm. In others, the trend is not to intervene, but to allow children to grow up intersex and decide their gender identity for themselves. In 2015, Malta became the first country to outlaw nonconsensual medical intervention for its intersex citizens.

Intersexuality has a long history of stigmatization. Around the world, intersex infants have been killed, their mothers accused of witchcraft, and their families shunned, considered cursed, and sometimes banished. In recent decades, intersex athletes have been disqualified from competitions for not being clearly male or female.

In ancient Roman law, people were male, female, or hermaphrodite—with legal rights and responsibilities corresponding to whichever gender traits appeared dominant. More recently, intersex issues have confounded European and American courts. Men have enjoyed more legal rights than women—voting, inheritance, property ownership—and intersex men pressed those rights while their legal adversaries argued they were actually women who didn't have them.

For a poignant window into intersex experience, read the Pulitzer Prize–winning novel *Middlesex* by Jeffrey Eugenides. Its protagonist starts life as a girl, Callie. During her adolescence, doctors discover she's intersex and advise surgery to make her more female. She flees and . . . I won't spoil the ending.

Recent research strongly suggests that a hero of the American Revolution was intersex—Casimir Pulaski, "father of the American cavalry."

In 1993, the Intersex Society of North America formed to combat intersex shame, discrimination, and nonconsensual surgery. In 2008, it was succeeded by the Accord Alliance (accordalliance.org).

Asexuality: Not Interested, Period

Many people feel erotic attractions but have little or no partner sex. They're nonsexual. Asexuality is different. The Asexual Visibility and Education Network (AVEN, asexuality.org)

354 Sizzling Sex for Life

defines it as feeling no sexual attraction to anyone, ever. However, asexuals may experience other forms of interpersonal attraction:

- **Aesthetic.** Feeling drawn to others based on their appearance.
- **Romantic.** Desire for love and intimacy apart from sex.
- **Sensual.** Desire for affectionate touch but not erotic play.
- **Gray-sexual.** The gray area between sexual and asexual. Gray-sexuals feel erotic attraction, but rarely.

Some asexual people masturbate, mostly men, but they have no interest in partner sex. Asexual folks don't feel repulsed by partner sex (aversion)—they simply have no interest.

Researchers wired the genitals of people who were sexually active, sex averse, and asexual, and showed them porn. Those who were sex averse recoiled. Heterosexuals and gays/lesbians became aroused when they viewed sex matching their preferences. The asexuals showed no reactions at all.

Sexologists first described asexuality in the late 1970s, but little research was published until the 1990s. It appears that around 1 percent of the population is asexual:

- In 1991, English researchers surveyed 13,765 UK adults and found that 0.9 percent had never had or wanted partner sex.
- In 2001, these same English scientists surveyed another 12,110 Brits—0.4 percent claimed lifelong abstinence.
- In 2004, another English team surveyed 18,000 UK adults. Those saying they'd never felt sexually attracted to anyone—1.05 percent.
- In 2010, Texas researchers surveyed 12,571 Americans. Just under 1 percent said they'd never experienced sexual attractions—0.8 percent of the women, 0.7 percent of the men.

Plenty of long-term couples have little or no sex. Horizontal romps are not necessary for emotional attachment. Compared with the general population, asexual people are more likely to be single, but depending on the study, 15–33 percent are cohabiting or married in straight or lesbian/gay/bi relationships. AVEN says asexuals can have successful long-term relationships without sex if their spouses can accommodate sexless relationships and if they share strong aesthetic, romantic, and/or sensual attraction.

Some asexual individuals have never had partner sex. But most tried it before giving it up. Compared with the general population, most report less childhood sex play, fewer sexual relationships, less sex in their relationships, and virginity loss later in life—for most people, sixteen to seventeen, but for the asexual population, around twenty-one.

Early sex researchers assumed everyone was sexual. In the 1990s, sexologists began focusing on desire and realized that some had little or none. They viewed desire as "normal," therefore its absence had to be "abnormal." Early editions of the American Psychiatric Association's guide to mental illness, the *Diagnostic and Statistical Manual of Mental Disorders* (DSM) included "sexual aversion disorder" and "hypoactive female desire disorder." But in the latest edition, DSM-5 (2013), these two diagnoses have been deleted. Some experts still call total lack of erotic interest abnormal, but increasingly sexologists consider asexuality a normal variation, with sexual orientation expanding from three categories to four: heterosexual, gay/lesbian, bisexual, and asexual. For more about asexuality, visit asexuality.org.

PART VI:
What Everyone Should Know about Pornography

CHAPTER 46:
The Main Problem with Porn: It Misleads Men about Themselves, Women, and Lovemaking

WHAT EXACTLY IS pornography? It involves explicit depictions of you-know-what, but beyond that, it's difficult to specify. So we fall back on what US Supreme Court Justice Potter Stewart said in 1964: "I can't define pornography—but I know it when I see it."

Some attack porn as disgusting, immoral, and misogynist, a contributor to rape, child sex abuse, teen sexual irresponsibility, and withdrawal into what some call "addiction." Others defend it as free speech, fantasy, and sex education.

Porn drives some women to despair. When they discover that their men indulge, they feel betrayed and deeply wounded. Some question the viability of their relationships.

If you detest porn, you have every right to your opinion. Unfortunately, porn so enrages some critics that they misinterpret or dismiss any research that challenges their beliefs.

I mean no disrespect to those who hate porn, but, on balance, the research shows it's not poison. For most men (and some women), it's simply a visual aid that enhances self-soothing masturbation. Solo sex requires fantasies, and men's own get stale. So they turn to internet porn, where a zillion fantasies are available for free.

A tiny proportion of men—and a minuscule proportion of women—develop problematic relationships to porn. But except for the anguish some women suffer, the best evidence shows that it causes no significant social harm. Porn is considerably less violent than many TV shows, movies, and video games. Since free porn exploded on the internet, US rates of child sex abuse, teen pregnancy, divorce, and sexual assault have all declined. And women porn actors are not disproportionate victims of child sex abuse.

Critics also contend that porn harms men by contributing to erection problems and destroying sexual interest in their partners. Actually, the huge majority of men view porn at least occasionally, many frequently, some daily, yet maintain loving relationships, have firm erections, and can't wait to play with their partners. As for addiction, a tiny proportion of men watch for hours a day, but most indulge for less than five minutes per session.

The main consequence of porn is not rape, divorce, erectile dysfunction, or child sex abuse, but masturbation. Most men masturbate much more than most women. Many women don't understand men's deep need to self-soothe by hand. Many women call masturbation fine for single men, but unnecessary—even infidelity—for those in couples: *I should meet all his sexual needs.*

Sorry, ladies, he was self-sexing long before he met you. As fantastic as you may be, as much as he may love you, the testosterone in his veins impels him to stroke just as the estrogen in yours may produce PMS, cramps, postpartum depression, and menopausal mood swings. Even frequent fabulous partner sex cannot satisfy most men's need to masturbate, which is, by definition, a solo pleasure.

The main problem with hardcore media is neither addiction nor any connection to social ills, but porn's primacy in men's sex education. Porn teaches sex all wrong. It's like the chase scenes in action movies—exciting and fun to watch, but not the way to drive. Porn presents a cartoon version of lovemaking. It's as realistic as the Roadrunner smashing Wile E. Coyote over the head with a sledgehammer and the latter suffering only momentary disorientation. Unfortunately, many men think porn is a documentary, a how-to sex manual. Far from it.

Our culture provides little real lovemaking education. So most men and some women turn to the ubiquitous medium available gratis on any internet-linked device—and make the huge mistake of trying to imitate it. Porn is socially benign, but sexually problematic.

Porn Teaches Sex All Wrong

The husband-wife team Jack and Marie Silva act in pornography, but their porn sex did not come naturally. As they discuss in *Marie and Jack: A Hardcore Love Story,* they had to learn it.

"Directors would say, 'Do this,' 'Do that,'" Jack explains, "and I'd think, *Really? You want that?*"

"Sex is our job," Marie says. "But it's nowhere near as pleasurable as our personal sex. Jack and I share a deep emotional connection. For sex to feel satisfying, I need more than hardcore action. I need emotional fulfillment with a man who wants to please me and knows how."

Occasionally, Marie and Jack slip into porn sex at home. "After a shoot," Jack explains, "I might try some porn move. Then one of us says, 'Wait. Let's make real love.'"

Porn presents male erotic fantasies fueled by more than a billion years of evolution. Everyone has fantasies. They're fine. In fact, sexologists encourage them. Fantasies enhance sex. In fantasy, everything is permitted and nothing is wrong—as long as you can distinguish between fantasy and reality. Unfortunately, many men have difficulty separating porn-inspired reveries from erotic authenticity. As a result, porn seriously misleads men about themselves, women, and lovemaking.

Here's what porn gets wrong:

- **Everyone is constantly sexual.** Search "porn" and you get two billion pages showing people in the throes. The implication is that everyone has sex very frequently. Most people don't. Studies by Australian and SUNY Albany researchers show that men consistently overestimate how frequently other men do it. They're convinced they don't get as much, that they have less sex than average. The nonstop sex in porn reinforces this misconception.
- **Everyone is hot to trot.** In porn, boy meets girl and almost immediately, she's on her knees, mouth open. In real sex, lovers have uniquely individual libidos. Some desire sex rarely if ever, others daily or more. Put two people with unique libidos together, and after the hot-and-heavy period, six months to a year, they're almost certain to fall out of sync on desired sexual frequency. Canadian researchers interviewed 117 long-term couples. Their top sexual complaint was conflict about sexual frequency, reported by 36 percent of the women and 39 percent of the men. Desire differences are also one of the leading reasons couples consult sex therapists. But in porn, desire differences are unheard of. Everyone is always eager to get it on.
- **No relationships, no intimacy.** Relationships require emotional intimacy, mutual self-revelation. That means ongoing conversations, negotiations, and conflict resolution.

But porn shows little more than fellatio and intercourse, with occasional cunnilingus. A good deal of porn doesn't even show faces, just organs grinding. No relationships, no emotional intimacy.

- **Little kissing.** For many men and women, kissing is crucial to enjoyment of lovemaking and sexual satisfaction. Porn rarely contains any.
- **Almost no whole-body caressing.** Sizzling sex is based on extended, whole-body loveplay. The sex in porn is almost all genital. Of course, genital play can bring great pleasure. But the genitals often don't work properly without lots of loving touch all over. Men who imitate porn are at high risk for premature ejaculation, difficulty ejaculating, and erectile dysfunction—not to mention disappointed, irritated women who decide their men are lousy lovers.
- **No coaching.** In porn, everyone's a mind reader. Everyone knows exactly what their partners want. In real sex, mutual coaching is vital. No one can read anyone else's erotic mind. To get the pleasure you want, you *must* speak up, ask for what you want, and provide coaching.

Hollywood Also Teaches Sex All Wrong

When movies and TV programs show intercourse, a few pumps bring both lovers to simultaneous orgasms. In real life, this is rare. Only one-quarter of women are consistently orgasmic during intercourse, and in every age group, around 30 percent of men suffer premature ejaculation, so only 70 percent of men last long enough to allow the 25 percent of women who orgasm during intercourse to get there. Hollywood sex is possible for, at most, only around 18 percent of couples—one in six. And many of the women in that modest percentage of couples prefer to have orgasms from cunnilingus.

- **Little use of lubricant.** Porn actors use lubricant by the gallon, but viewers rarely see it. The women appear to be perpetually wet, able to accept unusually large erections comfortably under any circumstances. Actually, even with loving, extended whole-body massage, many perfectly normal women don't produce much self-lubrication and *need* lube—saliva or commercial products.
- **Little safe sex.** Porn depicts effortless sexual abundance with no consequences whatsoever. Some porn includes condoms. But most ignores contraception and prevention of sexual infections.
- **Almost no disability.** Almost everyone in porn is blessed with excellent health. Very few have disabilities or chronic medical conditions. Meanwhile, many Americans—one in five (19 percent)—have disabilities that require sexual adjustments.
- **The men are hung like stallions.** Male porn actors are *selected* for huge endowments. They *really are* bigger than average. But porn penises are the standard by which men judge themselves, and it's seriously skewed toward humongous. No wonder so many men complain they're "too small."
- **The men raise instant erections.** A woman winks, the man unzips, and out pops firm pipe. This is total fiction. Men in their teens and twenties may be able to raise instant erections. But past thirty or so, that ability fades. For most men, firm erections require deep relaxation and gentle, playful, loving touch from head to toe. Porn ignores most men's real need for whole-body massage.

Porn sex is so alienating for the actors that before Viagra, many of the men had trouble getting it up. Crews often sat around "waiting for wood." These days, the men pop erection drugs like M&M's, and some still struggle with balky erections.

- **Erections never wilt.** Porn actors are rock hard from the moment Mr. Happy appears until ejaculation. That's possible for some young men, but after around forty, minor distractions—a siren on the street—may wilt erections, even during fellatio or intercourse.
- **The men last forever.** In porn, there's no premature ejaculation. In the real world, PE afflicts one-quarter to one-third of men of all ages. One reason for this—men imitating all-genital porn sex. Good ejaculatory control requires whole-body lovemaking rarely depicted in porn.
- **The men come on cue.** Men in porn never have ejaculatory difficulties. Here on Earth, many men have trouble working up to orgasm/ejaculation.
- **The women are exhibitionists.** Porn gals revel in strutting around naked. They have no qualms flashing anything anywhere. And they love sex in public. Actually, very few real women are exhibitionists, only around 2 percent. Most real women feel insecure about their bodies. Meanwhile, some men expect their lovers to prance around in the buff and can't understand why they roll their eyes.
- **The women can't wait to spread their legs.** In porn, boy meets girl, and they quickly proceed to intercourse. Porn encourages men to plunge in long before most women feel receptive. In real sex, most women need at least twenty minutes of kissing, cuddling, and whole-body massage before they feel ready for genital play. When men imitate porn, many women feel turned off, and wonder how their lovers can be so oblivious.
- **The women almost never have orgasms.** This is the *only* realistic element of porn. Hardcore action is overwhelmingly focused on the penis—sucking and fucking. After the man ejaculates—in porn lingo, "the money shot"—the sex is over. The women moan in the throes of supposed passion, but rarely, if ever, have orgasms. Porn presents male fantasies—sex anywhere and everywhere with anyone and everyone. But there's little interest in women's satisfaction. With the rushed, mechanical, nonsensual sex in porn, it's a rare woman who *could* come. No wonder so many men are in the dark about women's orgasms. In porn, they almost never see them.
- **Fellatio is universal.** The vast majority of porn contains extended—often endless—cock sucking. This vastly overstates the actual popularity of fellatio. While almost all men have received it, only around two-thirds have been sucked during the past year, and only one-third during the past month. Porn persuades men that other men get much more head.
- **The oral sex is too intense.** Porn features furious fellatio and machine-gun cunnilingus. Most real lovers prefer slower, gentler oral. Many clitorises are so sensitive to touch that direct tonguing, no matter how gentle, feels uncomfortable. Ask. If so, lick around her clit, not directly on it. You'd never know this watching porn.
- **Anal sex is vastly overrepresented.** A great deal of porn contains anal play: sphincter massage, licking, fingering, toy insertions, and penis-anus intercourse (PAI). Many men fantasize about anal, so it's no surprise that a good deal of porn includes it. But according to several studies, during the past year, fewer than 25 percent of couples have tried PAI, and during their last roll in the hay, only around 1 percent. Porn misleads men into thinking that anal sex is more popular than it is. In addition, porn actors on the receiving end of PAI use gobs of lubricant and often stretch themselves with butt plugs before going on camera. Viewers almost never see this.

- **Ass-to-mouth is hazardous.** In some porn, the guy pulls out of the girl's butt and she immediately sucks him. *Never do this.* Even if the recipient takes several enemas beforehand, ass-to-mouth can transfer bacteria and cause infection.
- **Sex toy play is often too rough.** In real lovemaking, partner sex toy play requires coaching. In porn, there's none.

Erectile Dysfunction: Has Internet Porn Increased Men's Risk?

Since the late 1990s, free porn has become ubiquitous on the internet. Some argue it has fueled a major increase in ED, notably US military researchers, who compared soldiers' ED rates before and after the arrival of internet porn and documented a significant increase. But if ED among soldiers has increased since the 1990s, these researchers ignored many other possible explanations:

- **War.** After the Vietnam War (1975), few American soldiers saw combat until the brief Gulf War (1990–91) and after that, until the conflicts in Afghanistan and Iraq (starting in 2001). Deployment to war zones is stressful, fear of death more so. Compared with most soldiers who served from 1975 to 2000, today's military personnel are under much more stress. Many fear for their lives. Severe anxiety is a major contributor to ED.
- **Posttraumatic stress disorder.** Researchers at the VA Medical Center in Houston have documented high rates of PTSD in combat veterans. One frequent symptom—sexual impairment.
- **Alcohol.** Soldiers in war zones often decompress with alcohol, a leading cause of erection problems.
- **Obesity and high blood pressure.** Since 1990, rates have risen in young men. Both contribute to ED.
- **Psychiatric medications.** Use of mood-altering drugs has increased. Many impair erection.
- **Reporting.** Internet porn became available around the time Viagra was approved. Viagra spurred discussion of ED, which encouraged more men—including more young men—to report it.

Contrary to the assertions of porn critics, a 2015 survey of 2,737 European men found "little evidence of any link between pornography and young men's sexual difficulties." And in a 2019 study of 1,498 young men, Bowling Green (Ohio) State University researchers found "no evidence of causal links between pornography use and ED."

But internet porn constantly miseducates men about sex, so why *hasn't* it caused more sex problems? Largely because men have *always* been miseducated about sex as a result of pre-internet porn, lingering Victorian beliefs, and banter among sexually clueless friends.

Obtaining porn used to be a challenge, but generations of men found it and mistook it for erotic instruction. Internet porn represents a *quantitative* increase in what's available, but no *qualitative* change in the sexual miseducation most men receive. As a result, the deluge of internet porn has not caused any new epidemic of ED.

- **Misrepresentations endlessly repeated.** Some of the earliest porn on film (1890s) is available on the internet (search "antique porn"). The clothing and hairstyles are nineteenth century, but the sex looks remarkably like contemporary porn. When big lies get repeated endlessly, they become persuasive. Viewers infer that rushed, mechanical, genitally fixated sex is the way sex should be.

Want sizzling sex? Review chapters 1–10, and do the *opposite* of what you see in porn.

Marie and Jack Silva do their best to leave porn sex at work. At home their lovemaking is very different. "There's a wonderful playfulness to our personal sex," Marie explains. "I love Jack's hands all over me. I don't come from intercourse, so he massages my clitoris by hand or does me orally. After the grind of sex at work, it's so nice to come home to the real thing."

Porn Has Legitimate Uses in Sex Education, Coaching, and Therapy

Porn is a cartoon, but cartoons can be educational. For some, porn provides valuable information.

- **Fundamentalists.** Several million Americans grow up as religious fundamentalists. The religion itself is irrelevant—what matters is the belief that sex is only for procreation, not pleasure. When fundamentalists who question the sex negativity of their upbringing view porn and see happy people enjoying themselves, it can feel liberating.
- **People who fear they're undesirable.** Internet porn features people of every imaginable adult age, race, ethnicity, size, shape, weight, and looks. Everyone turns someone on. That can be reassuring for those who fear no one could feel attracted to them.
- **The sexually averse.** Some people have difficulty imagining aspects of sexuality: self-sexing, oral, anal, BDSM, whatever. Porn shows them all and helps some conceive of what they'd considered inconceivable.
- **The single minded.** Some people make love in only one rigidly ritualized manner. Porn shows other ways to play.
- **Mental health professionals.** Since the 1970s, many mental health professionals have explored their sexual preconceptions in day-long Sexual Attitude Reassessment (SAR) seminars. SARs typically include some porn. University of Minnesota researchers surveyed 7,451 SAR alumni (1972–91). Which element did they consider most beneficial? The exposure to porn. Participants said it helped clarify their sexual values and thinking.
- **Sex therapy clients.** Many sex therapists never suggest clients view porn for all the reasons discussed in this chapter. But others assign it as homework. A Kansas State University researcher surveyed ninety-nine US sex therapists:
  - 81 percent recommended soft-core video erotica to clients, often *Sexplorations: The Better Sex Video Series.*
  - 30 percent suggested porn.

Researchers in the US and the Czech Republic surveyed 279 American and European sex therapists about their use of sexually explicit materials with clients. Three-quarters called them valuable for some clients.

CHAPTER 47:
The Deep Evolutionary Roots of Porn—and Another Art Form Many Women Love

T HE EARLIEST KNOWN art, forty-thousand-year-old cave paintings, shows human hands, the hunting of large mammals—and our ancestors getting it on. Many subsequent prehistoric rock carvings, petroglyphs, also look sexual. Petroglyph porn has been discovered on every inhabited continent. Samples can be viewed at Petroglyph National Monument near Albuquerque, New Mexico. Some of this art may have been used in religious fertility rituals, but much of it looks like the first porn. As a result, some social scientists suggest that enjoyment of hardcore sexual imagery may be hardwired into the human nervous system.

Why Sexual Reproduction?
For life's first billion years on Earth, there was no sex. Single-celled organisms reproduced by dividing. Sexual reproduction is more complicated. It's involved and awkward and may increase participants' vulnerability to predation. Nonetheless, sexual reproduction has thrived, so it must confer survival advantages. Biologists explain that sexual reproduction rearranges chromosomes, which increases genetic diversity and makes life more resilient, more adaptable to environmental changes.

Why endure the hassles and risks of sexual reproduction? Evolution made it pleasurable and blessed us with orgasms. It's not clear if all animals have orgasms, but our closest evolutionary relatives, the primates, do. The conventional wisdom says sex produces orgasms. But in evolutionary terms, the inverse is also true—orgasms produce sex. Climaxing feels so marvelous, we keep coming, literally, back for more sex.

Broadcasting Sperm versus Nurturing Children
Evolution impels us to send our genes into the next generation. But men and women accomplish this differently.

The most efficient route for men involves sex with as many women as possible—inseminating one, then quickly proceeding to the next, ad infinitum. The women themselves hardly matter, just their fertility, just reproduction. Evolution is neither civilized nor polite. It never had its consciousness raised. In evolutionary terms, women are sex objects, reproductive targets with bull's-eyes between their legs. Evolution has scant regard for relationships. In fact, for men, lasting ties to individual women create a reproductive disadvantage. Relationships interfere with pursuit of the next impregnation. If this seems crude and cruel, it is. Species survival isn't necessarily pretty.

The engine of human reproduction is testosterone. It surges during men's adolescence and ignites most men's double-espresso libidos. Hence the adage: *men have only one thing on their mind.* Testosterone focuses the male psyche on procreation.

Testosterone is also the hormone of war, rage, and rape. What if two men want the same woman? Testosterone spurs aggression and the drive to dominate that helps defeat competitors. What if women resist men's advances? The hormone increases muscle mass, making most men bigger and stronger than most women, and better able to overpower them.

Civilization, morality, and women's increasing economic and political power have partly corralled the savage beast in men's evolutionary souls. But many women would say *not much.*

Meanwhile, the best way for women to transmit their genes to the next generation is to bear a limited number of children and nurture them to sexual maturity. Child-rearing isn't easy. It takes time, energy, and resources. Women can raise children alone. But they increase their likelihood of gene transmission by joining forces with men or other women, usually the former. Consequently, beyond procreation, women have evolved an ancillary evolutionary mission—to domesticate barbaric men so they stick around long enough to help raise the kids.

Evolution has wired women to value long-term relationships. Of course, many men do, too, and some women care more about sexual pleasure than mothering. But in evolutionary terms, the stereotype holds true: *Men have relationships to gain sex. Women have sex to gain relationships.*

Most women enjoy lovemaking. But compared with typical men, they are less interested in the bedroom tango. Its possible result, pregnancy, saddles them with tremendous responsibility. Most women choose carefully before allowing men too near.

How Much of the Internet Is Porn?

The Broadway musical *Avenue Q* is a raunchy send-up of *Sesame Street.* One puppet character strikes it rich in online porn and leads the cast in the show's most rollicking number, "The Internet Is for Porn." Is it?

Antiporn groups, among them Internet Safety 101, estimate that as much as 30 percent of internet content is porn. Meanwhile, academic researchers have produced much lower estimates.

Computational neuroscientists Ogi Ogas, PhD, and Sai Gaddam, PhD, coauthors of *A Billion Wicked Thoughts: What the Internet Tells Us about Sex and Relationships,* explain that the proportion of the internet devoted to porn depends on the year. During the early internet (1996–99), the vast majority of users were young adult men. In 1999, 40 percent of web searchers involved porn. But as web demographics expanded to people of all ages, the proportion of internet content devoted to porn fell substantially.

Ogas and Gaddam analyzed the one million most visited websites and found that 42,337 were sex related, about 4 percent. They also tracked searches—porn accounted for 13 percent. Then they interviewed engineers at the major search engines. Their estimate of porn searches: 10–15 percent.

Meanwhile, in addition to oceans of free porn, American men spend an estimated $15 billion a year on sexually explicit websites, more than they spend on tickets to professional baseball, football, and basketball *combined.*

Men's Reproductive Wiring Crystallized: Porn

In addition to directing how the genders act, sex hormones also affect how we think. Evolution impels men to hunt women for sex. Men evolved to be perpetually on the prowl for *pussy*. The word has two meanings. Anatomically, it's the vagina. But when men say they *crave pussy*, they're not talking about the organ, but rather a primal, testosterone-fueled vision of pure sex—wild, ecstatic, nonstop fucking culminating in glorious ejaculations. That, in a nutshell, describes pornography.

In porn, there's only one thing on men's minds. The hardcore action is virtually nonstop. Prong A has a homing instinct for slot B. And there's always a happy ending.

The women's personalities—their lives, hopes, and dreams—are inconsequential. They're nonentities, sexual targets, interchangeable vaginas perpetually eager to be filled. Porn sex is so disembodied that a good deal shows no faces, just writhing flesh from neck to knees.

Compared with women, men tend to become more sexually aroused by visual imagery. When the genders view porn, men's brain scans light up much more. There's no shortage of pornographic prose (*Fanny Hill*, literotica.com, lushstories.com, etc.), but when men say "porn," they usually mean photos and videos with a laser focus on the genitals.

In porn, male acting boils down to two elements, huge erections and ejaculation on cue. Porn actors are hung like bulls. As for porn ejaculations, some shoot semen into vaginas ("creampies"), but quite often, the men unload on the women's faces ("facials"), breasts, bellies, or butts. Extravaginal ejaculations can't cause pregnancies, so why does so much porn feature them? In part, for dramatic climax—in both senses of the term. And in part because porn is unconcerned with fatherhood. It's all about male fantasies of effortless sexual abundance, shooting sperm everywhere, flooding the Earth with semen. One porn subgenre, "bukkake," even features groups of men who stroke over women and cover them in cream.

Some women complain that the gals in porn have such perfect bodies that by comparison, they feel flawed and insecure. Anyone who holds this view hasn't seen much internet porn. Visit any sample-aggregator site (PornHub.com, lobstertube.com, ixxx.com), and you find women of every imaginable legal age, race, ethnicity, weight, hair color, body type, breast and butt size, and pubic presentation: natural ("full bush"), trimmed, partly shaved, and bald. But no matter who the women are or how they look, they can't wait to get down and dirty anywhere and in any way: solo, coupled, threesomes, swinging, sex parties, and gangbangs. *Pussy galore.*

Of course, porn confounds and repulses many women. They call it misogynist, degrading, and assaultive. And through the lens of contemporary women's sensibilities, one can certainly make that case. But porn is fantasy.

When the urge strikes to self-soothe, men board a deeply subconscious runaway train barreling down primeval tracks toward another sticky, billion-year-old evolutionary climax.

Antiporn activists often divide men into two groups: good guys who shun porn and bad guys who get caught in its spiderweb and often become addicts. Actually, that's a false dichotomy. Hardly a man on Earth with internet access hasn't seen porn. University of Montreal researchers wanted to compare sexual attitudes among young adult men who either had or hadn't viewed porn. They couldn't find a single man who hadn't seen it, not one.

For millennia, virtually all men have seen porn:

- The walls of excavated brothels in Pompeii are covered with it, and sexually explicit art has also been uncovered in many of the buried city's homes.

- *The Song of Songs*, a.k.a. *The Song of Solomon* and *Canticles*, was incorporated into Jewish scripture during the second century. It's the only book of the Bible that does not mention God. Instead, it celebrates lovemaking. Some early rabbis denounced it as porn.
- *Memoirs of a Woman of Pleasure* or *Fanny Hill* by John Cleland, the first pornographic novel in English, was published in 1748 and has been continuously in print ever since.
- *Fanny Hill*'s success spurred publishers to release boatloads of pornographic novels and art, cheap books of crude drawings for the masses, and exquisitely detailed erotic art for the wealthy.
- Photography was invented in 1840, and almost immediately, photo porn debuted. It was very popular with soldiers during the Civil War.
- The Lumiere brothers screened the first motion picture in Paris in 1895. Immediately after, filmmakers began producing movie porn.

During the 1980s, I had a male friend who entered a Zen monastery a three-hour drive from anywhere down a barely passable dirt road. Every week, one monk spent all day driving to and from the nearest drugstore to replenish his brethren's toiletries—and buy *Playboy* and *Penthouse*, at the time often castigated as porn. Even monks dedicated to enlightenment feel the need to sand the dowel with help from visual aids.

Men's porn use has nothing to do with their villainy or virtue. Ladies, virtually every man you've ever known has whipped his willy to porn: your grandfathers, fathers, uncles, brothers, boyfriends, husbands, male friends, sons, and grandsons. Evolution has hardwired men's attraction to porn in the deepest, most instinctual recesses of the male soul.

A Snapshot of One of the World's Most Popular Porn Sites

It's PornHub.com. Alexa.com, the web traffic tracker, says that among the world's tens of millions of sites, PornHub ranks thirty-six. If we eliminate search engines (Google), web portals (Yahoo!), and shopping sites (Amazon), then PornHub is in the top ten, close to Wikipedia.

PornHub statistics for 2019:

- 33.5 billion total visitors, 92 million a day
- 30 billion category searches, 962 per second
- The audience: 71 percent men, 29 percent women
- Average age: 36
- PornHub discourages visits by minors, but many visit, claiming to be eighteen or older. Visitors by stated age:
  - 18–24: 26 percent
  - 25–34: 35 percent
  - 35–44: 17 percent
  - 45–54: 11 percent
  - 55–64: 7 percent
  - Over 65: 4 percent
- Average visit duration: ten minutes
- Highest-traffic times: 3:00–5:00 p.m. and 10:00 p.m. to 1:00 a.m.
- Most popular viewing devices:
  - Phones: 72 percent (and rising)
  - Desktop computers: 20 percent (and falling)
  - Tablets: 9 percent (holding steady)

In addition to PornHub, four more of the top 100 sites also present porn: XVideos.com (number 39), BongaCams.com (number 48), xHamster.com (number 76), and XNXX.com (number 91). In 2019, PornHub and these four accounted for more than *seventy-five billion* visits, the equivalent of ten annually for every person on Earth.

How Many Women View Porn? Why?

Using data harvested from Google Analytics, PornHub estimates that women comprised 29 percent of its audience in 2019. Most researchers estimate lower—5–15 percent—but even the lower estimate means that if you know twenty women, one to three view porn with some regularity.

Who are these women? Some are curious or highly sexual. But most watch with lovers, usually before or during sex. A great deal of porn shows men sexually dominating women. Antiporn feminists denounce this, but a surprisingly large proportion of women have submissive BDSM fantasies. Whether or not they actually play that way in real life, many enjoy video depictions of their sub fantasies.

While many women watch porn, few pay for it. According to CCBill, the online payment service used by most commercial porn sites, only 2 percent of payments get charged to credit cards with women's names.

Women's Reproductive Wiring Crystallized: Romance Fiction

Evolution has programmed women to invest their energy in enduring relationships with men who become their partners in child-rearing. But women often experience men as wild, unpredictable, sex-obsessed barbarians who resist domestication. Fortunately, canny women possess the tools to subdue the savage beast: intelligence, perseverance, and erotic charisma. Women deploy their smarts and sex appeal to hook mates, then use their wit, tenacity, and continuing willingness to do the deed to hang on to them. Their goal is to transform men's primordial quest for pussy into a firm commitment to single soul mates. That, in a nutshell, describes romance fiction.

Some commentators call romances "porn for women." Actually, the two are quite different—but complementary (page 369). Both spring from the same billion-year-old evolutionary imperative, species survival. Men's mission is to impregnate every woman on Earth. Women's is to corral Mr. Right and retain him long enough to nurture their children to maturity.

Compared with men, women tend to become less erotically aroused by visual cues. Sure, many if not most want men who look as they're endlessly described in romance fiction: tall, trim, strong, square-jawed, and broad shouldered (with little, if any, mention of penis size). But women also need to assess men for long-term relationship potential. For that, they need more than videos of their genitals. They must discover who their potential partners *truly are*—which requires information. Romance heroines invest a great deal of energy in studying their men, learning all they can about them, their *stories*. It's no coincidence that women tilt away from porn videos toward romances that delve into men's personalities.

Porn has prehistoric roots, but romance fiction dates from the 1740 publication of *Pamela, or Virtue Rewarded* by Samuel Richardson (1689–1761), a British printer. Richardson lived at the dawn of the Industrial Revolution, when the first cheap paperbacks appeared. As hordes of country peasants migrated to England's burgeoning cities to work in its new factories, increasingly literate wage-earning women developed a passion for reading—especially stories about girls like themselves winning rich, powerful men. They turned *Pamela* into the first wildly successful novel. The book became the template for the romance genre.

As *Pamela* begins, its impoverished namesake is maid to Lady B., who quickly dies. Her nasty son, Mr. B., inherits Pamela's services and quickly tries to seduce her. Despite his strength and rank, Pamela resists. Undaunted, Mr. B. stalks her, jumping out of her bedroom closet as she undresses. Still she resists. Pamela considers fleeing home to her parents but hesitates. Is she developing feelings for her crass but wealthy master? Mr. B. softens. He vows not to touch Pamela without her permission. But when she continues to withhold it, he explodes and banishes her to live with the abusive Mrs. Jewkes. Mr. B offers to rescue Pamela if she becomes his mistress, but she refuses. He visits and will not be denied. He forces Pamela into bed. But as he ravishes her, she faints. Mr. B. believes he's killed her and regrets the rape. He caresses Pamela tenderly, reviving her. He proclaims his love and they marry. Now a proper wife, Pamela willingly submits to her husband's sexual demands, and they live happily ever after.

In traditional romance fiction, the protagonist is always a woman. The plot always revolves around the many challenges she overcomes to win her man, who is always taller, stronger, richer, and more powerful. But he falls hard and must have her. She demurs. He often resorts to browbeating, stalking, blackmail, sexual harassment, and rape. She hates his pursuit but puts up with it. Eventually, he realizes he loves her and becomes a better, more sensitive man. Cue wedding bells.

Romance fiction is as popular with women as porn is with men. Romances are by far the bestselling category of fiction. Sales total more than $1 billion a year, accounting for 14 percent of the consumer book market (similar to the percentage of internet searches for porn).

Romances include varying amounts of sex, but even when utterly chaste, as in Jane Austen's *Pride and Prejudice* (1813), sexual tension abounds.

A great deal of romance fiction contains sexual harassment and attempted or completed rape. The heroines hate it but keep their eyes on the prize—domesticating powerful, unpredictable princes, industrialists, rock stars, pro athletes, military commanders, and so forth. The more threatening the man, the more he's inclined toward rape, the greater the heroine's triumph in taming him. His transformation from violent brute to loving husband proves her charm, power, and desirability.

Fast-forward to the 1960s, which produced the Pill and substantial acceptance of premarital sex. That era's social upheavals also added a new level of sexual explicitness—and assault—to romance fiction. In 1972, Kathleen Woodiwiss released *The Flame and the Flower*, the first of the "bodice-ripper" subgenre that quickly became wildly popular: "She felt his hardness searching, probing between her thighs, then entering. A half-gasp, half-shriek escaped her and a burning pain spread through her loins. . . ."

Still in print after more than forty years, *The Flame and the Flower* has sold more than five million copies. But those sales pale next to the *Fifty Shades of Grey* trilogy by E. L. James (2011). During its first eight years in print, it sold 150 million copies worldwide in fifty languages, the first book ever to reach that milestone. James's genius involved combining standard romance conventions with exquisitely detailed descriptions of BDSM, fantasies that excite a substantial proportion of women (and men).

In the real world, no women want to fall victim to sexual coercion. Yet evolution has primed both genders to have fantasies that involve it. Porn depicts a world where women are men's sex toys. Romances present a similar vision in a different guise. The protagonists are always subordinate to their chosen men, who often sexually force them. But eventually, they get what they want, loyal husbands and devoted fathers for their children.

Pornography versus Romance Fiction:
Two Sides of the Same Evolutionary Coin

Porn	Romance Fiction
Activates cues for male arousal.	Activates cues for female arousal.
Unrealistic about men, women, sex, and relationships.	Unrealistic about men, women, sex, and relationships.
Protagonist may be a man or woman.	Protagonist always a woman.
A major presence on the internet: PornHub, XVideos, etc.	A major presence on the internet: RomanceJunkies.com, AllAboutRomance.com, SmartBitchesTrashyBooks.com.
A guilty pleasure for many men.	A guilty pleasure for many women.
75–85 percent of the audience is male, 15–25 percent female.	85 percent of the audience is female, 15 percent male.
A male perspective.	A female perspective.
Minimal, if any, stories.	Elaborate stories.
Many subcategories: mature, Japanese, cars, office, wife swap, etc.	Many subcategories: contemporary, historical, time travel, etc.
May be set in any location or time.	May be set in any location or time.
Relationships minimal or nonexistent.	Forging a lasting relationship is the goal.
Entirely organized around sex, devoid of love and relationships.	Entirely organized around love, but with sexual tension or graphic sex.
Constant explicit sex with interchangeable, often faceless women.	Some sex, largely with Mr. Right.
Sexually experienced men, usually experienced women.	Sexually experienced men, less experienced women.
The women usually lack personalities.	The women are smart, resourceful, and persevering.
Except in some BDSM, the men are dominant, the women subordinate.	Leading men are always dominant, but heroines get their way.
Little sexual violence. Men sometimes force sex on women, who always submit.	Sexual violence is fairly common. Men may force sex on women, who sometimes submit.
All men are studs.	Leading men are studs and good providers.
Some condom use, but contraception and STI prevention largely ignored.	Contraception and STI prevention largely ignored.
The women rarely say "no."	Women initially say "no," but eventually say "yes."
The man ejaculates, the "money shot."	The couple marries and the woman enjoys socioeconomic gains.
The man ejaculates—a happy ending.	The couple marries—and lives happily ever after.
Socially controversial, scorned by many women.	Socially accepted, men voice no objections.

370 Sizzling Sex for Life

A Double Standard?

Women who demonize porn rarely critique romance fiction. Critics deplore porn for rein-forcing sexism. But they remain largely silent on the many ways romance fiction reinforces women's subordination to men. Critics condemn the sexual aggression in a small fraction of porn. But they don't seem bothered by the intimidation, sexual harassment, and rape in much romance fiction.

The real problem with porn is that it models sex and relationships all wrong. The same can be said for romance fiction. Both genres spring from the same primordial source, the evolu-tionary imperative to reproduce. And both are cartoons that revel in gender-specific fantasies.

During my almost fifty years of answering sex questions, many anguished women have despaired about their men's porn viewing. But I've never received a single inquiry from any man wondering about his gal's devotion to romance fiction. Men feel fine about women's erotic fantasies. But many women have major issues with men's.

CHAPTER 48:
How Much of Porn Is Violent? Does Porn Contribute to Sexual Assault?

IT'S A MANTRA among porn critics—88 percent of pornographic videos contain violence against women. This assertion has appeared in dozens of books, magazine articles, and online posts. If it's correct, the vast majority of porn meets the social science definition of violence: "Any behavior directed toward harming or injuring another who wants to avoid it."

One Study, Colossally Flawed

Does 88 percent of porn really depict violence against women? No way. Don't take my word for it. Just browse any site that aggregates porn clips (PornHub, lobstertube.com, ixxx.com). The large majority show lovers who look reasonably happy—at least not visibly unhappy—engaged in nonviolent, almost always consensual romps.

So what's the source of the 88-percent figure? A study by University of Arkansas researchers. And how did they come up with 88 percent? By completely misinterpreting consensual BDSM as violence.

The Arkansas team began with the 250 bestselling or most-rented porn videos in 2005. They randomly selected fifty for content analysis and scrutinized 304 scenes.

They found almost no:
- Kicking: 1 percent
- Verbal threats of violence: 1 percent
- Use of weapons: 1 percent
- Threats with weapons: 0 percent
- Punching: 0 percent
- Torture: 0 percent

However, many scenes contained:
- Spanking: 75 percent
- Gagging: 54 percent
- Verbal insults: 49 percent
- Slapping: 41 percent
- Hair-pulling: 37 percent
- Choking: 28 percent

Bridges, A., et al. "Aggression and Sexual Behavior in Best-Selling Pornography Videos: A Content Analysis Update." *Violence Against Women* 16 (2010): 1065.

371

The researchers called the second list violence against women. Actually, those activities are all hallmarks of completely consensual BDSM.

BDSM is not violent (chapter 44). There's no intent to harm, no wish to escape. Doms and subs engage in carefully scripted erotic theater. They negotiate scenes beforehand, agree on stop signals, and often solemnize their agreements with signed contracts. Doms' task is to take subs to their declared limits of sensation, but no further. Subs' task is to let go and allow the scene to unfold as agreed, secure in the knowledge that doms respect both their limits and their desire for possibly intense sensation.

A San Francisco State University researcher used internet kink sites to survey the practices of 1,580 women BDSM aficionados, age nineteen to seventy-two. They enjoyed:

- Spanking: 96 percent
- Hair-pulling: 93 percent
- Restraint, bondage: 88 percent
- Slapping, paddling, flogging: 84 percent
- Verbal insults: 67 percent

Rehor, J. E. "Sensual, Erotic, and Sexual Behaviors of Women from the 'Kink' Community." *Archives of Sexual Behavior* 44 (2015): 825.

The Arkansas group mistook standard elements of consensual BDSM for violence.

BDSM fantasies are popular. A survey of Canadian college students showed that 62 percent admitted fantasies of restraining a lover, and 65 percent fantasized being tied up. Indiana University researchers surveyed a representative sample of 2,021 American adults and found that many incorporate BDSM into partner sex occasionally or often: spanking (30 percent), dom/sub role-playing (22 percent), restraint (20 percent), and flogging (13 percent).

Commercial porn depicts BDSM because it sells. The Arkansas team selected their scenes from top commercial videos. It should come as no surprise that many included bondage, discipline, and sadomasochism.

If we eliminate the consensual, nonviolent BDSM from the Arkansas analysis, what's left? Actual violence in less than 1 percent of scenes—*hardly any violence at all.*

What's Violence?

In addition to the Arkansas report, five other studies have investigated violence against women in porn:

- Simon Fraser University, British Columbia: Violence in 36 percent of scenes
- Cal State University, San Bernardino: 23 percent
- Illinois Primary Health Care Association, Carbondale: 14 percent
- SUNY Stony Brook: 14 percent
- Queensland University, Australia: 2 percent

None come even close to 88 percent. Meanwhile, their findings vary considerably. Why? They defined *violence* differently.

Consider: a gang of big, tough, aggressive men get right in another man's face and without provocation strike repeated sharp blows to his head and chest. Most people would call that violence—assault. But if the men are football teammates and one has just scored a touchdown, the "assault" actually acknowledges a job well done—not violence, but congratulations. Violence must be judged not only by the action, but also by the context and the participants' intentions.

Of the five studies listed above, four repeated the Arkansas group's error, mistaking consensual BDSM for violence. Only the Queensland researcher, who found violence in just 2 percent of porn scenes, understood BDSM: "I did not count consensual BDSM as 'violence.' In BDSM scenes, consent is clear. BDSM involves no intent to harm and no motivation to avoid. All participants are explicitly willing."

If just 2 percent of porn contains violence against women, then compared with cop shows, action movies, and shoot-'em-up video games, porn contains considerably *less* violence.

Has Porn Become More Violent? Do Viewers Prefer Violent Porn?

Those who demonize porn often call current porn considerably more violent than its twentieth-century counterpart and claim that today's men gravitate toward increasing sexual violence. McGill University researchers analyzed 307 of the most popular videos uploaded to PornHub from 2008 through 2016. They attracted ten million views. During those nine years, there was *no* increase in violent content, and videos containing sexual violence became progressively *less popular*. In 2008, 13 percent of the most popular videos depicted violence against women. By 2016, the proportion had fallen to less than 3 percent.

Porn critics contend that over time, men who watch porn select increasingly violent videos. This analysis showed the opposite. The videos watched most contained only one-third as much violence as PornHub videos watched the least. Violent videos also received substantially fewer "likes." No credible evidence shows that porn viewers gravitate toward violent content. They actually click away from it.

The researchers concluded: "We found no increase over time in the number of videos depicting aggression. We found a downward trend in the number of videos containing nonconsensual aggression and a significant decrease in the average length of scenes containing it. Compared with videos containing no aggression, those with aggressive content were less likely to be viewed and less likely to receive favorable reviews from viewers. Pornography viewers prefer videos showing women's pleasure, not their brutalization."

Corroborating evidence comes from a study based on interviews with men who watch porn frequently. Most said they did not enjoy depictions of violence against women. When they came upon videos depicting violence, they had no wish to imitate it, and clicked away from it.

Is Porn Misogynist?

In 1969, the US Supreme Court ruled that in the privacy of their homes, Americans could view anything they wished, effectively legalizing porn. Appalled conservatives, among them President Richard Nixon, persuaded Congress to establish the Presidential Commission on Obscenity and Pornography, whose members included many social conservatives. The commission's report (1970) found "no evidence that exposure to explicit sexual materials plays a significant role in the causation of delinquent or criminal behavior." The commission recommended repealing all laws restricting access to porn.

During the late 1970s, home videocassette players became the rage, spurring a national explosion of video shops that rented movies—including tons of porn. That era also marked the beginning of the women's liberation movement, whose leaders changed the conversation about sex media. Social and religious conservatives had always condemned porn as immoral. The new antiporn feminists denounced it as misogynist, a violation of women's civil rights, a cause of sexual assault. In *Against Our Will: Men, Women, and Rape* (1980), Susan Brownmiller wrote, "Pornography represents hatred of women." The same year, feminist writer Robin Morgan declared, "Pornography is the theory. Rape is the practice." And feminist Andrea Dworkin called it "Dachau in the bedroom."

Soon after, President Ronald Reagan sponsored another investigation of porn, the Attorney General's Commission on Pornography, a.k.a. the Meese Commission. Its 1986 report called porn harmful. It cited studies showing that the large majority of men convicted of sex crimes have viewed porn—with some watching during their crimes—and that porn makes men more tolerant of violence against women and more willing to administer electric shocks to women.

Sexologists disparaged these findings:

- It's no surprise that rapists have watched porn. Virtually *all men* have, only a small fraction of whom commit sex crimes.
- The studies cited by the Meese Commission substantially overstated "aggression." After boys watch action movies, they engage in a bit more playful roughhousing that may look violent, but really isn't. And after couples watch porn, some men proclaim they're going to "take what's theirs" and then grab their lovers and throw them on the bed, actions both mutually understand as playful. But many of these studies would call the "taking" remark "verbal aggression," and the grabbing/throwing "violence."
- Finally, electric-shock experiments, while disturbing, don't necessarily reflect what happens in the real world.

Meanwhile, the weight of the evidence shows no association between porn and violence against women:

- Using the huge data set of the University of Chicago/National Opinion Research Center's General Social Survey, Canadian scientists investigated men's porn use and gender prejudice. Compared with men who rarely viewed porn, frequent consumers "held more egalitarian attitudes about women."
- Pennsylvania investigators compared porn viewing among sex offenders and men never involved in sex crimes. They found no differences.
- Australian researchers analyzed a dozen studies and concluded, "Our review fails to establish that pornography has any significantly detrimental effect on men's behavior."
- Scientists in Singapore surveyed the sexual histories and porn use of imprisoned rapists and men imprisoned for nonsexual crimes. The two groups viewed the same amount of porn.
- Canadian researchers surveyed 228 male sex offenders and fifty nonoffenders. There were no differences in the types of porn the two groups viewed—and compared with the control men, the sex offenders watched *less*.
- UCLA researchers surveyed recollections of porn use among law-abiding men and convicted rapists and child sex abusers. Throughout their lives, the sex criminals recalled consuming *less* porn.
- Finally, in a huge review, Toronto researchers analyzed ninety-two studies of porn and sexual violence. "There is little support for a causal link between pornography and sexual aggression."

So some studies suggest "more porn, *more* rape," others "more porn, *less* rape." Which is it?

This controversy has been fortuitously—but persuasively—resolved. Since the 1980s, more than two hundred million men around the world have participated in several "natural experiments" on porn and sexual assault. Natural experiments track real-world social changes and what actually happens as they unfold.

More Porn, *Less* Rape

Starting in the late 1990s, the internet became a tool used daily by much of the world's population. Suddenly, millions of porn videos became available for free to anyone with internet access.

If porn critics are correct, if more porn means more rape, then the rate of sexual assault should have started rising in the late 1990s, and it should have continued increasing during this century as the internet became ubiquitous and offered billions of porn pages—for free.

What actually happened? I tip my hat to the Justice Department's National Crime Victimization Survey (NCVS), which social scientists consider the best source of data, more credible than police and FBI statistics. According to the NCVS, since 1995, the US sexual assault rate has *fallen* 58 percent. As porn became more easily available, women's risk of rape fell by half. This finding reflects not some contrived study of a small group of undergraduates, but what actually happened in a nation of 320 million over more than twenty years.

Other natural experiments corroborate the US experience:

- In the 1970s, Denmark relaxed restrictions on pornography and the country quickly became a world center of porn production. Researchers compared arrest rates for sexual assault before and after the change. After porn became more accessible, arrests for rape decreased.
- Around the millennium, Japan, China, and Hong Kong relaxed laws restricting porn. Subsequently, in all three, sex crimes decreased.
- From 1948 to 1989, Czechoslovakia was a police state that punished possession of pornography with prison. Consequently, little was available. But in 1989, when the democratic Czech Republic emerged, porn was legalized and Czech men became enthusiastic consumers. Comparing sexual assault rates there during the decades before and after porn legalization, rapes decreased 38 percent and child sex abuse reports dropped 50 percent.

The porn bashers are mistaken. Porn doesn't incite men to sexual violence. The activity it provokes is masturbation. Porn appears to be a safety valve that gives men an alternative outlet for potentially assaultive sexual energy. Instead of attacking women, many potential assailants stay home and stroke to porn. Allegations that porn incites sexual assault are nonsense.

Porn, Alcohol, and Sexual Violence

Some rape victims recall assailants viewing porn before or during their attacks. The rapists usually indulged in something else as well—alcohol. University of Washington researchers showed porn to a large group of men, some of whom had consumed a few drinks. The nondrinkers showed no approval of or propensity toward violence against women. But many of the drinkers did. Compared with porn viewing, men's use of alcohol is much more predictive of sexual violence.

Successful Rape-Prevention Programs Do Not Discourage Porn

Many colleges and the US Navy have instituted rape-prevention programs that have reduced sexual assaults by 50–67 percent. These efforts involve:

- **Blunt talk.** Officials frequently and forcefully affirm that the institution has zero tolerance for sexual violence. They explain that most rapes are committed not by strangers, but by friends or acquaintances. For the women, they vividly describe the trauma of rape. For the men, they provide equally graphic descriptions of prison.
- **Designated party monitors.** Mix young adult partying and alcohol, and rape risk soars. Officials insist that friends appoint designated monitors who pledge to stay sober and intervene if things get out of hand.
- **Bystander intervention.** In addition to monitors, officials demand that *everyone* tune into situations that might lead to assaults and intervene to prevent them. *If you see something, do something.*

These programs don't mention porn. Yet they've quickly and consistently reduced rape rates by half to two-thirds.

CHAPTER 49:
Porn's Impact on Adolescents

MANY PARENTS HAVE trouble discussing sex with their children, and even the most comprehensive school sex-education programs have no measurable impact on teen sex. Meanwhile, porn is just a few taps/clicks away from teens and many view it regularly. This worries porn critics to no end.

Critics' Contentions Refuted

Detractors contend that preteens and teens experience unwanted exposure to porn. They insist that it sexualizes young people too early, ruins them for long-term relationships, and pushes young men toward sexism and sexual violence.

The best research rebuts all these assertions:

- Early teens age twelve to fourteen generally feel disgusted by sexually explicit media and quickly turn away from it.
- Even when they don't, unwanted exposure to porn doesn't cause harm any more than unwanted exposure to cooking shows causes obesity.
- Porn doesn't sexualize young people "too early." Most kids engage in childhood sex play years before they encounter porn. Of course, child sex play differs from hardcore action, but few children are completely sexually naive until they see porn.
- There's no evidence that porn ruins young people for long-term relationships. According to the National Center for Family and Marriage Research, the divorce rate peaked in 1980, long before internet porn became available. Since then it has steadily declined. In 2015, a generation after porn flooded the internet, the divorce rate fell to a *forty-year low*.
- There is an association between early porn viewing and early virginity loss. Porn critics say the former causes the latter. Not necessarily. Starting in childhood, some people are innately more sexual than others. Intrinsic sexual precociousness may instigate *both* porn viewing and early sexual initiation. Before internet porn, the most typical age for first intercourse was around seventeen. Since porn flooded the internet, that hasn't changed. In fact, compared to teens before the internet, today's adolescents are *less* sexually active (below).

More Reasons to Feel Reassured

Many studies show that adolescent porn exposure is no cause for alarm.

- A Texas Tech researcher surveyed 131 college men about their porn consumption and attitudes toward women. As their self-reported porn viewing increased, their sexism *decreased.*

- Scientists at the University of Zagreb, Croatia, surveyed 650 young adult men about their age at first porn exposure and their subsequent sexuality. "Early exposure had no effect."
- Another team of University of Zagreb researchers surveyed 1,005 young adult men about porn exposure and sexual irresponsibility. "Pornography use is not associated with sexual risk-taking."
- Swiss investigators surveyed 3,283 teen boys. "Pornography exposure, either willing or unwilling, is not associated with risky sexual behavior."
- Danish and Swedish studies show that while most teens turn to porn for information about the mechanics of sex, at the same time, they realize it's a cartoon—not a how-to manual, but fantasy.
- UCLA investigators asked pedophile and nonpedophile adolescents about their porn consumption. Compared with other teens, the sex offenders viewed "significantly less porn."

Since the Arrival of Internet Porn, Teens Have Become More Sexually Responsible

When research findings are contradictory, it's instructive to look beyond academia and explore what really happens out in the world. Actual teen behavior shows the porn bashers are mistaken. Porn has not unhinged adolescents.

If porn spurred teen sexual irresponsibility, then since the late 1990s when porn exploded on the internet, teens should have become more sexually active, and the teen birth rate should have risen. Neither happened. Both declined.

A team led by San Diego State University researchers surveyed 26,707 Americans, some born in the 1960s and '70s, who came of age before internet porn, and others born in the '80s and '90s, who grew up in a world glutted with it. The latter reported *less* partner sex.

In addition, according to the National Center for Health Statistics, the teen birth rate peaked in 1991, years before internet porn. Since then, it has *fallen* 70 percent.

The CDC's annual Youth Risk Behavior Survey corroborates these findings:

Sexual intercourse, ever
1997—the dawn of internet porn: 48%
2015—billions of free internet porn pages: 41%
Change: -7%

Sexual intercourse, previous three months
1997: 35%
2015: 30%
Change: -5%

Condom use, most recent intercourse
1997: 57%
2015: 57%
Change: none

Birth control pills prior to most recent intercourse
1997: 17%
2015: 18%
Change: +1%

Alcohol or other recreational drug use immediately prior to most recent intercourse
1997: 25%
2015: 21%
Change: -4%

Teens raped
2001: 8%
2015: 7%
Change: -1%

With porn just a tap away on phones, teens report less intercourse, less sexual assault, less alcohol use before sex, and no less use of contraception.

Teens have also become more responsible in other ways:

Seat belts
Always or almost always used them (previous year)
1997: 81%
2015: 94%
Change: +13%

Bicycle helmets
Always or almost always used them (previous year)
1997: 12%
2015: 19%
Change: +7%

Passenger of driver impaired by alcohol (previous month)
1997: 37%
2015: 20%
Change: -17%

Drove shortly after drinking alcohol (previous month)
1997: 17%
2015: 8%
Change: -9%

Carried a weapon (previous month)
1997: 18%
2015: 16%
Change -2%

Gotten into a fight (previous year)
1997: 37%
2015: 23%
Change: -14%

Considered suicide (previous year)
1997: 21%
2015: 18%
Change: -3%

Smoked cigarettes (previous month)
1997: 36%
2015: 11%
Change: -25%

Drank alcohol (previous month)
1997: 51%
2015: 33%
Change: -18%

Used marijuana (previous month)
1997: 26%
2015: 22%
Change: -4%

Despite the unprecedented availability of porn, the large majority of teens are doing fine—in fact, better than their pre-internet counterparts a generation ago. While some studies raise questions, real-world evidence shows that adolescents have not been perverted by porn.

Teaching Teens "Porn Literacy"

University of Pennsylvania investigators analyzed eighty-nine studies of porn's impact on teens. They found no social harm, and just one significant downside—"unrealistic sexual beliefs." As I argue in chapter 46, porn teaches sex all wrong, which increases risk of sexual disappointment for both men and women—not sexual violence or other social ills, but trouble between the sheets.

In 2016, a Boston University researcher surveyed students at a Massachusetts high school. Forty-five percent agreed that *porn offers a good way to learn about sex*. Then the researcher presented a ten-hour "Porn Literacy" curriculum. Its message: *Porn is unrealistic. Don't imitate it.* After the class, the proportion who still agreed that porn provides good sex education fell by more than half to just 18 percent.

This success is heartening, but it refutes chapter 15, where I argue that school sex education has no significant impact on teens. Contradiction? No. Studies of adolescent sexuality measure either attitudes or actions. Plenty of studies, including the test of the Porn Literacy curriculum, show that school can change teens' attitudes, at least in the short term. Where sex education fails is in the realm of actions, what teens actually do.

Sex education that actually impacts teens' actions usually comes from parents. If you're a parent anxious about porn's impact on your preteen and teenaged children, discuss your concerns with your kids. Ask what they've seen and how they feel about it. Don't forbid watching. Porn is just a tap away on any phone, and kids make their own media decisions. Instead, tell them how you feel. Speak from the heart. Remember, porn doesn't cause early sexualization, sexism, sexual irresponsibility, shunning of contraception, or violence against women, nor does it interfere with teens' ability to develop relationships. It has only two results—masturbation, which is normal and healthy, and unrealistic expectations about lovemaking, which you can discuss with them and help correct.

Parents who'd like help with these conversations can use the free resources provided by the Porn Conversation (ThePornConversation.org). I also recommend two other sites focused on teens: GoAskAlice.columbia.edu and Scarleteen.com.

Does Discussing Porn with Adolescents Encourage Them to View It?

If a friend touts a new restaurant, you might try it. Similarly, some parents believe that mentioning porn to adolescents encourages them to view it. Two studies have explored this issue:

- Croatian scientists asked 1,053 high school students if they watched porn. Six months later they asked again. Participants reported no significant increase in viewing.
- Using a similar approach, Dutch investigators surveyed 123 teens. "Questions about viewing pornography did not stimulate that behavior."

CHAPTER 50:
The Three Differences between Women Porn Actors and Other Women

M ANY CRITICS CONSIDER porn so abhorrent they can't imagine mentally healthy women willingly performing for its cameras. They assume the women actors must be victims of childhood traumatic sex abuse that made them easy prey for evil pornographers.

However, the only published survey of female porn actors' mental health paints a very different picture. Turns out they're remarkably similar to other women—with a few differences porn critics never mention.

Child Sex Abuse? Rape?
Several women porn actors have gone public with terrible memories of sexual trauma:

- Jenna Jameson: "As a young woman, I was gang-raped."
- Shelley Lubben: "Many girls in porn have been sexually abused."
- Traci Lords: "When I was ten, I was raped by a boy of sixteen. After that, my mother's boyfriend molested me. My entire childhood was shaped by sexual trauma that led me to porn."

These stories are chilling—but anecdotal. Other anecdotes differ. I've interviewed several women porn actors who swore they'd never suffered sexual trauma, including some who described happy childhoods in functional, loving, two-parent, middle-class families.

Do porn actresses really have disproportionate histories of sexual abuse? Until recently, that question could not be answered. Porn producers don't welcome researchers to shoots, so the women couldn't be interviewed at work. Off camera, women porn actors have proved equally elusive. Most are young and transient. Their video careers are usually part time and brief. They remain largely under the radar beyond researchers' reach.

"No Evidence of Disproportionate Sexual Abuse"
Sharon Mitchell (1956–) was a dancer and off-Broadway actor who debuted in porn in the mid-1970s. Unlike most women in porn, she made a career of it, appearing in more than six hundred films and eventually directing twenty-nine. In 1996, she quit and earned a PhD in sexology from the Institute for the Advanced Study of Human Sexuality in San Francisco.

During Mitchell's porn career, she contracted several sexual infections. She decided to help other performers avoid them. In 1998 in Los Angeles, she founded the Adult Industry Medical

Healthcare Foundation (AIMHF), an STI clinic focused on porn actors. By 2004, the clinic was administering 1,200 tests a month, and Mitchell was lauded as a public health pioneer. But in 2011, a security breach led to the release of personal information for about twelve thousand performers. Several sued, forcing the AIMHF to close.

Los Angeles County requires porn performers to be tested monthly for STIs and requires producers to employ only those whose most recent test was negative. For a dozen years, AIMHF was the go-to test site. Most porn actors visited regularly.

Mitchell was all too familiar with the stereotype that the women in porn are drug-addicted victims of sex abuse. She also knew there had never been a scientific survey of women porn actors. Assisted by psychologists at Texas Women's University, she launched one.

It wasn't easy, but Mitchell and her staff, including several other former women porn performers, eventually persuaded 177 female actors, average age twenty-six, to discuss their lives. The researchers also administered their questionnaire to 177 demographically similar women (matched controls).

Mitchell used a "convenience sample," women porn actors who visited her clinic and agreed to participate. Consequently, her study was less rigorous than surveys using representative samples. However, many studies use convenience samples, notably the enormous number that survey college undergraduates. The psychology journals would be mighty thin without them. While this study's sample is not ideal, it's well within the bounds of credible research.

The survey asked about childhood sexual abuse: "One of the most common stereotypes regarding pornography actresses is that they are victims of child sex abuse (CSA). We found no differences in reported history of CSA between the actresses and controls. Further, both groups reported CSA within the range found in other surveys of the general population. We found no evidence that porn actresses suffer more CSA than other women."

Three Differences

If porn actresses haven't suffered sexual trauma, why do they appear in porn? Top reasons included flexible hours, the glamor of movie work, and higher pay than they could otherwise earn.

The survey also explored the women's mental health. Compared with controls, three differences emerged: (1) The porn actors were more thrill-seeking. (2) They enjoyed sex more. (3) They reported significantly greater sexual satisfaction.

Some people are innately more sexual than others. A University of Chicago study shows that 6 percent of adult women are highly sexual, reporting partner sex four or more times a week. The US adult female population numbers 130 million. The highly sexual 6 percent comes to almost 8 million, way more than enough to populate porn.

However, many highly sexual women are not exhibitionists. How many women enjoy cavorting under lights in front of film crews? Quite a few.

Swedish researchers surveyed 2,450 Swedes, age eighteen to sixty. Women who reported exhibitionism (flashing genitals to strangers)—2.1 percent. If American and Swedish women are equally inclined toward exhibitionism, a good bet, then more than 2 million adult American women are open to it. Of course, momentary flashing differs from hours of hardcore action on camera. But if only 10 percent of exhibitionistic American women are open to appearing in porn, they would number some two hundred thousand, many times the number who act in porn.

Married American women number around 100 million. Sexologists generally estimate that 3 percent of married adults have visited swing clubs where they swap partners and play in groups. Many studies estimate higher, but if just 3 percent visit swing/sex clubs, that's three million women, way more than the porn industry employs.

In addition to flaunting their bodies, the survey revealed women porn actors to be sexual thrill-seekers:

- **Enjoyment.** Among control women, 33 percent said they enjoyed sex "very much"; among the porn performers, 69 percent. Corroborating evidence comes from a University of Miami, Florida, survey of 147 women adult entertainers. Compared with other women, they reported less likelihood of sex problems.
- **Precocious.** Currently, women's average age at first intercourse is seventeen. Among the performers, it was sixteen.
- **Bisexual.** Among controls, 7 percent claimed bisexuality; the performers, 67 percent.
- **More lovers.** During the year before being surveyed, the control women reported an average of 1.5 lovers. The performers reported 9.6 nonwork partners—often including multiple women.
- **Lovers' sexual experience.** In the control group, only 6 percent felt fine with mates who admitted ten or more previous lovers; the performers, 42 percent.
- **More drugs.** Compared with controls, the performers reported lifetime histories of using more alcohol, marijuana, tranquilizers, hallucinogens, ecstasy, cocaine, and amphetamines. But during the six months prior to the survey, they said they'd used only one drug significantly more frequently than controls; marijuana.

Psychologically Healthier

Even if women porn actors suffer no more sexual trauma than other women, their sexual exuberance and drug histories raise questions about their psychological health.

The researchers assessed this and found that compared with controls, the performers actually enjoyed *better* mental health. They reported greater self-esteem, more positive feelings about their lives, and more social support. The researchers concluded, "Performers are not psychologically impaired and appear more similar to other women than previously thought."

Of course, no single study is definitive. But this survey presents the only credible research to date. It shows that women porn actors are remarkably similar to other women—except they're greater thrill-seekers who like sex more and enjoy greater sexual satisfaction.

384 Sizzling Sex for Life

How *Not* to Appear in Porn

Guy meets gal. They click and join pelvises. Then he asks her to pose nude or have a go on video. She hesitates. He coaxes. She consents. Then they break up. If he's an ass or feels angry or betrayed, he might post those images without her consent on one of the many revenge-porn or ex-girlfriend sites. Or he might resort to "sextortion," threatening to post the videos if she doesn't provide sex or money.

Initially the term was *revenge* porn, but that's fading. The motive may not always be revenge. The more accurate label is *nonconsensual* porn.

As nonconsensual porn became an issue, an unlikely coalition of aggrieved women and porn producers fought it. The former include Holly Jacobs, whose videos were posted without her consent. She launched the Cyber Civil Rights Initiative to help victims lobby for protective legislation (CyberCivilRights.org).

Meanwhile, porn producers say nonconsensual porn is bad for their public relations. They insist on legal age and signed consent forms, but porn bashers charge that much commercial porn is nonconsensual. Producers want to stamp out nonconsensual porn to protect their reputations (and reduce competition).

As of 2019, forty-one states and the District of Columbia have criminalized internet posting of sexual images without models' written consent. Prosecutors around the country have forced several nonconsensual porn sites to shut down. Some of their owners have been imprisoned.

To avoid appearing in nonconsensual porn, either flatly refuse, or say, *I'd love to play on camera—on our tenth wedding anniversary.*

Nonconsensual porn usually involves new relationships. Initially, lovers have little basis to trust each other's discretion. If relationships unravel, despicable exes may post what you thought would remain forever private. But over time, long-term partners develop greater trust, and nonconsensual porn becomes less of a risk.

If he objects to waiting until your tenth anniversary, don't budge.

If he asks you to send him risqué images on Snapchat, saying he'll see them only briefly before they disappear forever, understand that there are many ways to preserve those images.

If he threatens to dump you over your refusal, you're better off without him.

Unfortunately, even those who have never disrobed for the camera might wind up in nonconsensual porn. It's possible to electronically graft one face onto another's body, for example, a porn performer's ("deep fakes"). At this writing, it takes considerable computer power and advanced tech skills to produce convincing deep fakes. But in the future, who knows?

CHAPTER 51:
Men, Porn, and the Controversy Surrounding "Sex Addiction"

EVEN BEFORE THE internet, most men saw pornography, during the twentieth century, in books, magazines, peep shows, and porn theaters. In 1964, US Supreme Court Justice Potter Stewart said he knew porn when he saw it. His statement implied he was fairly familiar with it. Of course he was. He was a man.

Today virtually every internet-connected adult man on Earth has seen porn. A University of Montreal researcher tried to find men who'd never seen any—and failed.

A huge number of websites present porn. Alexa.com, which analyzes web traffic, documents that in 2019, six of the world's top 100 sites featured it: PornHub.com (number 27), LiveJasmin.com (42), XVideos (46), xHamster (58), BongaCams (75), and XNXX (98). PornHub alone attracts 33.5 billion views a year. Add the five other top sites, and views likely total more than 70 billion. Add all the views the thousands of other porn sites attract, and total worldwide porn consumption probably tops 100 billion a year. Men account for around 70 percent of porn viewing—they log some 70 billion views a year. Of the world's population of 7.5 billion, some 4.4 billion are internet users, and around half of them are men, 2.2 billion. That works out to an average of thirty-two views a year for every internet-connected man on Earth, almost three a month, one porn session every ten days or so.

A University of Texas study agrees that men flock to internet porn. Using nationally representative survey data, it showed that almost half of US men age eighteen to thirty-nine (46 percent) intentionally view porn in any given week (as do 16 percent of women).

Some men view porn with their lovers, but the vast majority consume it solo for just one reason—to enhance the pleasure of masturbation. Shortly after men come, they click away—until the next time they feel that itch. Like Justice Stewart, the overwhelming majority of porn-watching men are functional, productive, and loving, not deviant, misogynist, or addicted.

Nature's One-Hand Tranquilizer

Most men masturbate substantially more than most women. University of Chicago researchers interviewed 3,159 men and women age eighteen to fifty-nine. The men stroked three times more often.

Why? Usually to relieve tension. Researchers at Dennison University in Ohio asked 249 young adults why they self-sexed. Among the women, 25 percent cited stress relief, the men 80 percent. Studies in Germany and at the University of California, San Francisco, corroborate this gender difference. They show that in women, sex has little impact on the stress hormone cortisol. But in men, sex significantly reduces cortisol levels. Men who feel tense look to sex for relief, and if partner sex is unavailable, they stroke solo.

Men joke about masturbation more than they seriously discuss it. But over the decades, I've been amazed how many men have spontaneously told me: *I've tugged so hard for so long, it's a miracle the thing's still attached.*

Why do men feel so driven to self-soothe? It's largely the result of testosterone, the hormone of irritability. In addition, testosterone grabs men by the balls and screams *Sex, SEX, SEX!* If they can play with lovers, they usually do. If not, they manage with two eyes on a screen and one hand between their legs.

Many women can relate. Currently, more than half of adult US women own vibrators. Some use them in partner play, but most—tens of millions—use their vibes exclusively for solo sex. For a decade, I worked with a sex toy marketer. The company's bestselling product by far: vibrators, in dozens of models.

Unless masturbation interferes with life responsibilities or partner lovemaking, there's nothing wrong with it, however frequently, even daily or more. If you feel distraught about sex with yourself, it's difficult to enjoy lovemaking with anyone else.

Unfortunately, many women can't comprehend men's eagerness to tickle the pickle. They don't appreciate how testosterone supercharges most men's libidos. Women who become transgender men express astonishment at how often they think about sex and feel driven to do something about it, usually solo.

Men use masturbation as Nature's tranquilizer. Life is a bitch. Things change so quickly. Change causes anxiety, which has become epidemic. In recent surveys, one-third of Americans say they feel chronically stressed.

When tense, the genders self-soothe differently. Many women masturbate, but estrogen also encourages them to converse with friends. Men also turn to friends, but testosterone pushes them into their "man caves"—the basement, garage, or bathroom—to jerk off. Before the internet, many boys discovered their first porn rummaging through their fathers' workbenches.

Screen Time: What's the Difference?

According to Nielsen, the media-tracking company, in 2016, the average American watched television (broadcast, cable, and streaming) thirty-five hours a week—almost the equivalent of full-time employment. Some viewers call themselves TV addicts, and websites offer tips for breaking the habit. But television provokes no outrage, no accusations of rending the social fabric.

NFL football games typically last three hours. During football season, many men spend Sunday afternoons and Sunday, Monday, and Thursday nights watching. If fans view two games on Sundays and all three night games, they watch fifteen hours a week. Many women call themselves "football widows," and websites offer support. But televised football prompts little hand-wringing.

Meanwhile, the University of Montreal study (above) shows that men typically watch porn for just five to seventeen minutes a day, and PornHub statistics show that only 1 percent watch an hour or more at a sitting—a small fraction of the time many men spend watching TV shows or televised football.

What's the difference between watching porn and other programming? Porn is explicitly sexual, and while watching, men self-sex, which some women consider appalling and the sex addiction industry calls pathological.

Meanwhile, whether single or coupled, masturbation is normal, natural, healthy, and the foundation of enjoyable partner lovemaking.

Men and Porn: Two Key Questions

When women discover that their men watch porn, some feel devastated and accuse them of "sex addiction." We owe the term to Patrick Carnes, PhD, and his 1983 book, *Out of the Shadows: Understanding Sexual Addiction*. It launched a cottage industry that now includes many books by Carnes and others; twelve-step groups (e.g., Sexaholics Anonymous); a research journal, *Sexual Addiction and Compulsivity* (founded by Carnes and colleagues); sex-addiction therapists (most credentialed by an organization founded by Carnes); and residential treatment centers (including Carnes's Gentle Path at the Meadows in Wickenberg, Arizona).

Supporters of the sex addiction paradigm say the affliction includes obsessive sexual thoughts, public flashing, serial one-nighters, extramarital affairs, group sex, and visits to sex workers. But today, with porn just a tap away on phones, the number one symptom of alleged male sex addiction is frequent masturbation to internet pornography.

Sex/porn addiction is controversial. But those who consider it a plague have scored one resounding victory. Since the millennium, the idea has become firmly rooted in popular culture.

Those distressed by sex addiction consider it as potentially disastrous as drug abuse. They tell heartrending tales of victims—overwhelmingly men—destroyed by out-of-control sex. They're quick to call it epidemic and link it to what Carnes calls the "deep undercurrent of sexual trauma in our culture": divorce, child sex abuse, teen promiscuity, contraceptive irresponsibility, and sexual assault. They contend that male porn addicts shirk their responsibilities and feel devastated by guilt, shame, social isolation, libido loss, and erectile dysfunction.

All of which raises two questions: How many men's sexuality/porn use is actually out of control? And does porn really cause social harm?

Out-of-Control Sexuality: How Big a Problem?

Most people would agree that heterosexual married couples who enjoy vaginal intercourse behind closed bedroom doors twice a month have their sexuality under control. Most would also agree that men repeatedly arrested for public masturbation while viewing porn on their phones on buses are out of control. But in between lies a vast realm of sexuality some might call problematic, while others insist it is normal and fine.

Porn critics allege that many men watch compulsively for hours on end. From Carnes's book, *In the Shadows of the Net: Breaking Free of Compulsive Online Sexual Behavior*: "The complaining partner is less and less a part of the using partner's life because the latter spends so much time on the Net." And in *The Porn Trap: Overcoming Problems Caused by Pornography*, Oregon psychotherapists Wendy and Larry Maltz argue that many porn viewers watch "for hours on a regular basis."

Actually, the overwhelming majority of men watch briefly. Here are Google Analytics data for PornHub, one of the world's largest porn sites:

Time spent on PornHub (2018) per visit	Site traffic share
0–5 minutes	52 percent
5–10 minutes	18 percent
10–20 minutes	16 percent
20–30 minutes	6 percent
30–60 minutes	5 percent
1–2 hours	1 percent
More than 2 hours	0.2 percent

PornHub figures.

Only one man in 100 watches for more than an hour at a time and only two per thousand stay longer than two hours. Most spend less than five minutes, 70 percent less than ten. Where's the social crisis?

A University of Montreal researcher surveyed men's viewing. Single guys averaged forty minutes three times a week (two hours total), married men 1.7 times a week for twenty minutes (thirty-four minutes total). That's five to seventeen minutes a day—and no threat to civilization.

New Zealand researchers surveyed 940 Kiwi adults. Thirteen percent of the men and 7 percent of the women said that sometime during the previous year, they'd *felt* sexually out of control. Why? Because of their sexual thoughts and fantasies. Apparently, they were unaware that erotic reveries—even if disturbing—are normal, healthy, and a key ingredient of sizzling sex.

There are no thought crimes. Erotic musings are not a social problem. The issue is sexual *actions*. Among the New Zealanders, fewer than 1 percent said they'd acted sexually out of control, that is, in life-disrupting ways—0.8 percent of the men, 0.6 percent of the women. Very few.

Only a tiny proportion of men disappear into a black hole of porn, a much smaller fraction than the sex addiction industry contends. Meanwhile, 99.8 percent of men tune in for a quick wank, then proceed with their productive, loving, mentally healthy lives.

However, if more than two hours of porn at a sitting signifies being out of control, and if 0.2 percent of US adult men do that, we have some 240,000 men who might have porn problems. Those plagued by sexual compulsivity—and their partners—suffer anguish, deserve sympathy, and need professional help (page 403). But they represent only a minute proportion of the population. The vast majority of men watch porn briefly and handle it just fine.

Problems Affecting Adult Men

Premature ejaculation	25–30 percent	Laumann, E. O. "Sexual Dysfunction in the United States." *Journal of the American Medical Association* 281 (1999): 537. The National Institute on Alcohol Abuse and Alcoholism. National Institute on Drug Abuse.
Alcoholism	7 percent	
Compulsive gambling	2 percent	
Heroin use	0.4 percent	
Out-of-control porn watching	0.2 percent	

Does Porn Cause Social Harm?

In chapters 48–50, I refute the allegations that porn recruits sexually abused women and contributes to violence, sexual assault, and teen sexual irresponsibility. In addition, critics charge that porn also causes:

Sexism. Porn critics allege it encourages objectification of women. Canadian researchers analyzed data from 25,646 adults (11,658 men and 13,988 women) from the General Social Survey, the largest ongoing study of Americans' attitudes and behavior. The findings spanned forty-one years, 1975–2016. Compared with respondents who shunned porn, those who viewed it expressed *more egalitarian* attitudes toward women.

The porn-related shift away from sexism was most evident among religious conservatives who believe women's place is in the home. Compared with religious conservatives who said they avoided porn, those who admitted watching expressed significantly more gender-egalitarian views.

Childhood sex abuse. Figures from the National Child Abuse and Neglect Data System show that from 1975 through 1990, childhood sex abuse steadily increased to twenty-three children per ten thousand population. But after 1990, it began declining, and by 2004, after porn flooded the internet, the rate had fallen by half to 11 per ten thousand.

Contraceptive irresponsibility. Critics contend that porn frays men's commitment to birth control. An Australian review of seventeen studies suggests this might be true. As men's porn consumption increased, they expressed less interest in contraception.

But if porn discourages birth control, abortions and adoptions should have increased since the late 1990s. Actually, both have declined. The abortion rate peaked in 1980, long before internet porn, and has fallen ever since. By 2014, it had dropped 48 percent. Adoptions have also declined from 65 per 100,000 US adults in 2001 to 49 per 100,000 in 2012. Porn-watching men may say they're less interested in contraception, but there's no evidence they're actually less involved in birth control.

Time with partners and families. Critics charge that porn seduces men away from loved ones. PornHub statistics show that's possible but rare. Plenty of people's jobs, work hours, and commute times interfere with partner and family availability. Do they have a mental disorder?

Infidelity. Porn haters assert it spurs adultery. Some research supports this. Using the authoritative General Social Survey, Indiana University investigators found that as men's porn consumption increased, so did their admissions of affairs and paying for sex.

However, this association is not proof of cause and effect. It's equally possible that other factors explain the link, for example, libido. As men's desire increases, so does their porn use *and* their willingness to step out. Sexual frankness may also explain the porn-infidelity link. Men who admit viewing porn may also be more forthcoming about affairs and commercial sex. No compelling evidence shows that porn *causes* infidelity. When men wank to porn, they're not chasing other women.

Anxiety, depression, substance abuse. Supporters of the addiction model assert that porn represents the slippery slope to mental illness. Several studies show that sex labeled "compulsive" is, indeed, associated with mood disorders and drug abuse. But again, this association is no demonstration of cause and effect.

Consider homosexuality. During the twentieth century, hundreds of studies linked being LGBTQ to anxiety, drug abuse, and psychiatric problems including suicide. Gay bashers insisted that homosexuality *caused* these problems. They developed "treatment" programs to convert LGBTQ folks back to the one true path, heterosexuality. Today we know that most LGBTQ mental health problems were caused not by disordered sexuality, but by being stigmatized—fired from jobs, shunned by family, assaulted, imprisoned, and sometimes murdered. Relentless bigotry can drive anyone crazy.

Now that Americans increasingly view orientations other than exclusively heterosexual as variations on normal, the LGBTQ population's mental health is approaching that of straight Americans. And many states have outlawed "conversion therapy."

The situation with sex addiction is similar. It usually has less to do with stroking and humping than with the anxiety, guilt, and shame many men and some women feel as a result of upbringings that condemned recreational sex.

Divorce. *The Porn Trap* claims that men's viewing contributes to many divorces. Any activity that becomes a chronic irritant may contribute to divorce—drinking, gambling, porn, whatever. But is porn a marriage killer?

The US divorce rate peaked in 1980. Since then, it has steadily fallen. Internet porn has not slowed the decline. By 2010, with porn ubiquitous, the divorce rate had fallen 40 percent from its peak. Porn may contribute to some divorces, but as internet porn has become ever-present, American couples have become substantially *less* likely to split up.

Loss of close relationships. *The Porn Trap* argues that men who view porn have difficulty maintaining intimate relationships. Many studies contradict this:

- English investigators assessed 164 men's social connections and porn use. "Regarding emotional closeness with partners, parents, and friends, we found no differences based on self-reported porn use." In fact, the men who viewed the most porn reported the closest social ties, "a craving for intimacy," not an escape from it.
- Idaho State University scientists showed erotic videos to forty-four heterosexual couples. The videos "increased men's desire to be close to their partners."
- The typical married man views porn about thirty minutes a week, and 99 percent watch for less than an hour at a time. That leaves plenty of time for close relationships.

Libido loss. *The Porn Trap* claims that porn strips men of desire for real partners. UCLA researchers surveyed the porn habits of 280 men. As their viewing increased, so did their desire for sex—both solo *and* partnered. Far from destroying libido, porn often spurs it.

Erectile dysfunction, orgasm difficulties. A few studies contend that internet porn has caused an epidemic of sex problems, particularly in young adult men. There's no question that porn miseducates men about sex or that porn-style sex contributes to sex problems. But men have been sexually miseducated for centuries. The internet has made porn more available, but there's been no *qualitative* change in men's sexual miseducation. When men develop porn-related erection difficulties, they're usually caused either by stroking before their postorgasm refractory periods have ended, or by the stress engendered by fundamentalist, sex-negative upbringings. Researchers at Bowling Green State University surveyed porn use and ED among 1,498 men. They found "no evidence of any causal link between pornography viewing and ED."

How Much Is "Too Much"?

In *Don't Call It Love: Recovery from Sexual Addiction*, Patrick Carnes notes that sex addiction involves sexual excess: "For days on end, sex addicts may spend most of their time in sexual stupors."

Carnes never quantifies "excessive," but Martin Kafka, MD, a Massachusetts psychiatrist, asserts that "hypersexual desire" may be indicated by "seven or more orgasms a week for at least six consecutive months after age fifteen." However, he acknowledges that this frequency constitutes a mental disorder only with significant personal distress and distraction from important responsibilities.

This sounds reasonable—until you get specific. Consider couples newly fallen in love. They often rock 'n' roll daily for at least six consecutive months, and while absorbed in each other may shirk important responsibilities and as a result, suffer distress. When they have tiffs, their disagreements may interfere with their jobs and social lives. Are they sex addicts?

Sexual Healing:
The Many Benefits of Solo and Partner Lovemaking

Beyond procreation, the sex addiction industry claims that sex offers one other bene-fit—marriage enhancement. That's true. Several studies show that compared with cou-ples who do it rarely, those who make love two to four times a month report happier, more stable marriages.

But those in a tizzy about sex addiction rarely mention the many other benefits of regular—even frequent—masturbation and partner sex:

- **Relaxation.** Orgasm is deeply relaxing. Deep relaxation helps treat many poten-tially serious conditions: anxiety, depression, high blood pressure, and heart dis-ease. Regular sex offers similar benefits. This is particularly true for men, who are more likely than women to use sex to manage stress.
- **Pain relief.** Sex reduces pain in two ways. It's distracting. While getting it on, people focus less on their suffering. In addition, sex is exercise. It releases endorphins, the body's own pain relievers. One of the nation's leading causes of chronic pain is osteoarthritis. The Arthritis Foundation recommends regular sex.
- **Mood elevation.** Got the blues? Sex often helps. Beyond relieving pain, the endorphins released during lovemaking also have antidepressant action.
- **Fitness.** Fitness includes strength, stamina, and flexibility. Men typically focus on strength and stamina, not flexibility. However, exercise physiologists agree that moving the joints through their full range of motion is crucial to fitness. Lovemaking enhances flexibility.
- **Sleep.** Sex often improves sleep, especially for men.
- **Blood pressure control.** All of the above help control blood pressure. A Scottish researcher found that regular sex helps reduce blood pressure.
- **Bladder control.** Many women suffer stress incontinence—urine leakage while coughing, sneezing, or laughing. The cause is weak urinary sphincter muscles that don't completely close. Doctors prescribe Kegel exercises to strengthen them. Orgasms help tone the same muscles.
- **Hot flashes.** A Nigerian study shows that lovemaking reduces this common menopausal discomfort.
- **Immune enhancement.** Regular moderate exercise boosts immune function. Sex is moderate exercise. Researchers at Wilkes-Barre University in Pennsylvania found that compared with couples who have little sex, those who twist the sheets once or twice weekly are less likely to catch colds. This is counterintuitive. Colds spread by close contact. Sex should increase risk. But the researchers found that something else outweighed the risk-elevation of close contact—the substantial immune boost lovemaking provides.
- **Prostate cancer prevention.** This disease may be sexually transmitted. As num-ber of STIs increases, so does risk. But frequent ejaculations help clear germs from men's genitourinary tracts. National Cancer Institute researchers asked twenty-nine thousand men, age forty-six to eighty-one, how often they ejacu-lated throughout life. Compared with those who estimated once or twice a week

since young adulthood, men who ejaculated daily were significantly less likely to develop the disease. *Honey, let's reduce my risk of prostate cancer tonight.*

- **Sperm quality.** An Australian fertility specialist asked 118 men with damaged sperm to ejaculate daily for a week. Their proportion of damaged sperm dropped significantly. Before attempting procreative intercourse, he advises daily ejaculations for at least a week.
- **Conception.** Successful fertilization depends, in part, on women retaining semen. British researchers have shown that women who have orgasms during or shortly after male ejaculation retain more.
- **Longevity.** Many of the above are associated with longer life. British scientists tracked nine hundred middle-aged men. Compared with those who had sex only once a month, those who did it twice a week lived significantly longer. Critics argued that the association might not be causal. Sexual frequency is a function of health. Perhaps the more sexual men were just healthier to begin with. That would explain their greater longevity. But the researchers statistically corrected for this and concluded that regular sex really does extend men's lives.

Frequent sex, solo or partnered, offers many health benefits the sex addiction industry ignores.

Consider dancing. Most people enjoy it. Many take dance classes for fun and fitness. And some become professionals and spend hours a day dancing for decades. Professional dancers often suffer personal, occupational, and social distress: injuries, audition heartbreaks, and extended periods away from loved ones. Do they have "compulsive hyperdancing disorder"?

Carnes concedes that sexuality varies considerably, and that "excessive" can't be defined quantitatively. Instead, he focuses on "the pattern . . . when out-of-control sexual behavior becomes the norm." In his view, addictive patterns include the following.

Inordinate time lost in sexual fantasies. He never defines inordinate. But researchers at Ohio State asked 283 college students to track how often they thought about sex. Men's median frequency was nineteen times a day, around once every waking hour, women's ten times, about once every two hours. With age, sexual thoughts usually decline, but most normal, mentally healthy people think about sex regularly.

Supporters of the sex addiction paradigm claim that as sexual thoughts increase, so do anxiety, guilt, shame, and addiction. But in this study, the men who thought about sex the most expressed the greatest sexual *comfort*. Sexual fantasies are normal, healthy, and contribute to sizzling sex.

However, sex fantasies spur masturbation, which advocates of the sex addiction model call pathological. Evidently, they haven't heard that solo sex, even daily, is normal, healthy, stress relieving, and how we explore our sexuality and resolve several sex problems.

Decades ago, I asked a friend how he was doing. "Great," he replied, "I have an orgasm every day." Some with his wife, but most solo. We laughed. As the years passed, whenever we chatted, he would say, "One a day." My friend is now elderly. We've shared that private joke for more than fifty years. I hasten to add that my buddy holds a PhD, is an authority in his field, makes an enviable income, was a tournament tennis player, has had a long, loving marriage, and has raised three children to functional adulthood. But the sex addiction industry would call him a compulsive masturbator, an addict.

Anonymous sex. This is the sex addiction industry's term for one-night stands. But sexual relationships need not be deeply committed to provide pleasure. The substantial majority of adults have enjoyed casual liaisons. Adam & Eve, the sex toy marketer, surveyed several thousand American adults. Two-thirds admitted one-time flings. The men averaged seven, the women, six. One-nighters may not be your cup of tea, but they're quite prevalent, usually pleasurable, and rarely cause lasting regret or anything pathological.

Having one relationship after another. The sex addiction industry recoils from serial partners, but the Adam & Eve survey shows that 88 percent of American adults—nine of ten—have had more than one:

Lifetime lovers	Proportion of respondents
One	12%
Two to five	24%
Six to ten	23%
Eleven to twenty-five	21%
More than twenty-five	20%

Adam & Eve. "Hooking Up: Casual Sex Facts."

Forty-one percent reported eleven or more partners. Are almost half of Americans sex addicts?

Group sex. Carnes calls group sex a symptom of sex addiction. But an Indiana University study of 2,021 adults shows that 10 percent of women and 18 percent of men admit participating in at least one threesome. Actual figures are probably higher. Around 5 percent of American couples have tried swinging, one in twenty. Far from being mentally disordered or addicted, Americans who experiment with group sex or engage in it frequently represent a snapshot of middle America—and they're no more likely than average to suffer mental illness.

Paying for sex. Whatever you think of prostitution, an estimated 15–20 percent of American men have paid for sex. Some visit sex workers compulsively, but for many, occasional paid sex helps reconcile an exuberant libido with chronic desire differences at home. It may not be admirable, but it's not necessarily out of control.

Frequent masturbation to porn. Supporters of the sex addiction model never define *frequent*, but they insist that regular self-sexing suggests addiction, especially when it involves porn. Rarely. Some men just have major libidos and enjoy tugging often, especially when stressed.

Using Facebook, researchers in Vancouver, British Columbia, recruited 14,396 adults, age eighteen to ninety-four, who completed a survey incorporating standard libido, sexual compulsivity, and personality assessments. Some had sought treatment for sex addiction. One-third—44 percent of the men, 22 percent of the women—reported sex, mostly solo, several times a week, frequencies the sex addiction industry would call compulsive and addicted. But among a broad range of personality and sexual variables, the researchers found only one difference between the most sexual third and everyone else—libido. The most sexual third wanted more sex, had more, and enjoyed it more. The researchers concluded that so-called sex addiction is "simply a marker of high sexual desire."

Everyone is sexually unique. There is no normal frequency, no conventional way to play. And if there's no normal, how can the sex addiction industry call so many people abnormal?

Gentlemen, You *Can* Get Aroused without Porn

Beyond enhancing masturbation, some older men stroke for another reason—to reassure themselves they can still become aroused. Older manhood brings not only erection problems, but for many, also difficulty feeling turned on. Many older men find arousal issues deeply upsetting. *My whole life I was hot to trot. Now I'm not. Who am I?* Some older men watch porn before partner sex to jump-start their arousal.

Porn works, but it's rarely necessary. A technique sex therapists recommend, "simmering," is equally effective. Simmering involves beginning the arousal process hours before sex by dreaming up brief, vivid erotic fantasies every hour or so. Much of porn involves only fellatio and intercourse. After a while, that can get boring. Scenes men dream up themselves may feel more arousing.

Initial loveplay is also arousing. Review chapters 4–10. Kissing, cuddling, wholebody massage, and oral sex spiced with novelty and fantasies are sufficiently arousing for most men to enjoy satisfying partner play.

I suggest experimenting. Schedule partner sex, and beforehand alternate using porn and your imagination. Chances are you don't need porn.

Many supporters of the sex addiction paradigm call frequent erotic fantasies problematic and a sign of addiction. But simmering involves frequent fantasies and sex therapists recommend it. Anticipating lovemaking enhances it and vivid fantasies add to erotic pleasure.

Brain Changes Identical to Drug Addicts?

Supporters of the sex addiction paradigm insist that whenever sex addicts do it, they exhibit brain changes identical to those of drug addicts—notably, surges of the neurotransmitter dopamine. Yes, heroin boosts dopamine, and so does sex. In fact, *every* pleasure boosts it, from petting kittens to a hole in one to winning the Lotto. Dopamine is the neurotransmitter of pleasure. For the large majority of people, sex is pleasurable so dopamine rises.

Considerable research shows that the brains of alleged sex addicts look *nothing like* those of drug addicts:

- University of New Mexico scientists assessed the brain function of fifty-two self-identified sex addicts without substance abuse issues. Their brains looked normal, nothing like those of drug addicts.
- Drug addicts experience breakdowns in brain mechanisms governing self-control. Brigham Young University researchers compared the self-control of thirty men in treatment for sex addiction and thirty controls. The two groups showed no differences.
- UCLA researchers performed brain scans on 122 people, some diagnosed as hypersexual. All their brains looked the same.

- The sex addiction industry claims that addiction-related brain changes cause erectile dysfunction. German investigators performed PET scans on two groups, men with normal erection function and men with ED who viewed tons of porn. Their brains looked the same.
- Finally, University of Minnesota investigators explored the brain function of a group of men, half of whom had been diagnosed as sexually compulsive. The two groups' brains were almost indistinguishable. The only difference was that the sex addicts showed more brain activity in areas indicative of anxiety.

Sex addiction reflects not brain derangement, but deep discomfort with recreational sex, particularly masturbation.

The Real Culprit in Sex Addiction: Sex-Negative Upbringing

Historically speaking, sex has come in three varieties: reproductive, relationship affirming (relational), and recreational. Humans have always engaged in all three, but from biblical times until the eighteenth century, the only religiously sanctioned justification was procreation. Lots of children made sense when most societies were agrarian and famine a constant threat. Kids were assets—more hands to work the fields.

After the Industrial Revolution, factory work and urbanization reduced family size, and religious thinking evolved. Reproduction remained God's favorite reason, but as farming yielded to wage labor, theologians decided the Almighty also approved of fewer children and relational sex to cement marriages.

Meanwhile, Western culture has always included an undercurrent of recreational carnality: sex work, consensual nonmonogamy, group play, same-gender couplings, and, for the past several centuries, BDSM. Civil and religious authorities often tolerated recreational play as long as it remained hidden—and unleashed periodic repression when they feared "perversion" threatened the social order.

When Alfred Kinsey published the first scientific studies of American sexuality (1948, 1953), his findings revealed that the large majority of Americans engaged in recreational sex, with many playing that way routinely. This shattered all illusions that Americans jiggled genitals only for God's two approved reasons.

Recreational sex is quite prevalent. Where would literature, movies, TV, gossip magazines, and popular song lyrics be without it? But religious fundamentalists insist that sex for fun is sinful, while cultural conservatives call it sex addiction.

Many people raised as religious or social conservatives feel deep distress about recreational organ grinding. They grow up hearing they should "save themselves" until marriage—but only 5 percent of Americans do. They also come of age believing masturbation is a ticket to Hell—but again, almost everyone strokes, many frequently, some daily or more.

Many men from conservative backgrounds wed women who share that upbringing. When sexually conservative women discover their men stroking to porn, some flip. *Sex addict!* For men who feel anxious and conflicted about sex to begin with, this accusation reinforces a lifetime of sexual bewilderment.

The sex addiction industry insists that among sex addicts, sexual feelings cause profound shame. Actually, sexual shame, anxiety, and guilt are usually the result of upbringings that condemn recreational eroticism. When those steeped in sexual fundamentalism play for fun, including self-sexing, many feel deeply distressed. But their anxiety, guilt, and shame stem not from the sex, but rather from authority figures who have relentlessly condemned it.

Most studies show that the best predictor of so-called sex addiction is an upbringing that demonizes recreational sex:

- Brigham Young University investigators surveyed 686 adults. Those who called themselves porn addicts were the most religious and expressed the most anxiety about sex.
- Scientists at the University of California, San Diego, compared 132 men who'd sought treatment for porn watching with 569 matched controls who watched the same amount of porn. There was only one difference between the two groups—religiosity.
- University of Oklahoma investigators asked parents (771 men, 904 women) how they felt about porn. Those most likely to revile it held the most fundamentalist religious views—and reported the greatest anxiety, guilt, and shame about viewing.
- Baylor University investigators surveyed 2,580 adults. Those who felt the most addicted to porn were the most religious.
- University of Texas researchers surveyed 1,913 Swedes about internet porn. The top predictor of distress—regular church attendance.
- Case Western Reserve scientists asked 2,232 adults if they felt addicted to internet porn. Most replied no, a few said yes. The latter were the most religious.
- In a survey of 2,279 adults, the same researchers found that as church attendance and prayer frequency increased, so did the belief that porn is "always wrong." But men expressing this view still watched a good deal, which triggered severe anxiety.

Speaking of anxiety, when sex-negative upbringing meets normal urges for self-sexing and other recreational eroticism, possible results include not only severe anxiety but also depression and other mental health issues.

Those who consider sex addiction a social crisis are mistaken. Excessive sex, whatever that may be, is rarely the problem. The real issues are the anxiety, guilt, and shame some feel about recreational sex, particularly its leading manifestation, men masturbating to porn. The best predictor of sex addiction is not time spent viewing porn, but depth of fundamentalist religious convictions.

"Promise Me You'll Stop Watching"

Some women make this demand and some men promise. But Palo Alto, California, sex therapist Marty Klein, PhD warns, "Never promise to stop watching porn unless you're 100 percent certain you can. If you're only 99 percent certain, don't promise. If you promise and get caught, you've broken a vow. Defending your porn watching may invite ugly conflict. But it's better to argue about that as moral equals than to pit a virtuous woman against a lying man." For help discussing porn, consult a sex therapist, ideally as a couple.

Are Sex and Porn Addictive?

At first glance, sex addiction appears plausible. If you can become addicted to alcohol, other drugs, and gambling, why not sex?

In addition, in contemporary America, many people use the term *addiction* quite loosely. Chocolate lovers are chocoholics. Coffee aficionados are java junkies. People joke about being addicted to exercise, bacon, shopping, the internet, romance fiction, and video games. But mention sex and the jesting ceases as sex addiction pundits decry the supposed scourge.

Medically, addiction refers to substance abuse. It has four hallmarks:

- **Tolerance.** The more addicts use, the more they need to obtain the desired effect.
- **Craving.** Gnawing desire compels addicts to organize their lives around their addictions.
- **Withdrawal distress.** If addicts stop using, they suffer. Caffeine withdrawal causes headaches. Alcohol withdrawal causes delirium tremens (DTs). Opioid withdrawal causes many problems.
- **Increasingly severe consequences.** The addiction hijacks addicts' lives, resulting in job loss, family and money woes, severe illness, and sometimes death.

However, the vast majority of those labeled sex addicts meet none of these criteria—including frequent viewers of porn.

No tolerance. If porn causes tolerance, over time, users would consume increasing amounts. But PornHub statistics (page 387) show that the large majority of men watch only briefly while stroking. When they come, they stop. The average American spends *five hours a day* watching TV, but only two porn viewers per thousand watch for more than two.

The sex addiction industry contends that as men slip into porn addiction, they become tolerant to conventional porn, and gravitate to more extreme genres: anal, BDSM, group sex, and violent porn. They call this tolerance.

Actually, porn depicting unconventional sex is not "extreme." Anal play, BDSM, and group sex are all perfectly normal and fairly prevalent, involving tens of millions of successful, loving, mentally healthy Americans, quite possibly the folks next door. Many porn viewers sample the enormous range of hardcore possibilities, but that's not tolerance. It usually reflects either curiosity or boredom. After viewing videos featuring wild, public, multiracial anal orgies, almost all men can still become aroused by watching one lone couple doing it in the missionary position in their bedroom. Where's the tolerance?

About violence: porn critics allege that over time, men seek out increasingly violent porn. McGill University researchers analyzed the most popular videos uploaded to PornHub from 2008 to 2016. In 2008, 13 percent depicted violence. By 2016, the proportion had *fallen* to less than 3 percent. Compared with nonviolent videos, those showing violence also received substantially fewer "likes." Men don't gravitate toward more violent content. They actually move away from it. Again, where's the tolerance?

No craving. There's a big difference between *craving* and *liking*. The vast majority of men like porn, but only an infinitesimal fraction come anywhere near organizing their lives around it. Alcoholics and drug addicts can't go a day without their substances. But if men have something better to do, they don't watch porn. Visits to PornHub decrease on all major holidays:

- New Year's Eve: views drop 38 percent
- Christmas Eve: -34 percent
- Super Bowl: -26 percent
- Christmas Day: -17 percent

- New Year's Day: -13 percent
- Thanksgiving: -13 percent

If the vast majority of men can't watch, they don't go bonkers. Very few men develop porn cravings that suggest addiction.

No withdrawal distress. When sports fans—mostly men—have responsibilities that preclude attending games, they feel bummed, but don't become unhinged. For the overwhelming majority of men, the same is true for porn. If it's available, they watch. If not, they function fine without it.

No increasingly severe consequences. Porn has two consequences—masturbation and disappointing partner lovemaking. Every so often, a man gets fired for wanking to porn at work. And when some women discover their men stroking to videos, they accuse them of sex addiction. But Brigham Young University researchers gave a standard personality test to 152 people who had been diagnosed—by themselves, partners, or mental health professionals—as hypersexual. "Our data fail to show any evidence supporting the notion that hypersexual patients experience addictive tendencies."

A tiny fraction of men exhibit sexual compulsivity. They—and their partners—need professional help (page 403). But to call frequent, even daily, masturbation to porn addictive mangles the term.

The Problems with SAFE
Even if frequent sex does not meet the medical definition of addiction, Carnes says it's still problematic based on four key signs, S-A-F-E, sex that's:

- **S**ecret
- **A**busive, that is, causes harm
- Used to avoid painful **F**eelings
- **E**mpty

Carnes's SAFE formula reflects a poor understanding of sexuality.

Secret. There's a big difference between *secret* and *private*. When people use the toilet, the huge majority do it alone with the bathroom door closed. That's not secret. It's private. The same goes for masturbation. Like toileting, it's private. People have every right to privacy.

Unless masturbation interferes with life responsibilities or partner sex, there's nothing wrong with it. In fact, for some sex problems, solo sex is therapeutic, notably premature ejaculation and inability to have orgasms. Mistaking privacy for secrecy and then demonizing it vilifies normal, healthy sexuality.

Meanwhile, some sex is, indeed, kept secret. Many LGBTQ folks are out with friends but not with their families or coworkers for fear of shunning. Or they're out in the US but not in some other countries for fear of assault and prison. Their sexual secrecy is not pathological. It's a healthy way to cope with potentially life-threatening bigotry.

Abusive. In *Don't Call It Love*, Carnes calls BDSM abusive: "Chains, whips, sadomasochism, receiving or causing pain to intensify sexual pleasure, willingly acting the powerless victim in sexual activity—how can these be pleasurable? For most of us, the combination of pain and sex is as repugnant as violence."

This reflects total ignorance of BDSM. Review chapter 44. There are no powerless victims. No one gets abused. Subs receive no sensation beyond their declared limits. Subs are always in control and free to stop play at any time. The millions of BDSM aficionados and tens of millions of BDSM fantasizers are as mentally healthy as the general population.

Used to avoid painful feelings. Life involves suffering. Both solo and partner sex are soothing. What's wrong with using sex to assuage pain? Would the sex addiction industry prefer people numb themselves with alcohol or antianxiety medication? Many mood-altering drugs are indisputably addictive and possibly lethal. Self-soothing with one hand is easier, cheaper, healthier, more convenient, and more fun.

Empty. According to the sex addiction industry, sex outside committed, monogamous relationships is empty. Of course, lovemaking in committed relationships may bring great pleasure and satisfaction—but not necessarily. For many longtime monogamous spouses, sex feels empty, if they make love at all. The vast majority of adult Americans have had one-night stands, brief flings, friends-with-benefits relationships, or other types of noncommitted sex. For the substantial majority, these experiences are enjoyable and instructional, not empty and addictive.

A Brief History of Sex Addiction

Starting in the 1950s, prior notions of "normal" sex and gender got upended. Kinsey showed that recreational and homosexual sex are quite common. Women entered the workforce in unprecedented numbers. The Pill and IUD separated sex from procreation as never before, freeing women to enjoy casual sex. The marriage rate fell. The divorce rate soared. Cohabitation flourished. The LGBTQ population emerged from the closet. The Supreme Court legalized abortion and porn. And in the mid-1970s, home video players became the rage, moving porn from seedy theaters into the nation's living rooms. Social and religious conservatives recoiled.

In the wake of these changes, in 1983, Patrick Carnes coined the term *sex addiction*. A disparate coalition quickly embraced it: social conservatives, religious fundamentalists, anti-porn feminists, talk show hosts, twelve-step veterans with sex issues, and some mental health professionals.

Five years later, in 1988, in their sex therapy textbook, *Sexual Desire Disorders*, Sandra Lieblum, PhD, and Raymond Rosen, PhD, both professors at the Robert Wood Johnson School of Medicine and Dentistry in New Jersey, expressed astonishment at the rise of the sex addiction model. They affirmed that in long careers specializing in treating desire problems, they'd seen only a handful of people actually sexually out of control.

Nonetheless, it didn't take long for the new scourge to become embedded in popular culture:

- Sex addiction flooded the internet. I searched the term—thirty-seven million hits.
- More than two dozen self-assessment questionnaires popped up, including the Sexual Addiction Scale, the Compulsive Sexual Behavior Inventory, and the Sexual Addiction Screening Test. They touch on compulsivity, but mostly measure sexual anxiety.
- Researchers flocked to study the new affliction. Before 1985, psychology and sexology journals rarely mentioned sexual compulsivity. By 2017, articles numbered more than twelve thousand.

- Celebrities stepped forward sheepishly admitting sex addiction—usually to bolster defense efforts during divorce proceedings.
- Celebrity confessions attracted media coverage—and not just in supermarket tabloids. The *New York Times* has published the term hundreds of times.

Today, many Americans believe sex addiction is real, prevalent, and devastating, with its leading manifestation—men stroking to porn. But the deeper one delves into sex addiction, the less one finds. Yes, a smattering of men develops issues with porn that make them and their partners miserable. But for most men suffering supposed sex addiction, the real issue is not porn, but the anxiety, guilt, and shame they've been raised to feel about masturbating—exacerbated by partner rage over their self-sexing to porn.

An old joke asks, why did the Puritan get so upset? *Somewhere someone was having fun.* Those unnerved by sex addiction are latter-day Puritans who condemn recreational sex as addictive. But recreation, that is, pleasure, is the number one reason Americans bump bellies. At its core, sex addiction represents a twenty-first-century reinvention of what used to be called "perversion," any sex the self-appointed arbiters of decency deemed unacceptable. But "perversion" is outdated. Addiction supplied a contemporary medical spin that may appeal to talk show hosts—but not to most mental health professionals.

Sex Addiction: Rejected by the Large Majority of Mental Health Authorities

In the US, the bible of mental illness is the American Psychiatric Association's *Diagnostic and Statistical Manual of Mental Disorders* (DSM). Its first edition, DSM-I (1952) listed excessive sex as a disorder—but only in women, "nymphomania." DSM-III (1980) added it in men, "satyriasis," after the constantly lusty satyrs in Greek mythology, or "Don Juan-ism," after the fictional Spanish libertine.

But since then, as researchers have documented the enormous diversity of normal, healthy sexuality, the professional consensus has shifted to the view that while a tiny fraction of the population struggles with sexual compulsivity, from a public health perspective, the sex addiction industry has made mountains of molehills.

To those outside the mental health professions, DSM machinations may seem obscure. In fact, the stakes are enormous—tens of millions of dollars a year. Without official DSM recognition, health insurers don't pay for treatment.

Starting in 2003, American mental health experts spent a decade producing DSM-5 (2013). The process involved thousands of stakeholders who debated tens of thousands of studies. Sexual conservatives lobbied hard to declare sex addiction an official disorder—but produced no compelling evidence that frequent, unconventional, or religiously proscribed sex, per se, solo or partnered, causes significant harm. Meanwhile, the sex-positive community countered with abundant research showing that, for the substantial majority of those diagnosed as sex addicts, the real issue is not their sexual activity but having been raised with sex-negative beliefs. DSM decision-makers rejected the Puritans' claims. DSM-5 does not mention hypersexuality or sex addiction, and it deleted all references of nymphomania, satyriasis, and Don Juan-ism.

"Sex addiction is as silly as thirst addiction, hunger addiction, or reading addiction," said the late Johns Hopkins psychologist John Money, PhD. "Sexual addictionology decrees that the only nonaddictive form of sexual expression is lifelong heterosexual monogamous marriage. Everything else is the gateway to sin, depravity, and addiction."

The organization that credentials US sexuality professionals agrees. The American Association of Sex Educators, Counselors, and Therapists (AASECT) "finds insufficient evidence to support sex/porn addiction as a mental health disorder and finds treatment methods for 'sexual addiction' poorly informed about human sexuality."

In addition to the DSM, the World Health Organization publishes a similar guide, the *International Classification of Diseases* (ICD). The latest edition, ICD-11, finalized in 2019, includes "compulsive sexual behavior disorder" (CSBD), which describes such activities as getting repeatedly arrested for public masturbation.

Those who support the addiction model claim the ICD's recognition of CSBD validates their beliefs. On the contrary, the ICD-11 says compulsive sexual behavior disorder:

- Is possible, but rare, much less prevalent than the sex addiction industry asserts
- Is not an addiction
- Should never be self-diagnosed, diagnosed by girlfriends or wives, or diagnosed based on internet checklists
- Should not be diagnosed when the sexual distress results merely from self-sexing to porn or from moral or religious conflicts about sex—which is the case with almost all purported sex addicts

Bottom line: the DSM, AASECT, the ICD, and the vast majority of mental health professionals worldwide reject the whole idea of sex addiction.

Worried You Might Have a Sex/Porn Problem?

Only two men per 1,000 watch porn for more than two hours at a sitting. That's a minute fraction of the population, but it's 240,000 American men. If you'd like to change your relationship to porn, read on.

Step 1. Why?

Why do you think you're sexually out of control?

- **Fantasies? Or Actions?** Are you worried about your thoughts, fantasies, and feelings? Or what you actually do? If only the former, you're normal. Everyone has erotic reveries. Some may be disturbing, but we're not responsible for our thoughts, only our actions. Accept your fantasies. Control your actions.
- **Upbringing?** Were you raised to believe that masturbation and casual sex are wrong? Harmful? Sinful? Actually, masturbation is by far the world's most popular type of sex. Decades of sex research show that solo sex is normal, healthy, and a key component of satisfying partner lovemaking. Except for the circumstances discussed below, masturbation causes no harm beyond possible genital chafing—use lubricant. Most mentally healthy men—and many women—masturbate regularly, some daily or more. Most Americans have engaged in recreational sex—and usually feel fine about it.
- **Who?** Who says you're out of control? You? Or your partner? If it's you, here's the test. Do your sexual actions significantly interfere with your life? Are you shirking school or work to be sexual? Have teachers, employers, or coworkers called your sexuality problematic? Have sexual pursuits placed you in physical danger? Have you been arrested for sexual actions? If so, proceed to steps 3 and 4.

If anyone else accuses you of sex addiction, ask why. That person may be mistaken. Ask your accuser to read part VII of this book. However, porn-critical girlfriends and wives raise one legitimate objection—men habitually stroking to porn while refusing to play with them.

Red Flag: Preferring Self-Sexing to Porn over Partner Lovemaking

I've received myriad questions from women in anguish because their men would rather stroke to porn than join them in bed. That's a problem. Unless both spouses agree to a sexless relationship, couples have a responsibility to negotiate regular lovemaking at a frequency both can live with.

Gentlemen, if your partner complains that you prefer solo sex to doing it with her, is it true? Do you? If so, why? Have you discussed your reasons with your mate? For help with this, consult a sex therapist.

Men may feel enthusiastic about partner sex but have solo orgasms shortly before their lovers suggest the prone dance. Because of the refractory period, men may not be able to get it up again soon after self-sexing. In that case, schedule partner sex in advance. With sex dates calendared, you can play solo at other times.

Independent of disagreements about porn, in long-term relationships, desire differences are virtually inevitable. To resolve them, sex therapists recommend negotiating a frequency and scheduling sex in advance. When porn is a sore point, scheduling becomes crucial. It reassures women that their men still desire them and are committed to making love. And it allows men to tug at other times.

Step 2. How?
According to the sex addiction industry, the leading sign of male sexual compulsivity is masturbation to porn. Among women, it's serial flings with a parade of partners.

Gentlemen, stroking to porn is rarely the real problem. It's usually the anxiety, guilt, and shame engendered by a sexually conservative upbringing compounded by partner condemnation.

Ladies, having lots of lovers is not necessarily pathological. Around 5 percent of normal, mentally healthy women—one in twenty—are highly sexual. Throughout history, many psychologically well-adjusted women have participated in consensual nonmonogamy and group sex. Today, several million American women affirmatively enjoy threesomes, swapping, and swinging, with millions more sufficiently curious to experiment. Some women just enjoy sex more than others, some considerably more.

Unless your sexual actions significantly derail your life, they're almost always fine. If they interfere with your daily responsibilities or primary relationship, proceed to steps 3 and 4.

Step 3. Convinced your actions are reckless?
Treat them as a habit you'd like to change. Start with self-help.

- **If at first . . .** Many people try to lose weight or quit smoking, drinking, or watching porn—and fail. Some conclude, *This habit is stronger than I am.* It probably isn't. Don't give up. Habit change is a learning process that often involves false starts. Persevere. Eventually, you're likely to craft an approach that works for you.

- **Itemize your triggers.** Triggers are the moments you feel pulled to indulge. What are they? Be specific. Triggers often include boredom, stress, loneliness, the end of the workday, or unstructured time. Once you understand your triggers, you can work to avoid them.
- **Ten minutes.** The next time you feel triggered, instead of slipping into your habit, for ten minutes, do something else—anything. Ten minutes isn't long. Even those in the grip of true addictions, for example, smoking, can usually manage to do something else for ten minutes. Call a friend. Take a walk. Read. Run an errand. Eat a snack. Watch TV. Answer messages—anything. Most men view porn on their phones. For ten minutes, put yours in a drawer and leave the room.
- **Another ten?** After ten minutes, decide if you feel up to postponing your habit another ten. If not, don't berate yourself. Some habits change slowly. You went ten minutes—congratulations. Your habit doesn't totally control you. Over time, extend one ten-minute period to several. You don't have to abstain from porn entirely. Just confine it to a smaller corner of your life.
- **Which substitutes work best?** Experiment to identify the activities that best allow you to avoid your habit. Work them into your daily life.
- **Relapses? Be kind to yourself.** Few people quit persistent habits the first time they try. If you relapse, analyze why you couldn't resist your trigger, and try again.
- **More tips?** Search "changing a habit."
- **I don't recommend these self-help groups: Sexaholics Anonymous, Sex Addicts Anonymous, Sex and Love Addicts Anonymous, and so forth.** On the plus side, they fill unstructured time and offer social support, both of which help with habit change. However, sex-focused anonymous groups have substantial drawbacks:
  - They embrace the addiction model, which has been rejected by the majority of mental health professionals.
  - They demonize recreational sex. From the Sexaholics Anonymous website: "For sexaholics, any sex with oneself or partners other than one's spouse is progressively addictive and destructive." Any sex with oneself is destructive? The vast majority of normal, healthy people masturbate throughout life, many frequently, some daily or more. Self-sexing is relaxing and pleasurable and offers valuable sexual and health benefits. Sex coaches and therapists encourage it and prescribe it as part of treatment for several sex problems. Any sex with nonspousal partners is potentially addictive? The overwhelming majority of Americans have engaged in nonspousal lovemaking. Only 5 percent of Americans are virgins at their weddings. Are 95 percent at risk for sexaholism?
  - Anecdotally, some claim benefit from sexual Anonymous groups, but others have insisted they gained nothing. In her memoir, *Getting Off: One Woman's Journey through Sex and Porn Addiction*, Erica Garza writes that Sex and Love Addicts Anonymous provided her no benefit. In fact, she sometimes became so aroused by participants' lurid confessions that after meetings she went home and masturbated.

Step 4. Still need help? Consult a mental health professional who uses cognitive behavioral therapy (CBT) or its offshoot, acceptance and commitment therapy (ACT). Fear of being out of control causes anxiety and efforts to find relief. When masturbation to porn causes anxiety, some men self-soothe with more masturbation to more porn. This creates a vicious cycle: stroking, anxiety, more stroking, and greater anxiety.

Were You Raised Fundamentalist Christian?

Reverend Beverly Dale is an ordained minister in the Disciples of Christ Christian church. She grew up in a devout family with parents and clergy who insisted that sex was "very, very bad." She came of age filled with sexual guilt and shame. She knew nothing about contraception and suffered an unplanned pregnancy. She did not have an orgasm for her first ten years of marriage.

Eventually, with the help of science-friendly clergy, she discovered sex-positive Christianity and made it a cornerstone of her own ministry. She is the founder of the Incarnation Institute for Sex and Faith (incarnationinstitute.org), which promotes sex-positive Christianity. In addition, she is the coauthor of *Advancing Sexual Health for the Christian Client* (with Rachel Keller, LCSW, also raised evangelical Christian). The book addresses therapists who work with fundamentalist clients, but it's accessible to all Christians burdened by guilt and shame about any aspect of sex—from solo play to recreational cavorting to unsatisfying marital lovemaking. The book cites Christian theology to correct sex-negative beliefs and embraces a joyous Christianity rooted in science-based sexual liberalism. I highly recommend it to any Christian who feels sex addicted. I also recommend *Sex, God, and the Conservative Church* by Tina Schermer Sellers, PhD.

Cognitive means thinking. CBT/ACT are simple yet powerful approaches to loosening the grip of anxiety-producing stressors by changing how we think about them. Mistaken thoughts can cause great distress. CBT/ACT corrects false beliefs. As a result, those in distress calm down and are often able to break their vicious cycles.

One type of mistaken thinking involves "catastrophizing," making a big deal out of minor annoyances. You miss a flight. Catastrophizers think, *My life is ruined.* Missing a flight can be a hassle, but there are other flights, and schedules can be rearranged. CBT/ACT therapists help people recognize catastrophizing and correct flawed thinking, which reduces their anxiety and any associated acting out.

Sexual catastrophizing includes these mistaken ideas:

- *Sexual thoughts and fantasies are wrong, harmful, sinful.*
- *Only bad people masturbate.*
- *Porn is evil.*

CBT/ACT therapists correct and decatastrophize them:

- There's nothing wrong with sexual thoughts and fantasies. Everyone has them. They're perfectly normal. They're a key element of sizzling sex. Accept your thoughts. Control your actions.
- Almost everyone masturbates, particularly men who feel stressed. Unless it interferes with life responsibilities or partner lovemaking, there's nothing wrong with it, even daily or more.
- Porn is not evil. It's a cartoon version of men's fantasies of effortless sexual abundance. Virtually every internet-connected man on Earth has seen porn, many frequently, some daily. It's okay to watch.

Several studies show that CBT/ACT works well for those who believe their sexuality is out of control:

- Utah State University researchers assessed the internet porn viewing of men who said it had destroyed their quality of life. They participated in eight ninety-minute sessions of ACT (twelve hours total). Afterward, their anxiety decreased significantly and so did their viewing. It remained low three months later.
- Swedish scientists used CBT to treat men suffering severe anxiety caused by their porn consumption. After seven sessions (seventeen hours total), their distress declined significantly. So did their porn viewing. It remained lower six months later.
- A Harvard researcher recruited twenty-eight adult men in distress because of pornography. Some were placed on a wait list. The rest received twelve sessions of ACT. The wait-list group showed scant change in porn viewing, but the ACT group reported significant reductions.
- Creighton University investigators took thirty-eight men convinced they were porn addicts to a rustic retreat center for eight days. They spent thirty-two hours in mindfulness meditation instruction and CBT. Their sexual anxiety and porn viewing decreased significantly.
- Swedish researchers identified 137 men diagnosed as "hypersexual." They placed sixty-seven on a wait list and enrolled the other seventy in a CBT program, seven 2.5-hour sessions over seven weeks (17.5 hours total). The wait-list group reported slightly reduced sexual distress, but sexual anguish in the CBT group plummeted—and remained low six months later.

To find a CBT therapist near you visit the National Association of Cognitive-Behavioral Therapists (nacbt.org). To find an ACT professional, visit psychologytoday.com/us/therapists/acceptance-and-commitment-therapy-act.

Or consult a sex therapist credentialed by AASECT. Many offer CBT/ACT. Their training incorporates current sex research, so they have the knowledge to correct mistaken sexual beliefs. They appreciate the great diversity of normal, healthy sexuality. They do not condemn masturbation. They understand that while sex may cause problems, for the vast majority of people, lovemaking—solo or partnered, however frequent—usually brings pleasure, not addiction. To find an AASECT-certified sex therapist near you, visit aasect.org.

In my opinion, you're unlikely to benefit from sex addiction therapy provided by certified sex addiction therapists (CSATs) credentialed by the International Institute for Trauma and Addiction Professionals (IITAP), founded by Carnes with training reflecting his beliefs. Here's why:

- Successful treatment of perceived sexual compulsivity involves reducing anxiety. But the label "sex addict" often increases it. The label itself is counterproductive.
- Successful treatment of perceived sexual compulsivity involves correcting mistaken beliefs about sex. As shown throughout this chapter, supporters of the sex addiction model hold sexual beliefs that are seriously mistaken. How can they help correct anyone else's erroneous thinking? The large majority of mental health professionals reject the very idea of sex addiction.

If you feel troubled by out-of-control sexuality, I hope you and your partner get therapy that provides lasting relief. But porn ranks among men's top internet destinations, and only two men per thousand watch anywhere near compulsively. Porn does not contribute to the many social ills often blamed on it. For at least 998 of every 1,000 men, masturbation to internet porn has nothing to do with misogyny, infidelity, child sex abuse, sex trafficking, or sexual violence against women. It's simply a visual aid for brief interludes of self-soothing—and that's all.

CHAPTER 52:
The Anguish Some Women Feel about Porn

A SURPRISINGLY LARGE NUMBER of women watch pornography. PornHub, one of the world's largest porn sites, reports that women comprised 29 percent of its 2018 audience. Women visitors logged ten billion views, the equivalent of several that year for every internet-connected woman on Earth. Most porn-viewing women watch with partners before lovemaking or as background while playing. But some watch the way men do, as a visual aid during self-sexing. Half of adult American women own vibrators. Most use them solo.

Other women feel ambivalent about porn. They have difficulty comprehending why men watch and may fret about its impact. But they're not antiporn crusaders.

And some women detest porn and consider it an abomination. When they discover that their partners watch, they feel rejected, degraded, and betrayed.

"I Thought I Knew Him . . ."

The sex addiction industry asserts that when men view porn, the women in their lives suffer anguish. One oft-cited study agrees: Illinois State University researchers visited internet relationship sites and collected 100 posts by women who'd discovered their men had viewed porn (often by spying on their phone and computer browsing histories). They felt traumatized. Many called their men's porn habits "betrayal" or "infidelity," proof that their lovers no longer desired them. They also grieved the loss of their men's affection, sexual interest, and intimacy and trust in their relationships. Many said their men's porn habits made them feel ugly, undesirable, and worthless. They called their men sick, perverted, degenerate, and addicted. Most lamented, *I thought I knew him, but now I realize I never did. Who is he?*

Most Women Feel Okay

Clearly, some women consider porn poison. But those in the study just mentioned were far from representative. How do most women feel?

A study by University of Arkansas investigators suggests an answer. They recruited participants from websites aimed at women and surveyed the first 100 who responded. This sample, self-selected and rather small, is far from ideal. But this study represents the best evidence to date. It shows that most women don't feel devastated by their men's porn viewing:

Survey statement	Agree*	Disagree*
My partner's porn use proves he's mentally ill.	11%	86%
His porn use means our relationship has serious problems.	17%	74%
He no longer desires me.	17%	74%
His porn use shows he no longer cares about me or our relationship.	21%	75%
Since learning he watches, our intimacy has suffered.	30%	62%
His porn use has hurt my self-esteem.	34%	56%
His porn use has nothing to do with me.	65%	25%
My partner cares very much about me.	82%	9%
I feel no need for him to keep his porn use secret.	85%	9%
My partner and I enjoy watching porn together.	36%	50%

*Some didn't respond to all statements, so rows don't add up to 100 percent.

Bridges, A. J., et al. "Romantic Partners' Use of Pornography: Its Significance for Women." *Journal of Sex and Marital Therapy* 29 (2003): 1.

Only around one-quarter of respondents expressed distress about their men's porn viewing. The other three-quarters might not like it, but they didn't feel betrayed or degraded, nor did they consider porn a threat to their relationships. One-third said they watched with their men, which lends credence to PornHub's analysis that women comprise 29 percent of its audience.

A Canadian study corroborates these findings. Researchers at the University of Western Ontario surveyed the impact of porn on 215 couples in which the men watched alone or with their partners. Most of the women said porn had "no negative effects" on their relationship. Some said it offered benefits—more sexual communication, experimentation, and comfort. Very few said porn threatened their relationships.

Does Men's Porn Use Betray Their Partners?
Nothing I write is likely to alter the sentiments of women convinced that porn is the work of Satan. This section addresses women who may feel ambivalent but remain open minded.

Betrayal? Infidelity? If couples swear monogamy and one subsequently joins genitals with someone else, that's infidelity, a betrayal. But adultery requires twisting of sheets. Men who tug to porn have no sexual contact with anyone but themselves. How is that infidelity? As long as solo sex doesn't interfere with life responsibilities or partner lovemaking (below), everyone has a right to self-sexing.

Half of American women own vibrators, and most of them are coupled. Are the tens of millions of women who masturbate with vibes betraying their husbands? I don't think so. In a crazy world, they're simply self-soothing.

Many women love sex-drenched romance fiction that ignites erotic fantasies—and self-sexing. Are they betraying their men?

"I should satisfy all his sexual needs." Some women say they object to porn, when they actually object to their partners masturbating. That's what a University of Oklahoma researcher found when he analyzed two nationally representative surveys of twelve thousand Americans. Initially, when considering the impact of porn on relationship happiness, it appeared that as men's porn use increased, women's relationship satisfaction decreased. But when the analysis included male masturbation, the women objections to porn, per se, evaporated. What they really objected to—their men stroking.

Some women believe that once men say "I do," they should instantly lose all desire to masturbate. Sorry, ladies, he was one-handing it long before he met you. Why stop going to the beach once you've visited the mountains?

Masturbation and partner lovemaking are both sexual, but they're quite different. In partner sex, lovers must please each other, negotiate livable frequencies and repertoires, and work to overcome inevitable differences. Partner lovemaking can feel sublime, but it also takes effort and involves negotiations that may prove daunting. Solo sex is easier. The only person you have to please is yourself. Women can't possibly meet men's need to masturbate, which is, by definition, a solitary pleasure.

Demeaning? Porn shows a great deal more fellatio than cunnilingus. That isn't fair and might be considered demeaning. Many women *need* oral sex to have orgasms. When men imitate porn, many women don't come.

But porn isn't real sex. It presents testosterone-fueled male erotic fantasies. It's a cartoon. Saying that porn degrades women is like saying *The Simpsons* demeans families.

Almost all porn-watching men cherish their mates and have no wish to traumatize them. Most porn shows women who appear to be enjoying themselves. How is that degrading?

"I can't compete with those women." Many women feel deeply insecure about their bodies. They believe that by watching porn, their men have rejected them for better bodies.

I sympathize with those who have body insecurities. I've experienced them myself. My wife loves to watch professional basketball—every NBA player is bigger, taller, stronger, younger, and more athletic than yours truly. But I don't feel threatened by her hoop dreams. It's entertainment, an innocent diversion that has no implications for our marriage. The same goes for porn. Women are no more in competition with the women in porn than I am with NBA players.

"He must not want me." When men watch porn, some of their lovers feel undesirable, rejected. Actually, the vast majority of porn-viewing men love their partners and desire them:

- Idaho State University scientists showed porn to forty-four heterosexual couples. The men's top response—"more desire for their partners."
- English investigators quizzed 164 men about their porn habits, then surveyed their social connections. The men who watched the most porn reported the *closest* social ties. The researchers concluded that men who view porn "crave intimacy," not escape from it.

"I can't compete with porn for his attention." People in committed relationships don't spend every moment together. During their free time, women read, shop, exercise, watch TV, check messages, and visit with friends. Are they ignoring their men? Healthy relationships involve negotiating time spent together and apart. Porn may be one of men's top internet destinations, but it still allows plenty of time for their partners.

"He'd Rather Masturbate to Porn than Make Love with Me"

That's a real problem. In sexual relationships, couples have a responsibility to accommodate each other's needs for regular lovemaking at frequencies both can live with. After the brief hot-and-heavy period, couples' libidos almost always diverge. When this causes conflict, sex coaches and therapists recommend scheduling sex in advance. That way both people know they'll make love and when.

If porn is an issue, scheduling becomes even more necessary. With scheduled sex, women can feel reassured that their men still want to make love with them, and both are free to play alone at other times—with men watching porn if they like.

Sex Videos that Arouse Women

Some women wouldn't watch porn in a million years. Others watch with their men. And some might feel open to viewing but feel turned off by standard porn. If you're among this latter group, consider feminist pornography.

The first feminist porn producer was Candida Royalle (Candice Vadala, 1950–2015). After appearing in twenty-five conventional porn films (1975–80), she tired of the male point of view and decided to produce sex videos with a woman's touch. In 1984, she founded Femme Productions (in the HBO series *The Deuce*, the porn director, Candy, is loosely based on Vadala).

Femme videos contain plenty of hardcore action, but the characters do more together than just hump. They converse, laugh, and have some semblance of relationships. The sex is less preoccupied with the genitals, and there's as much cunnilingus as fellatio.

Two studies have compared men's and women's reactions to standard porn versus Femme videos:

- Researchers at the University of Connecticut showed 395 students (200 men, 195 women) three typical porn videos and three from Femme. The men loved all six. The women disliked the standard porn but enjoyed the Femme programs—and were more likely to make love after viewing them.
- At the University of Amsterdam, Dutch scientists showed forty-seven women standard porn or a Femme program. They frowned on the former but felt aroused by the latter.

Femme videos are available from Amazon.com, or visit these sites:
- FeministPornGuide.com.
- Good Vibrations after Dark (goodvibesblog.com/good-vibrations-after-dark-feminist-porn-on-demand)
- BrightDesire.com
- ErikaLust.com
- Make Love Not Porn (makelovenotporn.com). This site is nothing like conventional porn. It's real lovemaking in all of its splendid diversity. Compared with standard porn (largely fellatio and intercourse), MLNP offers much broader, more creative, more authentic lovemaking.

Watching together invites women to remind men that standard porn is a cartoon that should not be imitated. Viewing together also helps women coach men on the erotic moves they actually enjoy. Most women prefer the *opposite* of porn, not just sucking and fucking, but leisurely, playful, whole-body massage that eventually includes the genitals.

One Final Question

If you're a woman who despises porn, you have every right to your opinion. One-quarter of women feel similarly. But whether or not they like porn or watch any, three-quarters of women don't feel particularly distressed that their men watch. Which raises a question for women who insist that porn is poison. Why do you think most women feel differently?

Help for Women Distressed about Men's Porn Viewing

If your man's porn habits are driving you crazy, consider cognitive behavioral therapy (CBT) or acceptance and commitment therapy (ACT). Both have shown real benefit for men troubled by their porn use. I bet they'd also help women in distress about porn (page 403).

Acknowledgments

I FEEL ESPECIALLY INDEBTED to the more than fifty million readers of my PsychologyToday.com blog, "All about Sex," and the more than two million visitors to the Q&A site I publish, GreatSexGuidance.com. Their comments and questions have demonstrated over and over again that each of us is sexually unique.

Deepest thanks to my longtime literary agent, Amy Rennert of the Amy Rennert Agency, for forty-plus years of friendship, and for having faith in a project other agents might have dismissed as too ambitious.

Much appreciation to everyone at Skyhorse Publishing, especially my marvelous editor, Leah Zarra, and cover designer, Daniel Brount.

Many thanks to my editors at PsychologyToday.com: Hara Marano, Lybi Ma, and Kaja Perina.

Sincere thanks to my ace tech consultant, Frank Colin, for managing GreatSexGuidance.com and repeatedly rescuing me from computer hell.

I feel particularly indebted to sex therapist and author Marty Klein, PhD, whose decades of friendship and profound insights have added tremendously to my understanding of sexuality.

Special thanks to longtime sexologist friends for their support and guidance: Patti Britton, PhD, MPH, Betty Dodson, PhD, Joan Price, David Steinberg, and Louanne Weston, PhD.

Major kudos to the world's sex researchers, notably Debby Herbenick, PhD, and her colleagues at Indiana University; Rosemary Basson, MD, Lori Brotto, PhD, and their colleagues at the University of British Columbia; and the University of Chicago's National Opinion Research Center.

Equal gratitude to the editors and publishers of the nation's sex research journals, particularly *Sexual Medicine*, the *Journal of Sex Research*, the *Journal of Sexual Medicine*, the *Journal of Sex and Marital Therapy*, *Archives of Sexual Behavior*, and the *American Journal of Sexuality Education*. What a shame the news media spotlight so little sex research. I hope this book brings important sexological findings to a wider audience.

Heartfelt thanks to the legion of sex educators, counselors, coaches, therapists, researchers, journalists, and friends, both living and deceased, whose invaluable perspectives contributed to this book: Kelly J. Ace, PhD, JD, Isadora Allman, MFT, CST, Lonnie Barbach, PhD, Ellen Barnard, MSW, CSE, Ellen Bass, Myisha Battle, Mieke Beckman, LMSW, CST, Alicia Beltran, LCPC, CST, Robert Berend, PhD, Laurie Betito, PhD, Vena Blanchard, PhD, Joani Blank, Stephen Braveman, LMFT, Susie "Sexpert" Bright, Patrick Carnes, PhD, Rebecca Chalker, Bill Clark, Cheryl Cohen, Eli Coleman, PhD, Heather Corinna, Martha Cornog, Theresa Crenshaw, MD, Erica Curci, Rev. Beverly Dale, Laura Davis, Melanie Davis, PhD, Joseph Dhara, LMFT, Bill Dillingham, Rick DiNapoli, DO, Gail Dines, PhD, Paul Dohearty, Braxton Dutson, LCSW, CST, Carol Ellison, PhD, Madelyn Esposito-Smith, LPC, CST, Adrianna Fernandez, Helen Fisher, PhD, Sai Gaddam, PhD, John Gagnon, PhD, Cindy Gallop, Sandor Gardos, PhD, Mimi Gelb, LMFT, CST, Kim Glenn, CST, Pippa Gordon,

Staci Haines, Andrew Hancock, PhD, CST, Charla Hathaway, Julia Heiman, David Hersh, PhD, Erica Hungerford, MS, Shere Hite, Duncan James, Cacilda Jetha, MD, Paul Joannides, PhD, Virginia Johnson, Barbara and Michael Jonas, Helen Singer Kaplan, MD, PhD, Ian Kerner, PhD, Katie Kleinsasser, Elizabeth Rae Larson, PhD, Nava Lerner, Judith Levine, Amy Levinson, Mike Lew, David Ley, PhD, Sandra Leiblum, PhD, Sandra Lindholm PsyD, CST, Elizabeth Lloyd, Joseph LoPiccolo, PhD, Edward Loumann, PhD, Priscila Magossi, PhD, Thomas Maier, Rachel Maines, Wendy and Larry Maltz, LCSW, Amy Marsh, EdD, William Masters, MD, Juliane Maxwald, LP, Barry and Emily McCarthy, PhD, Kate McNulty, LCSW, CST, Heather McPherson, LMFT, CST, Michael Metz, PhD, Lisa Meyers, LCSW, CST, Laurie Mintz, PhD, Nazanin Moali, PhD, CST, Jack Morin, PhD, Stephanie Mitelman, CSE, Charles Moser, MD, Emily Nagoski, PhD, Rachel Needle, PsyD, Linda Newhart Lotz, MSW, PhD, Zita Nickeson, MEd, Kimberly Nelson, PhD, Ogi Ogas, PhD, Gina Ogden, PhD, Peggy Orenstein, Norelyn Parker, PhD, Esther Perel, LMFT, Jim Peterson, Steve Purser, Carol Queen, June Reinisch, PhD, Elizabeth Rintoul, Stella Resnick, PhD, Mary Roach, Desirée N. Robinson, LCSW-C, ACS, Deborah Rogow, Ray Rosen, PhD, Cynthia Lief Ruberg, LPCC-S, CST-S, Christopher Ryan, PhD, Dan Savage, Mark Schoen, PhD, Anne Semans, Rickey Siegel, PhD, Michael Singer, PhD, Stephen Snyder, MD, Seth Stephens-Davidowitz, PhD, Kenneth Ray Stubbs, Reay Tannahill, Tristan Taormino, Rebecca Teng, MD, Anni Tuikka, CST, Jennifer Valli, PhD, James Wadley, PhD, Cheryl Walker, APC, Laurie Watson, PhD, Linda Weiner, LCSW, Beverly Whipple, PhD, Jennifer Wiessner, LCSW, Diana Wiley, PhD, Barbara Wilhite, MFT, Cathy Winks, Kelly Wise, Ph.D., CST, Jay Wiseman, Hank Wuh, MD, and Bernie Zilbergeld, PhD.

A tip of the hat to my attorney, Bert Krages.

Heartfelt thanks to my brother, David "Deke" Castleman, the world's most hawkeyed editor.

Many thanks to my children, Jeff and Maya Castleman, for showing me how challenging—and rewarding—it can be to discuss sex with one's offspring.

Much appreciation to my dear friend David Fenton, my editor long ago at the *Ann Arbor Sun*. In 1974, with Valentine's Day approaching, he cajoled me into writing my first article about lovemaking.

Finally, perpetual thanks to my wife of almost fifty years, Anne Simons, MD. When David asked me to write that first sex piece, "How to Make Love," I refused. I was twenty-four. What did I know? But Anne urged me to tackle the subject. "Who knows?" she quipped. "You might learn something. . . ."

About the Author:
The World's Most Popular Sex Writer

DURING A CAREER spanning almost fifty years, medical journalist Michael Castleman has become the most popular sex writer on Earth. His twice-monthly blog, "All about Sex," launched in 2009 on PsychologyToday.com, attracts 700,000 views a month, and has amassed more than fifty million total views. The Q&A website he's published since 2010, GreatSexGuidance.com, has garnered more than two million.

Library Journal has called Castleman "one of the nation's top health writers." His eighteen consumer health titles include two previous sexuality guides, *Great Sex* (2004) and *Sexual Solutions* (1980), which have sold more than 600,000 copies in several languages. His other books include *The New Healing Herbs, Building Bone Vitality, Nature's Cures, An Aspirin a Day,* and many more.

From 1991 through 1995, Castleman answered the sex questions for *Playboy*'s "Advisor" column, then American men's most widely read source of sex information. From 1997 through 2007, he wrote a monthly sex research newsletter that circulated to one hundred thousand customers of Xandria, then a major sex toy marketer. His UC Berkeley journalism master's thesis, "Uncovering the Condom Industry," formed the basis for *Consumer Reports*' first-ever analysis of condoms (1980). He was also a founder of the nation's first birth control clinic for men (1976).

For the past five decades, he's written about sexuality for dozens of magazines and websites, including WebMD, *Reader's Digest, Cosmopolitan, Self, Psychology Today, Family Circle,* Salon. com, *Men's Health,* and *Men's Journal.*

Finally, he has answered more than twelve thousand sex questions—and occasionally still gets new ones.

Bibliography and References

Bibliography
The 160 books are listed at greatsexguidance.com/bibliography/.

Journal Citations
The more than 2,500 studies can be found at greatsexguidance.com/references/.

Index

#

9½ Weeks, 34
The 40-Year-Old Virgin, 143
The 120 Days of Sodom (Francoise),
339

A

AARP, xxii, 219
ABC News, 150
abdominal tenderness, 124
abductions, child, 80
abortion, 123–124
abstinence, 5, 99, 102, 105
and athletes, 14
statistics, 143
Accord Alliance, 353
acetaminophen, 207
acne, 117, 120, 295
acupuncture, 246, 307
Adam & Eve, 393
Adams, Abigail, 59–60
Adams, John, 59–60
addiction, 204. *See also* Sex addiction
craving, 397–398
increasingly severe consequences,
397–398
tolerance, 397
withdrawal distress, 397–398
Addy, 294–296
adolescence, 78. *See also* Teen
adrenaline, 13
AdultFriendFinder.com, 333
Adult Industry Medical Healthcare
Foundation (AIMHF), 381–382
adult play, 5–6
Advanced Study of Human Sexuality,
382–383
*Advancing Sexual Health for the
Christian Client* (Dale and Keller),
404
Advil, 207, 223
affair. *See* Cheating
affection, 171
AFL-CIO, 160
afterglow, 39–41
creating, 45
*Against Our Will: Men, Women, and
Rape* (Brownmiller), 159, 373
age and sex, 215–224, 297
aches and pains, 223
arousal, 219
best sex of your life, 222–223
body anxiety, 216
condoms, 219
elder abuse, 223–224
erectile dysfunction (ED), 254,
258–259

erection changes, 261–262
evolution, 220
history, 215
insertion, 219
maintaining sizzling sex, 222
male body changes, 218
masturbation, 220
nursing homes, 223–224
orgasm/ejaculation (O/E)
problems, 247
orgasm without erection, 218–219
outercourse, 218–219
premature ejaculation (PE), 245
problems with sex by age, 217
sexually transmitted infections
(STIs), 219
solo *vs.* partner sex, 220–221
statistics, 215–217
widowed women, 221
"Aggression and Sexual Behavior in
Best-Selling Pornography Videos:
A Content Analysis Update"
(Bridges), 371
aging, 6, 8, 248. *See also* Age and sex
Ailey, Alvin, 351
alcohol, 8, 13, 45–46, 140, 153, 198,
248–249, 255–257, 290, 330,
336, 343, 361, 375
central nervous system depressant,
201
and consent, 29
and hookups, 147–148
and pregnancy, 174–175
and sex through lifespan, 147
and sexual assault, 155–156
and sexual problems, 201
sobriety, 241
teens, 378
alcoholism, 388
Aleve, 202, 207, 223
Alexa.com, 385
*Allies in Healing: When the Person You
Love Was Sexually Abused as a Child*
(Davis), 92
alprostadil, 268
Amazon.com, 314
American Association of Sex
Educators, Counselors, and
Therapists (AASECT), xv, 226–
228, 401, 405
American Association of University
Women, 160
American Institute of Bisexuality, 351
American Journal of Public Health,
103
American Psychiatric Association, 18,
339, 354, 400

American Psychological Association,
13
American Revolution, 332, 353
American Society of Plastic Surgery,
277
American Urological Association
(AUA), 258
Amnesty International, 187
amphetamines, 204
amyl nitrate, 263
anabolic steroids, 256
Anafranil, 203
anal beads, 318–319, 326
anal itching, 128
anal play, 6, 38, 55, 250, 312. *See also*
Anilingus
one wants it, the other doesn't, 328
teen, 101
uninformed, 308
Anal Pleasure and Health (Morin),
325
anal sex, 322–329
and AIDS, 323
anatomy, 324–325
control by recipient, 327–328
and enemas, 325
and hemorrhoids, 324
history, 322
and HIV, 324
hygiene, 325
lubrication, 324–327
and orgasm, 328
pain, 327
popularity of, 322–324
pornography, 360–361
receiving and homosexuality,
328–329
safety, 361
sex coach, 329
sex therapy, 329
solo, 325–326
statistics, 345
anal toys, 317. *See also* Anal beads;
Butt plugs
androgens, 8, 291, 295
patches, 295
anemia, 117
anesthesia reactions, 122–123
anesthetics, topical, 246
angelica root, 208
angiotensin converting enzyme
(ACE), 202
anilingus, 323, 326, 345
anorexia and pregnancy, 174
antianxiety drugs, 291
antibiotics, 130
anticipation, 40

antidepressants, 46, 203, 245–246, 248, 255, 291
  and gingko, 206
  and pregnancy, 174
  and sexual problems, 201
antihistamines, 202
antihypertensives, 202–203
Anti-Slavery International, 187
antiviral drugs, 130–132
anus, 38
  lubrication, 318
anxiety, 14, 35, 136, 204, 285, 291, 297, 305, 308, 388, 396, 405
  sexual, 220
aphrodisiacs, 206–208
  cocoa and chocolate, 206
  coffee, 206
  damiana, 206
  and erection medication, 264
  ginkgo, 206
  ginseng, 207
  guarana, 206
  maca, 207
  maté, 206
  muira puama, 207
  Yohimbine, 207
  Zestra, 208
Aphrodyne, 267
Apollo, 34
appetite loss, 132
Archives of Sexual Behavior, 4, 149–150, 345, 372
ArginMax, 206, 267
Aristophanes, 233
Aristotle, 284
Arizona State University, 158, 291
Arnot, Bob, 14
arousal, 219, 293, 358. See also Desire and arousal issues
  excitement, 241
  female, 48, 278
  four phase process in men, 241
  lack of, 48
  orgasm/ejaculation, 241
  plateau, 241
  resolution, 241
  slow, 66
  without pornography, 394
The Art of Sex Coaching (Britton), 226
Asexual Visibility and Education Network (AVEN), 353–354
Ash Wednesday, 331
asking for what you want, 41–46
aspirin, 207, 223, 267
"A Study of Sexuality and Health among Older Adults in the United States" (Lindau), 18
atherosclerosis, 255, 263
atherosclerotic plaque, 11
Atromid, 204
attachment, 60
Attorney General's Commission on Pornography (Meese Commission), 374
attraction, 5, 35, 42, 82, 206, 261, 349, 354, 366
Auburn University, 127
Augustus, Flavius, 95
Austen, Jane, 368
avanafil. See Stendra
Avenue Q, 364

aversion to sex, 227
Avodart, 256

B
baby, sex after, 175–176
  anxiety, 175
  depression, 175
  hiatus, 176
  hormonal changes, 175
  nursing, 175
  priorities, 175
  sleep schedule, 175
  vaginal pain, 176
Baby and Child Care (Spock), 78
Bacchanalia, 331
Bacchus, 331
backache, 124
bacterial vaginosis (BV), 73, 276
  and pregnancy, 174
baldness, 204
balls, blue, 138
Barbach, Lonnie, xv
Barber, L. L., 150
Barbie, 287
Barrymore, Drew, 351
Bartholin's glands, 284
basal body temperature (BBT), 115
baseball analogy, 137
Bass, Ellen, 91
Bassinger, Kim, 34
Basson, Rosemary, 170–171, 278, 296
bathing together, 218, 261
baths, hot, 13
Battered Wives (Martin), 159
Baylor University, 396
BBW/BBM, 11–12
BDSM, 5–6, 64, 67, 304, 323, 327, 338–346, 398. See also Nipple clamps
  alcohol, 343
  blindfolds, 344. 168
  bondage, 334, 338, 340, 343, 345, 372
  clubs, 334
  communication, 346
  consent, 342
  contracts, 346
  detering sexual assault, 342
  discipline, 338
  domination-submission (D/s), 6, 338
  exhibitionism, 345
  hair pulling, 338, 344–346, 371
  history of, 339
  and intimacy, 344, 346
  limits, 346
  masochism, 339
  mental health, 341
  popularity in fantasy, 339–340
  pornography, 372
  role play, 6, 345
  rules, 343
  sadism, 339
  sadomasochism (SM), 338–339
  safe words, 342–343, 346
  spanking, 6, 168, 218, 321, 345–346, 371–372
  starting, 343–344
  statistics, 345–346
  submissive in charge, 343

toys, 317, 321
  trust, 338
  varieties, 338–339
  vs kink, 338
  whipping/flogging, 6, 321, 338, 340, 345–346, 348, 372
  and women, 345–346
Beach Boys, 221
Becoming Orgasmic: A Sexual and Personal Growth Program for Women (Heiman and LoPiccolo), 250, 302
Beigi, M., 289
"Beliefs about Women's Vibrator Use: Results from a Nationally Representative Probability Survey in the United States" (Herbenick), 312
Bemoan, Rob, 14
benign prostate hyperplasia (BPH), 256
ben-wa balls, 9, 317, 319
Berkowitz, Eric, 96
Bernstein, Leonard, 351
Bible, 3–4, 16, 26, 95, 182, 215, 349, 366
A Billion Wicked Thoughts: What the Internet Tells Us about Sex and Relationships (Ogas and Gaddam), 364
biofeedback, 307
birth control, 107–124
  abortion, 123–124
  barrier, 113–114
  cervical cap, 112–114, 129
  charting, 107, 114
  condoms for men, 110–111, 114, 129, 131, 140, 151. See also Condoms
  contraceptive irresponsibility, 389
  diaphragm, 107, 112–114, 129, 151
  effectiveness, 107–108
  emergency, 121
  female condoms, 129
  fertility awareness, 114–115
  hormonal, 290–291
  implant, 120
  injected/Dept-Provera, 118–119
  internal condoms, 111–112
  intrauterine devices (IUDs), 117–118, 128, 399
  IUD, 107, 109
  libido, 290–291
  menopause, 213
  morning after, 109
  NuvaRing, 119
  outercourse, 107, 109, 114, 127
  patch/Ortho Evra, 119–120
  pill, 48, 115–117, 128, 151, 291, 293, 305, 378, 399
  responsibility for, 107
  spermicide, 107, 111–113
  sponge, 113–114
  tubal ligation, 123
  vasectomy, 122
  withdrawal, 109
Bisexual Center, 350
"Bisexual Chic: Anyone Goes" (Newsweek), 350
bisexuality, 348–350

coming out twice, 351
history, 349
myths, 350
pornography, 383
prejudice, 350
promiscuity, 350
Bisson, M. A., 149
Bivocals, 350
Bivona, Jenny, 68–69
black cohosh, 213
bladder, 248, 254, 312
control, 391
bleeding, 267
blindfolds, 168, 344
blindness, 130
blood
clotting, 115, 117, 119–120, 264
flow, 11, 13, 48, 206, 211, 218, 235
pressure, 48, 116–117, 120, 218, 255, 263, 267, 391, 3617
Bloomberg News, 215
Blumberg, Eric, 289
body
anxiety, ways to minimize, 216
image, 290, 297
bondage. *See* BDSM
bone density loss, 118, 120
BongaCams.com, 367, 385
Bono, Chaz, 3
Bono, Sonny, 3
The Book of Love, Laughter, and Romance (Jonas and Jonas), 62, 181
books about sex for kids, 81–84
anatomy, 82–83
borage seed, 208
Borgia, Cesare, 331
Boston University, 13, 127, 379
Boston Women's Health Collective, xv
Bowling Green State University, 389
Boys and Girls Clubs, 103
breakups, 150
breast. *See also* Cancer, breast
discomfort, 118
enlargement, 204
how to caress, 277
mammary intercourse, 345
pain, 120
play, 137
size, 117, 279
surgery, cosmetic, 277
tenderness, 117, 119–121, 204
breast fascination
fashion, 277
men's, 275, 277, 284
women, 277
breastfeeding, 116
breast tenderness, 116
breathing, deep, 33, 242
bremelanotide, 294–295
Brennan, Peter, 78
Brents, Barbara, 187
Bridges, A., 371, 407
Brigham Young University, 164, 394, 396, 398
BrightDesire.com, 410
British Medical Journal, 215
Britton, Patti, 44, 226
brothels, 331

Brownmiller, Susan, 159, 373
Brown University, 11–13
bruising, 267
bupropion. *See* Wellbutrin
Buss, D. M., 4
butt plugs, 318–319, 326

C

caffeine, 238
calcium citrate supplements, 306
Calgary University, 153–154
California Health Interview Survey, 348
California State University, 324–325
Cal State Los Angeles, 232, 275
Cal State San Marcos, 14
Cal State University, 372
cancer, 13, 35, 305. *See also* Prostate cancer
breast, 115–117, 195–196, 205, 214, 294
cervical, 73, 118, 129, 276
endometrial, 117–120
lung, 14, 255
ovarian, 117, 120
penile, 73
uterine, 197
canes. *See* BDSM
cannabis, 147, 202
high-CBD, 207, 223
and pregnancy, 175
Canticles, 366
cardiovascular system, 8, 11, 13, 192, 205
Carell, Steve, 143, 227
Carey, A. G., 145
Carey, M. P., 148
Carnegie Mellon University, 35
Carnes, Patrick, 387, 392–393, 398–399
Carnival, 331
Case Western Reserve University, 396
catastrophizing, 404
CCBill, 367
Celexa, 203, 255
celibacy, 146
Center for Sexual Health, 265
Centers for Disease Control and Prevention (CDC), xviii, 102, 104, 126, 154, 276, 323, 378
cervix, 234
cervical mucus, 115, 118–120, 276
chafing, 308
Chalker, Rebecca, 279
Chamberlain,. Wilt, 14
Chapin, Henry Dwight, 30
Chapman University, 298
cheating, 61, 165, 245, 274
and pornography, 389
and STIs, 125
Cher, 3
chest pain, 116
Child Pornography Prevention Act, 79
children. *See also* Teen; Toddlers and preschoolers
protecting, 81
and sex play, xx, 6, 77
children, talking to about sex, 81–82
answering questions, 82
books for kids, 84

brevity, 82
continue talking, 82
guiding them to enjoy sex, 84
masturbation, 83
oral sex, 84
orgasm, 83
practice, 82
silence, 81
ways to make love, 83
your manner, 82
child sexual abuse, xviii, 298. *See also* Pedophilia
see also pornography, child
decline of, 87
dissociation, 88
flashbacks, 89
gender, 87
impact of, 88–89
loss of control, 88
and masturbation, 16
and pornography, 389
and pornography actresses, xviii, 381–382
repulsed by sex, 88
sexual recklessness, 88
and silence, 81
statistics, 86
and trust, 88
child sexual abuse recovery, 86–93
anger, 91
believing, 91
celibacy, 89
cognitive behavioral therapy (CBT), 91
confronting abuser, 92
flashbacks, 91
grief, 91
healing, 87–88
healing path, 89
how men can help survivors, 92–93
masturbation, 89–90, 93
men, 87
mindfulness meditation (MM), 91
not your fault, 91
realization, 91
recalling, 91
rediscovering partner lovemaking, 91
resolution, 92
self-forgiveness, 92
somatic therapy, 89
speaking up, 91
stages, 91–92
talk therapy, 89
triggers, 91
chills, 124, 132
Chlamydia trachomatis, 128
cholesterol, 12, 116, 204, 218, 255
chordee, 237
chronic illness and sex, 189–198
breast cancer, 195–196
coaching, 190
diabetes, 191
diabetic erectile dysfunction, 192
expanding definition of sex, 189
heart attack, 193
hysterectomy, 197–198
information and support, 189–190
lubricants and sex toys, 190
osteoarthritis (OA), 190–191

prostate cancer, 193–195
staying healthy, 190
therapy, 190
Cialis, 192, 195, 215, 240, 263–264.
    See Viagra
cimetidine, 202
Cimicifuga racemosa, 213
Cipralex, 203
circumcision, 73–76
    AIDS prevention, 73
    erectile dysfunction, 75
    female health, 73
    impact on sex, 74
    penile cancer, 73
    phimosis, 73
    and religion, 73–74
    sensitivity, 74–75
    sexual impairment, 74
    urinary tract infection, 73
cirrhosis, 115
cisgender (cis), xix, 3
Citracal, 306
Civil War, 151
Cleland, John, 365
Cleveland Clinic, 192
Clift, Montgomery, 351
"Clinical and Biopsychosocial
    Determinants of Sexual
    Dysfunction in Middle-Aged
    Men and Older Australian Men"
    (Martin), 253
Clinton, Bill, 134
The Clitoral Truth (Chalker), 279
clitoris, xxii, 37, 105, 141, 208, 279
    caressing, 280
    clitoral enlargement, 295
    clitoral kisses, 300
    clitoral shaft, 279
    clitoral stimulation, 141, 243
    clitoral system, 279–282
    clitoral system, development, 279
    clitoral system, history, 281
    crura, 37
    glans, 282
    and pleasure, 237
    sensitivity, 12, 54, 201
    shaft, 37
    size, 281
The Clouds (Aristophanes), 233
coaching, 302, 306, 313, 359
    professional, 226
coaching, mutual, 42, 138, 141–142,
    191, 222
    afterglow, creating, 45
    asking questions, 45
    chronic illness, 190
    compliments, 44
    and masturbation, 46
    and sexual quality, 179
    sexual quality over time, 178
    "yes," 45
cocaine, 174, 204
cock rings, 236, 317, 319
cohabitation, 178
coital alignment technique (CAT),
    301–302
colds, avoiding through sex, 190
Cole, Martin John, 143
coleus, 208
colonial New England, 151
Columbia University, 104

Coming Home, 198–200
commitment, 149
communication, 42, 349
communism, 332
"A Comparative Study of Sexual
    Dysfunctions before and after
    Menopause" (Beigi and Fahami),
    289
Compulsive Sexual Behavior
    Inventory, 399
concentration problems, 211
conception, 392
Concordia University, xvii
condoms, xiv, 49, 57, 105–106,
    110–111
    advantages, 111
    and aging, 219
    carrying, 140
    disadvantages, 111
    estimated use, 111
    and fellatio, 110
    internal, 111–112
    interruption, 110
    male willingness to use, 110
    myths about, 110–111
    and sensation, 99, 110
    side effects, 111
    and spermicide, 111
    and STIs, 110
    teens, xxii, 103, 378
    types, 110
    using, 111
cone biopsy, 129
Conroy, Pat, 161
consent, 25–29, 288
    affirmative consent, 27
    affirmative consent and sexual
        assault, 27
    and alcohol, 29, 153
    and better sex, 28
    body language, 29
    history of, 25–27
    and mixed messages, 29
    "no means no," 27
    and nonmonogamy, 334
    nonverbal, 27
    and rape, 26
    and sexual assault, 153–154
consent, age of, 94–98
    child marriage, 96–97
    current, 96
    history, 95–96
    statutory rape laws, 94–95
constipation, 295
Consumer Reports, xiv
contact lenses, 117
continuous positive airway-pressure
    machine (CPAP), 15
contraception. *See* Birth control
Contraceptive Technology (Hatcher),
    108, 290
Coolidge, Calvin, 59
Cooper, M. I., 150
Copen, C. E., 348
Corinna, Heather, 106
Cornell, 192, 264, 269
cortisol, 13, 35, 385
cougars, 97
counseling, relationship, 293, 306

*The Courage to Heal: A Guide for
    Women of Child Sexual Abuse* (Bass
    and Davis), 87, 91
courtship, ongoing, 296
Cowper's gland, 48
cramping, 124, 128, 295
cranberries, 127
Creighton University, 405
Crime and Punishment (Dostoevsky),
    185
Crimes Against Children Research
    Center, 86
crones, 215
cryosurgery, 129
cryptococcal meningitis, 132
C-tactile fibers, 31
cuddling, 39–40, 217–218, 327, 394
    and sexual quality, 179
cunnilingus, xxi, 138, 141, 218,
    273–274, 299–300, 315, 326,
    409. *See also* Oral sex
    and anal play, 55
    anticipation, 53
    coaching, 53
    combined with massage, 54
    gentleness, 53
    and hand massage, 54
    man's guide to, 52–54
    and menstruation, 54
    and orgasm, 179, 298
    positioning, 53
    and sexual quality, 179
    and spermicides, 112
    statistics, 345–346
    technique, 53–54
    teen, 101
Curtis, Jamie Lee, 185
Cyber Civil Rights Initiative, 384
cycling, 258

D
Dale, Beverly, 404
Damiana aphrodisiaca, 206
Dangerfield, Rodney, 66, 183
Danocrine, 204
Darkness to Light, 86
Dartmouth, 5
dating. *See* Hookups and dating
David (Michelangelo), 233
Davis, Laura, 87–88, 91–92
Davison, Audrey, 223
daydreams, 64
Dean, Alisha, 94
Deep Throat, 57
dehydroepiandrosterone (DHEA),
    295, 307
Delafield, Alice, 30
Deliverance (Dickey), 161
dementia, 132, 214, 294
D'Emilio, John, 77
Dennison University, 385
Densen-Gerber, Judianne, 79
depression, 14, 35, 116–118, 120,
    205, 238, 248, 255, 291, 305,
    308, 388
de Sade, Marquis, 339
desire, 10, 204
    and arousal issues, 59
desire, women's, 288–296
    age, 290
    alcohol, 290

birth control pill, 291
body image, 290
boosting, 293
drugs, 294–295
exercise, 293
and good sex, order of, 296
health, mental, 293
health, physical, 293
highly sexual women, 288–290
history, 288
hormonal contraception, 290–291
illness, 291
income drop, 291
instruction about risk factors, 293
low androgens, 291
low desire risk factors, 290–291
menopause, sudden, 290
and menopause, 292
and menstrual cycle, 291–292
mindfulness meditation, 293
mood-altering drugs, 293
mood-altering medications, 291
novelty, 294
prevalence of, 289
progressive muscle relaxation
    (PMR) exercises, 293
relationship counseling, 293
relationship duration, 290
relationship misery, 290
risk factors, 293
scheduling, 294
and seasons, 292
sedentary lifestyle, 290
self-help, 294
sexual abuse or assault, 291
slow to develop, 296
stress, anxiety and depression, 291
stress, work, 292
talk, 294
thoughts, 294
time, 294
touch, 294
vaginal dryness and pain, 291
weight loss, 293
desire differences, 164–172, 227
affairs, 165
and affection, 171
age, 165
child sex abuse or sexual trauma,
    165
communicating about, 169
complacency, 167
compromise, 169–170
contempt, avoiding, 169
cost of, 167
count your blessings, 168
divorce, 165
education, 165
familiarity, 167
flexibility, 168
and gender, 167
good will, 171
happiness, 165
health, 165
hot-and-heavy period ending,
    166–167
humor, 169
individual differences, 165
"I" statements, 169
libido, unchanging nature of, 169
listening, 169

long-term cohabitation, 165
negotiating sexual frequency, 168
not in the mood, 170
options, 169
power, experiencing, 168–169
pregnancy, 165
relationship problems, 167
relationship stage, 165
religion, 165
remarriage, 165
reporting differences, 166
responsibilities, 167
routines, 166
scheduling sex, 170–172
separating from love, 169
shared housework, 165
single parenthood, 165
succinctness, 169
talking to friends, 168
teammates, 169
therapy for, 172
things that don't influence it, 164
things that influence it, 165
what you really want, 168
who controls the sex, 167–168
working on other issues, 169
young children, 165
The Deuce, 410
DeVito, Danny, 313
Devon, Molly, 343
diabetes, 12–13, 48, 116, 191, 238,
    248–249, 263, 265
blood sugar control, 192
diabetic erectile dysfunction, 192
diabetic vaginal dryness and
    orgasm problems, 193
erection medication, 192
healthy lifestyle, 193
lubricants, 193
sex therapy, 192–193
vacuum constricting device
    (VCD), 192
vibrators, 193
Diagnostic and Statistical Manual of
    Mental Disorder (DSM), 18, 339,
    354, 400–401
Dialantin, 204
Diamox, 204
diarrhea, 121, 128, 295
Dickey, James, 161
Dickinson, Robert, 282–283, 297
diet, 8, 11–12, 218, 235, 257, 324
low-oxalate, 306–307
Mediterranean, 11
and menopause, 212
and pregnancy, 174
vegetarian, 11, 18
Digoxin, 204
dildo, 288, 317, 319
anal, 318–319
strap-on, 267, 319–320
teledildonics/cyberdildonics, 23
Dionysus, 331
dirty old men, 215
disabilities, 6, 198–200, 359
children with disabilities and
    sex, 85
and desire, 199
masturbation, 199
myths, 198–199
orgasm, 200

privacy, 199
and real sex, 199
and sexuality, 198–199
sizzling sex, 199
surrogate partners, 200
and virginity, 144
discharge, 118, 124
divorce, 61
and pornography, 389
rate, xxii, 377
dizziness, 267
Dodson, Betty, 31, 36, 234, 237, 327
"Does Drinking Lead to Sex? Daily
    Alcohol-Sex Behaviors and
    Expectancies among College
    Students" (Patrick and Maggs),
    147
Don't Call It Love (Carnes), 398
dopamine, 35, 60, 64
boosting, 61
Dostoevsky, Fyodor, 185
douching, 54, 112
dangers of, 276
droit du seigneur, 95–96
drugs, 45–46, 48, 201–209
abuse, 255
antidepressants, 203
aphrodisiacs, 206–208
blood pressure medication,
    202–203
narcotics, cocaine, amphetamines,
    204
other prescription drugs, 204
over-the-counter, 202
pain relievers, 207, 223
seizure medications, 204
testosterone replacement, 204–205
tranquilizers, antianxiety, and
    psychiatric drugs, 203
Tribulus terrestris, 208–209
Duke University, 11–12
Duncan, Isadore, 351
Durex, 340
dutasteride, 204, 256
Dwrokin, Andrea, 374
dysparunia, 46, 304

E
E. coli, 326
Economic Polic Institute, 159
Edison, Thomas, 14
education level, 297, 300, 336
Effexor, 203
ego, male, 43
Egypt, 330–331
Eichel, Edward, 301
ejaculation, 241, 365
difficulties, 204
ejaculatory control, 244
female, 38, 54, 280–281, 284
male, 38
problems, 220
retrograde, 58, 248–249
surgery to prevent, 58
and vasectomy, 122
elder abuse, 223–224
Elders, Jocelyn, 18
ella, 121
embryonic cells, 37
Emory University, 105
"An Enchanting Evening," 180

Endocrine Society, 205
endometriosis, 117, 120, 204, 305
endorphins, 35
enemas, 325
Enlightenment, 288
epispadias, 55–56
Equal Employment Opportunity
  Commission (EEOC), 157–158,
  160
Equal Rights Advocates, 160
erectile dysfunction (ED), xvi, 11–12,
  14–15, 31, 74–75, 205, 207–208,
  211, 218–220, 248–249, 252
  acute illness or injury, 255
  and age, 253–254
  alcohol, 255–256
  Alprostadil, 268
  anabolic steroids, 256
  antidepressants, 255
  asking for touch, 266
  atherosclerosis, 255
  benign prostate hyperplasia (BPH)
    drugs, 256
  communication, 266
  depression, 255
  diabetes, 192, 256
  dildos, strap-on, 267
  fantasies, 266
  ginkgo, 267
  ginseng, 267
  healthy lifestyle, 266
  Kegel exercises, 267
  L-arginine, 267
  low-intensity shockwave therapy
    (LIST), 268
  maca, 268
  male and female views, 260
  and masturbation, 20
  most common problem, 238
  neurological disorders, 256
  obesity, 256
  obstructive sleep apnea, 256
  penile implants, 268–269
  penis extenders or prosthetic penis
    attachments (PPAs), 267
  penis pumps/vacuum constriction
    devices, 266
  penis rings, 266
  periodontitis, 256
  pornography, 361, 389
  prostate cancer, 193–195
  prostate cancer treatments, 256
  prostate enlargement, 256
  risk factors, 255–257
  saffron, 268
  sedentary lifestyle, 256
  sex coaching, 267
  sex therapy, 267
  statistics, 252–253
  stress, 255
  tobacco, 255
  and tobacco, 201
  treatments, 266–268
  vitamin D deficiency, 256–257
  Yohimbine, 267
erection, 365
  alcohol, 257
  bathing or showering, 261
  changes with age, 261–262
  cycling, 258
  diet, 257

dissatisfaction, 253
dissatisfaction enhancing
  lovemaking, 262
and doctor appointments,
  262–263
dreams, 254
exercise, 257
failure, 259–260
flossing, 257
impairment, 202–203, 205
impairment and aging, 258–259
loss, 203
love nest, 261
maintaining firm, 257
mechanics of, 254
medical history, 262
medication, 262–265
men as sex machines, 259
morning, 254–255
myths, 259–260
obstructive sleep apnea, 257
and orgasm, 260
oxygen, 254
patience, 261
pornography, 359–360
problems, 217, 227
psychological history, 262
quality time, 261
quickies and spontaneous sex, 261
and refractory period (RP), 262
sex coaching, 262
sex therapy, 262
sexual arousal, 254
sexual performance, 259
stress management, 257
testosterone measurements,
  262–263
tests, 262
tobacco, 257
urination, 254
vitamin D, 257
weak, 20
weight, 257
women and porn, 260–261
and women's satisfaction, 260
erection medication, 263–265
  advantages, 263
  cost, 265
  and damaged relationships, 265
  disadvantages, 263–264
  effectiveness, 264–265
  fatality, 263
  instant erections, 265
  on the internet, 269
  not aphrodisiacs, 265
  popularity, 264
  side effects, 265
  upset the status quo, 266
  use by older men, 264
ErikaLust.com, 410
erotic pleasure, 4
Eschenbach, David, 276
Esidrix, 202
Eskalith, 203
estrogen, 48, 116, 119, 210–211,
  294, 357
  hormone replacement therapy
    (HRT), 205
  hormone therapy (HRT), 204
  topical, 213
  vaginal cream, 295

The Ethical Slut: A Practical Guide to
  Polyamory, Open Relationships, and
  Other Adventures (Hardy), 334
Eugenides, Jeffrey, 353
evening primrose, 208
evolution, 220, 363–364
exercise, 8–10, 12–13, 235, 241,
  257, 293, 324
  aerobic, 9, 13
  menopause, 213
  regularity, 10
exhibitionism, 345, 360, 382
experimenting, 394
exploitation of women, 147–148
eyes, dry, 116

F
Facebook, 159, 393
Fahami, F., 289
Fanny Hill (Cleland), 365
fantasies, 6, 46, 64–69, 217, 266,
  394
  accepting, 66
  adjusting, 242
  BDSM, 339–340
  and dopamine, 64
  and guilt, 66
  guilt avoidance, 68
  and hypnosis, 67
  as meditation, 64
  and mental health, 64
  most popular, 65–66
  partial fulfillment, 67
  pornography, 69
  rape/force, 67–69
  realizing, 67
  sexual desirability, 68
  sexual openness, 68–69
  sharing, 66–67
  simmering, 66
  time lost to due to pornography,
    392–393
  and visualization, 67
  vs. reality, 64
fatigue, 12, 116–117, 120–121,
  124, 205
FBI, 94
fellatio, 55–58, 218, 273–274, 319,
  409. See also Oral sex
  coaching, 56
  and condoms, 110
  ejaculation in mouth, 57–58
  gagging, 55, 57
  guided, 250
  and hygiene, 55–56
  and massage, 56
  and sexual quality, 179
  statistics, 345
  stop-start, 244
  technique, 56
  teen, 101
  and teeth, 56
  uncircumcised men, 73
Female Sexual Pain Disorders
  (Goldstein), 305
FeministPornGuide.com, 410
Femme Productions, 410
fertility, 254
  awareness, 108, 114–115, 121
fertilization, 114
fetus. See Pregnancy

fetuses, multiple, 174
fever, 118, 124, 132
fibroids, 116–117, 197
Field, Tiffany, 35
Fielder, R. L., 148
Fifty Shades of Grey (James), 232, 340–341, 346, 368
Fifty Shades of Kink (Taormino), 343
Finasteride, 204, 256
fingering, 297–298
Finkelhor, David, 86–87
Fisher, Helen, 60–61
fitness, 391
The Flame and the Flower (Woodiwiss), 368
Fleet, 325
Fleischhauer-Hardt, Helga, 79
Fleshlight, 250, 319
flibanserin, 294–295
floggers, 321. *See also* BDSM
Florey Adelaid Male Aging Study (FAMAS), 253
flossing, 257
fluid retention, 267
flushing, 263, 265, 267, 296
folic acid, 246
Fonda, Jane, 198–200
Food and Drug Administration, xx, 204, 207, 252, 295
foreplay, 31, 36
    extended, 32
    rushed, 31
foreskin, 218
Fortune and Men's Eyes (Herbert), 161
For Yourself: The Fulfillment of Female Sexuality (Barbach), xv
Francoise, Donatien Alphonse, 339
Freedman, Estelle B., 77
Free University of Berlin, 186
frequency of sex, 5, 273
Freud, Sigmund, 18, 38, 78, 239, 281, 299, 339
Friday, Nancy, 64
friends with benefits (FWB), 149
fruits and vegetables, 11
Fualaau, Vili, 97
fungus, 204

G

G6PD enzyme deficiency, 126
Gaddam, Sai, 364
Galen, 279, 284
gallbladder disease, 116, 119
gambling, 388
Garbo, Greta, 351
Garcia, J. R., 146
gardening, 13
garlic, 267
Gates, G. J., 348
gay. *See* LGBTQ
gender, xix
    affirming surgery, 3
    identity, 351–354
General Social Survey (GSS), 111, 145, 348, 374, 388
Genesis, 4, 16, 25, 185
genital irritation, 128
genital itching or burning, 128–129
genital warts. *See* Human papillomavirus infection (HPV)
Gentle Path in the Meadows, 387

Georgia State University, 156
Giardia, 326
ginkgo, 267
ginseng, 267
glands, swollen, 132
glans, 244
Global Alliance Against Trafficking in Women, 187
Goldstein, Andrew, 305
Good Morning America, xiv
Good Vibrations after Dark, 410
Google, 159, 167, 231
Google Analytics, 367
Gould, Terry, 332
Grafenberg, Ernst, 282–283
Graham, Sylvester, 18
Grant, Hugh, 185
Granville, Joseph Mortimer, 314
Gray, John, 273
Great Sex (Castleman), xv–xvi
GreatSexGuidance.com, xvi, 134, 218, 328
Gregor, Thomas, 182
group sex, 393
    parties, 234
G-spot, 37, 280–283
    caressing, 283
    and ejaculation, 284
    intercourse, 283
    locating, 283
    orgasm, 299
The G-Spot and Other Recent Discoveries about Human Sexuality (Ladas, Whipple, and Perry), 283
Guardian, 348
Guelph University, 153–154
guilt, 396
gum disease, 256
Guttmacher Institute, 104

H

hags, 215
Haines, Staci, 88–91
Hall, G. Stanley, 78
hall passes, 183
hand jobs, xx, 83, 101, 105, 107, 109, 127, 134, 137–138, 174, 184, 236, 252, 298, 300, 302, 335, 345–346
    dry hand, 244
    lubricated, 244
    and pregnancy, 174
    statistics, 345
Handman, Heidi, 78
happiness, 5
Hardy, Janet W., 334
Harry, Debbie, 351
Harvard, 21, 194, 212, 405
Hastert, Dennis, 81
Hatcher, R.A., 108
having sex *vs.* making love, 142
Hawkes, John, 144, 200
hay fever, 202
headaches, 116, 118, 120, 263, 265, 267, 296
Healing Sex: A Mind-Body Approach (Haines), 88, 90
health, mental, 19, 21, 65. 69, 175, 226, 277, 288, 293, 334, 339, 352, 381–382, 389, 396, 398, 401
    BDSM, 341

female porn actresses, 382–383
    and nonmonogamy, 334
health, poor health and sexual quality, 179
Healy, Dylan, 94
hearing and vision loss, 263
heart
    disease, 115–116, 122, 205, 214, 294
    rate, 267
heart attacks, 10, 117, 119–120, 264–265
    healthy lifestyle, 193
    lifestyle, 193
    make love regularly, 193
    sex after, 193
    sex therapy, 193
    talk to doctor, 193
heartburn, 202
Hebrew Home, 223
Heche, Anne, 351
heels, high, 278
Heiman, Julia, 250, 302
hemorrhoids, 129, 324, 327
    and pregnancy, 175
hepatitis, 115
Herbenick, D., 18, 24, 216, 312
Herbert, John, 161
heroin, 388
Herpalieve, 131
herpes, 73, 308
heterosexuality, xix, 6
hickeys. *See* BDSM
Hill, James, 12
Hippocrates, 35
Hirsch, Alan, 34
Hitachi, 316
Hitachi's Magic Wand, 314
Hite, Shere, xv
The Hite Report: A Nationwide Study of Female Sexuality (Hite), xv
Holiday, Billie, 351
Hollywood, 359
honesty, 66, 67, 140
honeymoon cystitis, 127
"Hooking Up: Casual Sex Facts" (Adam & Eve), 393
"Hook-Up Behavior: A Biopsychosocial Perspective" (Garcia and Reiber), 146
hookups and dating, 145–152
    activity during, 146
    alcohol, 147–148
    celibacy, 145–146
    and commitment, 149
    exploitation of women, 147–148
    friends with benefits (FWB), 149
    history, 151
    intercourse frequency, 146
    reasons for, 148
    regrets, 148
Hope Springs, 227
hormone replacement therapy (HRT), 213–214, 294
hormones, 3, 13, 35, 60, 352
hot flashes, 210, 391
    dietary changes, 212
    minimizing, 211–213
    soy foods, 211–212
    vitamin E, 212
How I Was Born, 82

How Many People are Lesbian, Gay, Bisexual, and Transgender? (Gates), 348
Human Sexual Inadequacy (Masters and Johnson), xiv
Hunt, Helen, 144, 200
Hyde, Z., 220
hydrochlorothiazide, 202
Hydrodiuril, 202
hymen, 135–136
    checking your own, 139
    imperforate, 136, 305
    piercing, 135
hypersexual, 405
hyperthyroidism, 238, 241
hypnosis, 67, 307
hypospadias, 55–56, 237
hypothalamus, 60
hysterectomy, 197–198, 211, 285
    arousal, 197
    impact of, 197
    lubrication, 197
    sexual satisfaction after, 197
hysteria, 313–314

I

IAXX.com, 371
ibuprofen, 207, 223
Idaho State University, 341, 389, 409
Illinois Primary Health Care Association, 372
Illinois State University, 407
illness and injury, acute, 189, 255, 291, 293
imagery, guided, 213
immunoglobulin A (IgA), 190
impotence, 252
Incarnation Institute for Sex and Faith, 404
income, 297
    drop, 291
Indiana University, 6, 18, 22, 24, 49, 101, 131, 134, 297–298, 308, 311, 313, 321–323, 327, 333, 340, 393
individuation, 102
Industrial Revolution, 95–96, 367, 395
infidelity. *See also* Cheating; Monogamy
    definition, 184
    prevalence, 183–185
insertion
    deep penetration, 237
    shallow, 236
    slow, 236–237
    too deep, 308
insomnia, 295
intercourse
    age at first, 273
    mock, 302
    rushed, 307
    stop-start, 244
interest in sex, 217
    lack of, 220
International Classification of Diseases (ICD, World Health Organization), 401
International Institute for Trauma and Addiction Professionals (IITAP), 405

International Labor Organization, xix
International Professional Surrogates Association (IPSA), 144, 200
internet, xvi, 364
Internet Safety 101, 364
Intersex Society of North America, 353
interstitial cystitis, 305
intestinal upset, 208
In the Shadows of the Net: Breaking Free of Compulsive Online Sexual Behavior (Carnes), 387
intimacy, xiii, xviii, 4–5, 23–24, 37, 92, 139, 180, 199, 202, 211, 240, 247, 249, 278, 280, 320, 322–323, 328–330, 335, 344–346, 354, 358, 390, 407–409
Intimate Matters (D'Emilio and Freedman), 77
Intrarosa, 307
irritability, 116–117, 120, 267
irritable bowel syndrome, 305
"Is 10% of the Population Really Gay?" (*Guardian,* Spiegelhalter), 348

J

James, E. L., 232, 340–341, 346, 368
Jameson, Jenna, 381
Johns Hopkins University, 400
Johnson, Virginia, xiv, xviii, xx, 47, 144, 226, 240–241, 244, 278–279, 281, 284, 288
Jonas, Barbara, 62, 180–181
Jonas, Michael, 62, 180–181
Jones, Lisa, 86–87
Jones, Tommy Lee, 227
Jong, Erica, 183
Joplin, Janis, 351
Joshua, 185
Journal of Bisexuality, 350
Journal of Nursing and Midwifery Research, 289
Journal of Sex, 145
Journal of Sex and Marital Therapy, 148, 312, 407
Journal of Sexual Medicine, 216–217, 220, 252–253, 289, 312
Journal of Social Evolutionary, and Cultural Psychology 2, 146
Journal of the American Medical Association, 135, 388
Judah, 185
Justine (Francoise), 339

K

Kahlo, Frida, 351
Kahr, Brett, 65
Kama Sutra, 51, 239, 284, 339
Kanka, Megan, 79
Kaufman, Miriam, 200
Keaton, Diane, 193
Keeler, Christine, 332
Keener, Catherine, 143
Kegel, Arnold, 9
Kegel exercises, 9, 195, 218, 248–249, 267, 280, 285, 307, 319
Keller, Rachel, 404
Kellogg, John Harvey, 18
Kerner, Ian, 55

Ketoconazole, 204
key parties, 332
kink, xv, 61, 64, 67, 83, 85, 107, 109, 168, 174, 218, 232, 252, 259, 340–342, 345–346, 372
    vs BDSM, 338
Kinsey, Alfred, 16, 52, 83, 184, 240, 284, 297, 339, 347–349, 395
kissing, xxi, 34–36, 105, 137, 217–218, 296, 327, 346, 359, 394
    in animals, 35
    and breath, 35
    coaching about, 44
    and compatibility, 35
    French, 35–36
    and hormones, 35
    and pregnancy, 174
    and sexual quality, 179
Kissinger, Henry, 341
Klein, Marty, 396
Kleinfelter syndrome, 353
Kowalski, Heather, 94

L

Ladas, Alice Kahn, 281–283
Lady Gaga, 351
Lancet, 10
L-arginine, 207, 267
lasers, 129
Las Vegas, 5
latex allergy, 111
laughter, 13, 61, 142, 216
Laumann, E. O., 18, 217, 252, 388
Lee-Gartner, Kerrin, 14
lemon balm tea, 131
Lenox Hill Hospital, 191
lesbian. *See* LGBTQ
lesions, 130
Letourneau, Mary Kay, 97
Levine, T. R., 149
levirate marriage, 16–17
Levitra, 192, 215, 240, 263–264. *See* Cialis
levonorgestrel, 118
Lew, Mike, 87
Lewinsky, Monica, 134
Lexapro, 203
LGBTQ, xix, 6, 328–329, 399. *See also* Bisexuality; Transgender
    activities, 349
    asexuality, 353–354
    communication, 349
    gender neutral, 352–353
    intersex, 353
    lesbian until graduation (LUG), 349
    libido, 349
    nonbinary, 352–353
    orgasm, 349
    queer, 352–353
    satisfaction, 349
    sexual satisfaction, 348–349
    statistics, 347
Liber, 331
libido, 3, 12–15, 116–120, 202, 204–205, 207–208, 211, 220, 227, 289, 349
    changing partner's, 169
    and desire differences, 170
    and hormones, 3, 175
    loss, 389

low, xvii, 59
and pregnancy, 173
and ultra-strenuous workouts, 12
women. See Desire, women's
Lieblum, Sandra, 399
life expectancy, 210
The Lifestyle: A Look at the Erotic Rites of Swingers (Gould), 332
Lindau, S. T., 18
lingerie, 317
full coverage, 318
guide to buying for women, 317–318
modeling, 318
silky, 318
skimpy, 317–318
liquid nitrogen, 129
literotica.com, 365
Lithonate, 203
LivesJasmin.com, 385
Livy, 331
lobstertube.com, 371
Lohan, Lindsey, 351
longevity, 392
LoPiccolo, Joseph, 250, 302
Lords, Traci (Nora Kuzman), 78–79, 381
Los Angeles Police Department, 158
Los Angeles Times, 79
Lot, 25–26
love, 5, 142
Lovehoney, 317
lovemaking the way women enjoy, xv, xvi
loveplay, 36
and lubrication, 48
Lubben, Shelley, 381
lubricants, 33, 40, 47–50, 127, 138, 140, 193, 197, 208, 213, 219, 243, 250, 296, 307–308, 317, 320, 325–327, 359
anal sex, 324
and anus, 318
and chronic illness, 190
and condoms, 49
history of, 48–49
and men, 49
oil-based, 50
petroleum-based, 50
popularity of, 49
and pregnancy, 175
silicone-based, 50
types, 50
and vibrators, 315–316
water-based, 50
and women, 49
lubrication, 236, 285, 293. See also Vagina, lubrication
lushstories.com, 365
Lusi tribe, 182
lust, 5
Lustral, 203
Luvox, 203, 255
lysine, 131

M
maca, 268
MacBeth (Shakespeare), 13, 201
Maggs, J. L., 147
Magic Wand, 314

"The Maiden Tribute of Modern Babylon" (Stead), 96
Maier, Thomas, xviii
maintaining sizzling sex, 179
children, getting away from, 179
coaching, 179
honoring monogamy, 179
kiss and cuddle, 179
marriage, 179
novelty, 179
oral sex, 179
scheduling, 179
staying healthy, 179
MakeLoveNotPorn.com, 410
male pattern baldness, 295
MaleSurvivor.org, 87
Maltz, Larry, 387, 389
Maltz, Wendy, 387, 389
Mansfield, Jane, 277
Mardi Gras, 331
marital harmony, 4
marriage
age, 151
child, 96–97
married love, 60, 63
and sexual satisfaction, 179
Martin, Del, 159
Martin, S., 253
Massachusetts Male Aging Study, 258
massage, 13, 16, 105
deep tissue, 32
hand, 141
lotion, 33
Swedish, 32
massage, mutual whole-body, 30–41, 191, 217–218, 226, 236, 242, 252, 280, 296, 301, 327, 394
and arousal, 32–33
and breathing, 33
health benefits, 35
pregnancy, 174
and sight, 33
and smell, 34
and sound, 34
and taste, 34
and vibrators, 315
mastectomy, 196
Masters, William, xiv, xviii, xx, 47, 144, 226, 240–241, 244, 278–279, 281, 284, 288
Masters of Sex, 144
Masters of Sex (Maier), xviii
masturbation, 16–24, 93, 137–138, 199, 313–314, 409
and age, 19–20, 220
boys, 6
and cancer, 16
and childhood sexual abuse, 16
children, 77–78, 83
circle jerks, 21
couples vs. singles, 20
demographics, 19
and deviance, 18
dry hand, 242–243
for each other, 24
and erectile dysfunction, 20
female orgasm, 298
frequency, 18–19
girls, 6
healing from sex abuse, 89–90
lubricated hand, 243

men, 21–22, 385–386
mental health problems, 21
mutual, 200
myths and truths, 20–22
with pelvis, 249
pornography, xvi, 357, 393–394, 409–410
preference for, 24, 402
and premature ejaculation, 16, 22
and prostate cancer, 20–21
and refractory period (RP), 262
and relationships, 22–23
remote sex, 23
before sex, 245
showing how you masturbate, 249–250
statistics, 274, 345–346
stigmatism, 16
style, 248
talking about, 143
teen, 101
teledildonics/cyberdildonics, 23
terms for, 17
transitioning to sex, 142
and using up sexuality, 20
weak erections, 20
women, 22
Match.com, 177
May Day, 331
Mayo Clinic, 198
McBride, Will, 79
McGill University, 373, 397
McMartin Preschool, 79
McMaster University, 102–103
meditation, 13, 64, 91
mindfulness meditation (MM), 91, 293
Megan's Laws, 79–80
Melbourne Women's Midlife Health Project (MWMHP), 292
Melissa officinalis, 131
Mellaril, 203
Memoirs of a Woman of Pleasure (Cleland), 366
Memorial Sloan Kettering, 195
menarche, 95
menopause, 47, 54, 210–214, 305
chemical or surgical, 211
concentration problems, 211
contraception, 213
and desire, 292
exercise, 213
herbal medicine, 213
hormone replacement controversy, 213–214
hot flashes, 210
how men can help, 211–214
mood changes, 210–211
pain during intercourse, 211
process, 210–211
reduced libido, 211
relaxation, 212–213
sleep problems, 211
sudden, 290
vaginal atrophy, 210–211
vaginal dryness, 210–211, 213
menstruation, 48, 54, 114, 117–118, 120, 210
cycle and orgasm, 303
increased flow, 295
irregular, 120

menstrual cramps, 120
menstrual cycle and desire, 291–292
Meston, C. M., 4
Metamucil, 324
Methodone, 204
Michelangelo, Leonardo, 233
Michigan State University, 74, 149
Microsoft, 159
Middlesex (Eugenides), 353
migraines, 116
Miller, Philip, 343
Mills, Wilbur, 185
mind-reading, 42
Mineo, Sal, 351
Minnelli, Liza, 313
Minnesota Vikings, 14
Mintezol, 204
Mintz, Laurie, xvii
misogyny, 373–375
missing children, 80
Mitchell, Sharon, 382–383
Money, John, 400
monogamish, 183
monogamy, 61, 115. *See also*
    Infidelity
    history of, 182–183
    honoring, 179
    naturalness of, 182–183
Monroe, Marilyn, 351
Monto, A. M., 145
mood
    changes, 210–211
    elevation, 391
    setting, 222
Morgan, Robert, 373
Morin, Jack, 325
Mormons, 332
Moses, 215
Mothers Against Driving Drunk, 156
Motrin, 207, 223
Mount Sinai School of Medicine, 276
MSNBC.com, 232
Müllerian ducts, 37
multiple sclerosis, 248–249
muscle
    aches, 124
    atrophy, 205
music, 13
*My Secret Garden: Women's Sexual
    Fantasies* (Friday), 64
Mysoline, 204

N
naproxen, 202, 207, 223
nasal congestion, 263, 265
National Association of Adult
    Survivors of Child Abuse, 86
National Association of Cognitive-
    Behavioral Therapists, 405
National Cancer Institute (NCI), 21,
    194, 391
National Center for Family and
    Marriage Research, 377
National Center for Health Statistics,
    100, 348, 351, 378
National Child Abuse and Neglect
    Data System, 86
National Coalition for Sexual
    Freedom, 340

National Crime Victimization Survey,
    86, 161, 375
National Health and Social Life
    Survey, 137–138, 178
National Health Statistics Report, 348
National Institute of Environmental
    Health, 174
National Institutes of Health, 213
National Opinion Research Center,
    374
National Sexual Assault Hotline, 28
National Sexual Health Survey
    (NSHS), 80–81
National Survey of Family Growth,
    104, 143, 323, 348
National Survey of Sexual Attitudes
    and Lifestyles, 348
National Survey of Sexual Health &
    Behavior, 348
National Weight Control Registry
    (NWCR), 12
National Women's Law Center, 157,
    160
Native Americans, 332
nausea, 116–117, 119–121, 295–296
Nawrot, T. S. et al, 10
NBC News, 222
necking, 151
"Negotiating a Friends with Benefits
    Relationship" (Bisson and Levine),
    149
Neisseria gonorrhoreae, 129
nerve damage, 13, 263–264
nervousness, 118, 267
nervous system, 8, 11, 31
neurological problems, 248–249, 256
neuropathy, 192
"A New Standard of Sexual Behavior?
    Are Claims Associated with the
    'Hookup Culture' Supported
    by the General Social Survey?"
    (Monto and Carey), 145
Newsweek, 350
New York Medical College, 342
New York Times, 59, 65, 400
New York Times Magazine, 332
New York Yankees, 14
Nexplanon, 120
Next Choice, 121
NFL, 386
niacin, 204
Nicholson, Jack, 193
Nielsen, 386
night sweats, 132
Nin, Anais, 183
nipples, 38, 303
    clamps, 38, 321, 338–339
nitric oxide, 207, 267
Nixon, Richard, 373
Nizoral, 204
non-Hodgkins lymphoma, 132
nonmonogamy, 6, 182–183, 330–
    337. *See also* Cheating; Polyamory
    BDSM clubs, 334
    coercion, 332
    exploring consensual, 334–337
    foursomes, 338
    ground rules, 335
    history, 330–332
    mental health, 334
    open relationships, 333

safe sex, 335
safe words, 335
sex clubs, 333, 335
spousal presence, 335
spring fever, 330
statistics, 333
swinging, 333, 335
threesomes, 337–338
women enjoying groups of men,
    336
nonoxynol-9, 112
normality, 6–7
North American Swing Club
    Association (NASCA), 332–333
North Carolina State University, 104
Northeastern University, 146, 158,
    197
Northwestern University, 197
novelties, 317
novelty, 59–63, 217, 222, 294, 296,
    394
    and aging, 62–63
    and courtship, 63
    falling in love, 59–60
    nonsexual, 62
    persuading a partner to try, 61–62
    surprise dates, 62
    time or place, 61
    tips for creating, 61
Noyes, John Humphrey, 332
nitric oxide, 207
nursing, 175
nursing homes, 223–224
nymphomaniac, 289, 400

O
obesity, 9, 11–13, 116, 256, 3617
    and pregnancy, 174
obsessive-compulsive disorder, 60
Odette, Fran, 200
Odyssey House, 79
Ogas, Ogi, 364
The OH in Ohio, 313
Ohio State University, 174
Old Dominion University, 78
Olivier, Laurence, 351
Onan, 16–18
*Onanism, A Treatise on the Diseases
    Produced by Masturbation* (Tissot),
    17
"On Self-Pollution" (Graham), 18
oophorectomy, 211
oral sex, 6, 51–58, 127, 137, 217,
    252, 273–274, 297–298, 326. *See
    also* Cunnilingus; Fellatio
    history of, 51–52
    popularity of, 52
    pornography, 360
    and pregnancy, 174
    and sexual quality, 179
    talking to children about, 84
    teen, 101
Oretic, 202
orgasm, 200, 241, 251. *See also*
    Orgasm, female
    anal sex, 328
    and antidepressants, 46
    clitoral, 38–39, 45, 279
    context, 39
    contractions, 38
    delayed, 202–204

diabetic problems, 193
and drugs, 39, 45–46
dry, 248
duration, 39
ejaculation, 38
erections, 260
evolution, 363
faked, men, 247
female, 38, 278
gap between men and women,
   297–298
giving, 43
as goal, 39
as goal of sex, 297
G-spot, 38–39, 283
male, xxi, 38
male, statistics, 297
more intense, 218
multiple, 38, 303
novelty, 39
number of in life, 20
pornography, 360, 389
and pregnancy, 173–174
premature in women, 246
refractory period, 38
responsibility for, 251–252
simultaneous, 141–142
stimulation, 39
straight vs. LGBTQ, 349
talking to children about, 83
time for, 45–46
unable to, 217
vaginal, 38–39, 141, 281
ways to speed up, 45–46
without erection, 195, 218–219
orgasm, female, xxi–xxii, 9, 297–303
and a ball, 302
beliefs, 297
boosting likelihood of, 301–302
clitoral, 299
coaching, 302
coital alignment technique (CAT),
   301–302
and conception, 303
cunnilingus, 298
demographics, 297, 300
faking it, 300
G-spot, 299
help for difficulties, 302
hormones, 303
masturbation, 298
and mate selection, 303
and menstrual cycle, 303
mock intercourse, 302
pelvic contractions, 299
pelvic motion, 301
pornography, 360
positions, 301
reasons for, 303
reasons for difficulty, 297
recognizing, 300–301
relationships, 297
sex coaching, 302
sex therapy, 302
sexual trauma, 298
vaginal, 299
vaginal intercourse, 298
vibrator, 302
vulvar massage and fingering, 298
women not having, 178

orgasm/ejaculation (O/E) problems,
   247–251
age, 247
aging, 248
alcohol, 248–249
causes, 248–249
checkup, 249
curing, 249–250
delivery boy attitude, 248
depression/antidepressant
   medication, 248
drug side effects, 248
guided fellatio, 250
infections, 248
masturbation style, 248
masturbation with pelvis, 249
neurological problems, 248
positions, 250
showing how you masturbate,
   249–250
stimulation needed, 249
stress, 248
stroking, 250
surgery for prostate enlargement,
   248–249
women's fault, 249
Orgasmic Women: 13 Self-Loving
   Divas, 301
osteoarthritis (OA), 190–191
bathing or showering, 191
coaching, 191
joint replacement, 191
massage, 191
medicine, 191
pillows, 191
scheduling sex, 191
therapy, 191
vibrators, 191
osteoporosis, 120, 214
Our Bodies, Ourselves (Boston
   Women's Health Collective), xv
outercourse, xx, 107–109, 114, 127,
   218–219, 222–223, 245, 252,
   259–260, 285, 308
Out of the Shadows: Understanding
   Sexual Addiction (Carnes), 387
ovarian cysts, 117, 120
ovulation, 114–115, 118, 120, 210,
   291
oxalate irritation, 305
   low-oxalate diet, 306–307
Oxford English Dictionary, 149
oxytocin, 31, 35, 60, 303

P
Pacheco, Richard, 234
pads, 127
pain, 12, 35, 297
   abdominal, 116, 118, 122–124,
      128
   during intercourse, 128, 211,
      217, 291
   leg, 116
   men's sexual, 308
   pelvic, 197
   relief, 391
   reliever, 202, 207
   sexual, 46, 227
   vaginal, 176
pain, women's sexual, 304–308
   abuse recovery, 306

acupuncture, 307
birth control pills, 305
checkup, 305–306
coaching, 306
cognitive behavioral therapy, 306
imperforate hymen, 305
insertion too deep, 308
Intrarosa, 307
lack of lubrication, 307–308
lovemaking, adjusting, 307–308
low-oxalate diet, 306
medical conditions, 305
menopause, 305
oxalate irritation, 305
pelvic floor physiotherapy, 307
porn-style pounding, 308
relationship counseling or therapy,
   306
relationship turmoil, 305
relaxation regimen, 306–307
rushed intercourse, 307
sexually transmitted infections
   (STIs), 305
sexual trauma, 306
silence about, 304
statistics, 304–305
treatment, 306–307
uninformed anal play, 308
vaginal infection, 305
vaginismus, 305
vaginismus treatment, 307
vulvar skin conditions, 305
vulvar vestibulitis (VV), 305
vulvar vestibulitis (VV) treatment,
   307
Pall Mall Gazette, 96
Pamela or Virtue Rewarded
   (Richardson), 367–368
Panasonic, 316
Pap test, 117, 129
paraplegia, 248–249
parasites, 204
paraurethral glands, 280
parenting and sex, 176–177. See also
   Baby, sex after; Teen
babysitters, 176
discussing kids, 176
nap times, 176
new limits, 176
regular lovemaking improves
   parenting, 176–177
and sex quality, 178
single parents, 177
sleepovers, 176
time away from children, 179
partners, number of, 145–146, 393
patience, 261
Patrick, M. E., 147
Paxil, 203, 245, 255
pedophilia, xviii, 79–81
   gender, 80
   gender of perpetrator, 97
   perpetrators, 80
   proximity and authority, 81
peer pressure, 137
pelvic exams, 130
pelvic floor muscles, 9, 218, 248–
   249, 280, 285, 324
   and orgasm, 299
pelvic floor physiotherapy, 307

pelvic inflammatory disease (PID), 117, 119–120, 125, 130, 276
pelvic pain, chronic, 304
pelvic radiation, 285
penetration, 237
penile-anal intercourse (PAI). *See* Anal sex
penis. *See also* Penis size
  birth defects, 55–56
  corona, 56
  extenders, 267
  frenulum, 56
  glans, 37, 73
  penile discharge, 128, 130
  penile implants, 195, 268–269
  preoccupation with, 75
  prosthetic penis attachments (PPAs), 267
  pumps, 236, 266
  pus, 128
  rings, 266
  self-consciousness about, 55
  shaft, 37, 56
  shrinking, 218
  size insecurity, 231–232, 359
  sleeve, 250, 317
penis size, 231–237
  averages, 232–233
  birth defects, 237
  blood flow, 235
  committed relationship, 235
  diet, 235
  enlargement scams, 231
  exercise, 235
  history, 233
  making peace with, 237
  making the most of, 235–236
  and pleasing women, 236–237
  and pot belly, 236
  problems with large size, 234
  relaxation, 235
  size and shoe size, 231
  slow down, 235
  stress, 235
  surgical enlargement, 234–235
  tobacco, 235
  toys to boost, 236
  trimming pubic hair, 236
  warmth, 235
  why men think they are too small, 233–234
  women's feelings, 232
penis-vagina intercourse (PVI), 134, 137
Penn State, 105
Penthouse, 287
performance anxiety, 142, 217, 238
perineum, 280
periodontitis, 256
Perkins, Anthony, 351
Perry, John, 281–283
Petroglyph National Monument, 363
pets, 13
Peyronie's disease, 308
Pfizer, 294
Phenobarbital, 204
phenylethylamine (PEA), 206
pheromones, 35
phimosis, 73, 308
physical appearance, 5
phytoestrogen, 211, 213–214

pillows, 237
Pistor, Fanny, 339
pituitary problems, 48
placenta previa, 174
Plan B, 121
Planned Parenthood, 104, 107, 151
Playboy, xv, 287
  Advisor, xv
pneumocystis carinii pneumonia (PCP), 132
Polomo, John, 94
polyamory, 182, 334
polygamy, 182, 332
population, 221
PornHub.com, 234, 261, 299, 366–367, 371, 385–387, 397, 407
pornography, xvi, xxi, 141, 219, 233, 250, 264, 274, 287, 336, 357–411
  addiction, 396–398
  and adolescents, 377–380
  alcohol, 375
  anal sex, 360–361
  anguish women feel about, 407–411
  anonymous sex, 393
  anxiety, depression, and substance abuse, 388
  arousal without, 394
  audience, 260–261
  BDSM, 340, 372–373
  as betrayal, 407–409
  bodies, 365
  bukkake, 365
  caressing, 359
  changing your relationship to, 401–406
  child, 78–79
  and child sex abuse, 389
  coaching, 359
  constant arousal, 358
  contraceptive irresponsibility, 389
  definition, 357
  demeaning, 409
  desire, 358
  determining if you have a problem, 401–402
  disability, 359
  divorce, 389
  drugs, 383
  ejaculation, 365
  erectile dysfunction (ED), 361, 389
  erections, 359–360, 365
  exhibitionism, 360, 382
  as fantasy, 69
  female actresses marital status, 382–383
  female actresses mental health, 382–383
  gangbangs, 336
  group sex, 393
  health testing, 382
  history, 363, 365–366
  how much is too much, 390, 392
  increase in violence, 373
  infidelity, 389
  internet, 364, 366–367
  kissing, 359
  legitimate uses, 362
  libido loss, 389
  loss of close relationships, 389

  lubricant, 359
  masturbation, 357, 393–394, 409–410
  and men, xxi, xxii
  and men's fantasies, 179
  and men's reproductive wiring, 365–366
  misleading, 357–362
  misogyny, 373–375
  movies, 52
  nonconsensual, 384
  one relationship after another, 393
  oral sex, 360, 409
  orgasm, 360
  orgasm difficulties, 389
  penis size, 359
  petroglyph, 363
  porn literacy for teens, 379–380
  pounding, 308
  promise to stop watching, 396
  prostitution, 393
  and rape, 375
  relationships and intimacy, 358–359
  revenge, 384
  romance fiction, 367–370
  safe sex, 359
  self-help for, 402–403
  and sex addiction, 387
  sexism, 388
  sex toys, 361
  sites, 385
  social harm, 388–390
  and social woes, xxii
  talking about with teens, 380
  teaches sex wrong, 358–362
  teens and sexual responsibility, 378–379
  that arouses women, 410
  time lost to sexual fantasies, 392–393
  time with family and partners, 389
  and the vagina, 37
  viewing time, 386–388
  and violence, xviii
  violence against women, 371–376
  violence against women, defined, 372–373
  watching together, 410
  women, 360
  women porn actors, 381–384
  women viewers, 367, 407
The Porn Trap: Overcoming Problems Caused by Pornography (Maltz and Maltz), 387, 389
Posey, Parker, 313
positions, 141, 250
  missionary, 141, 237, 250, 285
  and orgasm, 141
  and pregnancy, 175
  rear entry, 141, 234, 237, 301, 308
  spooning, 301
  woman-on-top, 141, 301
postpartum depression (PPD), 175
prasterone, 307
pre-ejaculatory fluid, 48, 109
pregnancy, 117
  age, 174
  ectopic, 117, 120, 276
  and libido, 173
  lubricants, 175

orgasm, 173
positions, 175
premature labor or harm to fetus from sex, 173–174
premature labor triggers, 174
sex after, 175–176
premature ejaculation (PE), xiv, xvi, xx, 16, 22, 31, 217, 220, 248–249, 388
acupuncture, 246
adjusting fantasies, 242
affairs, 245
checkup, 241
curing, 238–246
deep breathing, 242
diagnosis of, 238
and distraction, 241
drugs, 240
dry hand job, 244
dry hand masturbation, 242–243
ejaculatory control, 241
exercise, 241
as a habit, 240–241
herbs, 246
history, 239–240
how to last longer, 241–245
how woman feel, 240
if she's reluctant to help, 245
low-dose antidepressants, 245–246
lubricated hand job, 244
masturbation before, 245
new partner, 244
proceeding to partner sex, 243
recurrence, 245
risk factors, 239
self-help, 238
sex coaching, 245
sex workers, 245
sobriety, 241
squeeze, 244
stop-start fellatio, 244
stop-start intercourse, 244
stroke with lubricated hand, 243
supplements, 246
therapy, 245
time, 244
topical anesthetics, 246
whole-body massage, 242
women's preferences, 246
premenstrual syndrome, 117, 120
Presidential Commission on Obscenity and Pornography, 373
preterm delivery, 276
Pretty Woman, 185
"Prevalence and Characteristics of Sexual Hookups among First-Semester Female College Students" (Fielder and Carey), 148
"Prevalence and Characteristics of Vibrator Use by Women in the United States: Results from a Nationally Representative Study" (Herbenick), 312
"Prevalence and Predictors of Sexual Desire, Sexually Related Personal Distress and Hypoactive Sexual Desire Dysfunction in a Community-Based Sample of Midlife Women" (Worsley), 289

"Prevalence and Predictors of Sexual Problems in Men Aged 75-95 Years: A Population-Based Study" (Hyde), 220
priapism, 203, 263, 308
Price, Joan, 216, 221
Pride and Prejudice (Austen), 368
Primidone, 204
The Prince of Tides (Conroy), 161
procreation, 3–4
prodrome, 131
Profumo, John, 332
progestin, 118–119
progressive muscle relaxation (PMR) exercises, 293
progressive sexual play, 137
prolactin, 303
Prolixin, 203
Propecia, 256
Proscar, 256
prostaglandin E, 268
prostate cancer, 16, 20–21, 122, 193–195, 205, 220
age, 194
brachytherapy, 193
erectile dysfunction (ED), 193–195
hormone therapy, 256
morning erections, 194
penile implants, 195
pretreatment sexual function, 194
prevention, 391–392
prostate-specific antigen (PSA), 194
radiation, 193, 256
surgery, 193–195, 256
treatments, 256
prostatectomy, 256
prostate enlargement, 204, 256
surgery, 248–249
prostate gland, 218
prostate-specific antigen (PSA), 220
prostatitis, 238, 241, 248, 308
prostitution, 393. *See also* Sex workers
Protection of Children against Sexual Exploitation Act (P-CASE), 79
Prozac, 203, 245, 255
Pscyhopathia Sexualis (*Sexual Pathology*, von Krafft-Ebing), 339
psychiatric medications, 3617
Psychology of Addictive Behavior, 147
Psychology Today, xvi
psyllium, 324
puberty, 95
pubic hair, 236, 282
grooming, 286–287
pubic lice, 287
"Public Health Importance of Triggers of Myocardial Infarction: A Comparative Risk Assessment" (Nawrot), 10
pubococcygeus (PC) muscle, 9, 280
Pulaski, Casimir, 353
puncture vine, 208

Q
Queens College, 150
Queensland University, 372
queer. *See* LGBTQ
quickies, 31, 40–41, 261

R
ranitidine, 202
rape
alcohol, 375
and consent, 26
fantasies, 67–69
and female porn actresses, 381–382
marital, 26
and pornography, 375
prevention programs, 376
statistics, 161
statutory, 94–95
teens, 378
Rape, Abuse, and Incest National Network (RAINN), 86
rape, information for partner of victim, 161–163
accusations, avoiding, 162
couple counseling, 162
decisions, 162
fun, arranging, 162
help, encouraging her to get, 162
help for yourself, 162
how to help with recovery, 161–162
listening, 162
nonsexual sexuality, 162
reassure her of love, 162
revenge, 162
support, 161–162
rash, 132
ratio, male-female, 221
Rayhons, Donna, 223–224
Rayhons, Henry, 224
Reagan, Ronald, 374
rebound sex, 150
"Rebound Sex: Motives and Behaviors Following a Relationship Breakup" (Barber and Cooper), 150
recreation, 5
rectum, 324
Reeves, Keanu, 193
refractory period (RP), 38, 262
Rehor, J. E., 345, 372
Reiber, C., 146
Reingold, Daniel, 223
Reinisch, J. M., 135
relationship, 305
duration, 290
loss of close relationship, 389
misery, 290
one relationship after another, 393
therapy, 293, 306
turmoil, 305
relaxation, 8, 46, 235, 327, 391
regimen, 306–307
religion, 73–74, 297, 300, 362, 395–396
fundamentalist Christian, 404
Remeron, 203
Remifemin, 213
Renaissance, 331
restraints, 321
Revactin, 207
rhythm, 237
Richardson, Samuel, 367
Richmond, James Cook, 23
rimming, 326, 345
Rivera, Geraldo, xiv

Roaring Twenties, 151
Roberts, Julia, 185
Robert Wood Johnson School of Medicine, 399
Rockefeller, Nelson, 10
role play, 345
romance fiction, 367–370
 history, 367–368
 pornography vs romance fiction, 369
Romanticism, 96
"Romantic Partners' Use of Pornography: Its Significance for Women" (Bridges), 407
Rome, ancient, 26, 331, 353
Romeo and Juliet (Shakespeare), 95
Rosen, Raymond, 399
Rourke, Mickey, 34
Royalle, Candida (Candice Vadala), 410
Rudd, Paul, 313
Rutgers, 184–185, 292

S
safe words, 335, 342–343, 346
saffron, 268
saliva, 213, 308, 325
Salmonella, 326
Sanders, S.A., 135
San Diego State University, 378
San Francisco State University, 345, 372
Savage, Dan, 183
Scarleteen.com, 106
scheduled sex, 179, 191, 222, 294, 394
Screw the Roses, Send Me Thorns (Miller and Devon), 343
scrotum, 37, 56
Sears and Robuck Catalog, 314
seasons, 292
sedentary lifestyle, 13, 218, 256, 290
Seinfeld, 134
selective serotonin reuptake inhibitors (SSRIs), 255
self-defense training, 154
self-esteem, 12
self-harm, 255
self-help and lovemaking, xvi–xvii
self-sexing. *See* Masturbation
Sellers, Tina Schermer, 404
Semans, Anne, 173, 176–177
semen, 38, 48, 57, 249, 365. *See also* Sperm
 calories, 57
 contents, 58
 and diet, 58
 less, 218
 swallowing, 57, 345
 taste of, improving, 58
sensate focus, 226
"Sensual, Erotic, and Sexual Behaviors of Women from the 'Kink' Community" (Rehor), 345, 372
serotonin, 35, 60
serotonin reuptake inhibitors (SSRIs), 203
Seroxat, 203
Sesame Street, 364
The Sessions, 144, 200

seven-year itch, 61
sex
 anonymous, 393
 benefits of, 391–392
 and calories, 10
 clubs, 182
 crime registration, 79
 deviant, 5, 7
 and heart attacks, 10
 negativity, xvii–xviii, 5
 not pleasurable, 217
 parties, 67
 positivity, xvii–xviii
 premarital history, 151
 premarital rates, 104
 reasons for, 3–5, 170–171
 solo. *See* Masturbation
 surrogate. *See* Surrogate partner therapy
 thinking about, 100
 trafficking, xix
 unconventional, 6
 uniqueness, xix
 vanilla, 345–346
Sex, God, and the Conservative Church (Sellers), 404
S.E.X: The All-You-Need-to-Know Sexuality Guide to Get you through Your Teens and Twenties (Corinna), 106
sex abuse. *See* Child sexual abuse
sex addiction, xxii, 289, 387, 396–398
 abusive, 398–399
 brain changes, 394–395
 celebrity, 400
 coining of term, 399
 empty, 398–399
 and group sex, 393
 history, 399–400
 mental health authorities, 400–401
 professional help, 403
 relapses, 403
 S.A.F.E., 398
 secret, 398
 self-help, 402–403
 self-help groups, 403
 sex-negative upbringing, 395–396
 substitutes, 403
 ten minutes, 403
 triggers, 403
 used to avoid painful feelings, 398–399
Sex Addicts Anonymous, 403
Sex after Grief (Price), 221
Sexaholics Anonymous, 387, 403
Sex and Love Addicts Anonymous, 403
Sex and Punishment: Four Thousand Years of Judging Desire (Berkowitz), 96
sex coaching, 143, 245, 262, 267, 302, 329. *See also* Sex therapy
Sex Coach University, 226
sex education, xx, 99–106, 226
 and a, 134
 abstinence, 99, 102, 105
 comprehensive, 99, 103, 105
 condoms, 106
 consent, 106
 lubrication, 106

 and parents, 100, 103–104, 106
 for parents, 105
 peer pressure, 137
 pleasure, 106
The Sex Handbook: Information and Help for Minors (Handman and Brennan), 78
sexism, 388
sex problems, 225–228
 defining, 225–226
 massage, 226
 self-help, 226
 sex coaching, 226
 sex education, 226
 sex therapy, 226–228
 statistics, 225
sex therapy, 172, 226–228, 245–246, 252, 262, 267, 329, 362, 402. *See also* Sex coaching
 aversion or virginity, 227
 certification, xviii
 desire differences, 227
 erection problems, 227
 libido, 227
 women's sexual pain, 227
sex toys, 190, 218, 236, 252, 259, 296. *See also* Ben-wa balls; Butt plugs; Cock rings; Dildo
sexual abuse recovery, 306
Sexual Addiction and Compulsivity, 387
Sexual Addiction Scale, 399
Sexual Addiction Screening Test, 399
sexual assault, 291
 and affirmative consent, 27
 and age, 38
 and BDSM, 342
 and fantasy, 67–69
 rate, xxii
sexual assault and harassment, preventing, 153–160, 376
 affirmative consent, 153–154
 alcohol, 155–156, 201
 arbitration, 159
 authority to receive complaints, 159
 blunt talk, 376
 bystanders, 154, 156, 160, 376
 civil rights, 158
 designated party monitors, 376
 false accusations, 158
 focus on young men, 156–157
 gag orders, 159–160
 middle and high school programs, 157
 naiveté, 154
 ongoing blunt talk, 159
 power/prestige, 154
 prevention programs, 155–156
 rape victims asking for it, 155
 risk for, 154–155
 self-defense training, 154
 serial rapists, 157
 silence, 158
 statistics, 154
 strength in numbers, 159
 triggers, 153–155
 workplace, 157–158
 workplace culture change, 159–160

Sexual Attitude Reassessment (SAR) seminars, 362
"Sexual Behavior, Sexual Attraction, and Sexual Orientation among Adults Aged 18-41 in the United States: Data from the 2011-2013 National Survey of Family Growth" (Copen), 348
Sexual Behavior in the Human Male (Kinsey), 240
"Sexual Behavior in the United States: Results from a National Probability Sample of Men and Women Ages 14-94" (Hebenick), 18, 24, 216
Sexual Desire Disorders (Lieblum and Rosen), 399
"Sexual Dysfunction among Older Adults: Prevalence and Risk Factors from a Nationally Representative U.S. Probability Sample of Men and Women 57-85 Years of Age" (Laumann), 217, 252
"Sexual Dysfunction in the United States (Laumann), 388
sexual harassment. *See* Sexual assault and harassment, preventing
sexual infections, 57
sexuality
  male *vs.* female, 273–274
  and orientation, xix
sexually transmitted infections (STIs), 99, 103–104, 106, 109, 111, 117–123, 125–133, 219, 241, 248, 287, 305, 336, 381
  and age, 126
  AIDS, xvi, 18, 99, 103, 112, 350
  AIDS and anal sex, 323
  and cheating, 125
  chlamydia, 73, 117, 125, 128, 276
  chlamydia and pregnancy, 174
  communication about, 125
  and condoms, 110
  gonorrhea, 117, 125, 129–130
  gonorrhea and pregnancy, 174
  herpes, 125, 130–132
  human immunodeficiency virus (HIV), 125, 128, 132–133, 323–324
  human papillomavirus (HPV), 73, 125, 128–129
  and pregnancy, 174
  and spermicide, 112
  syphilis, 125, 132
  treatment, 126
  trichomoniasis, 73, 125, 128, 276
  trichomoniasis and pregnancy, 174
  urinary tract infections (UTIs), 126–127
sexual medicine practitioners, 228
Sexual Medicine Society of North America, 228, 285
"Sexual Orientation and Health among U.S. Adults: National Health Interview Survey" (Ward), 348
sexual performance, 259
sexual quality and time, 178–181
  books, 180
  children at home, 178
  coaching, 178

cohabitation, 178
gender, 178
genital preoccupation, 178
maintaining quality, 179
oral sex, 179
playing games, 180
poor health, 179
reasons for erosion, 178
routine, 178
ruts, 179
straight vs LGBTQ, 180
women not having orgasms, 178
sexual regret, 274
sexual response cycle, female, 278–279
  arousal, 278
  orgasm, 278
  plateau, 278
  resolution, 278
sexual satisfaction, 273, 293
  straight vs LGBTQ, 348–349
Sexual Solutions (Castleman), xv
sexual trauma, 306
sex workers, 6, 143–144, 245. *See also* Prostitution
  girlfriend experience (GFE), 187
  legalization, 187
  rate of use, 186
  why men pay for sex, 185–188
Sexy Mama: Keeping Your Sex Life Alive While Raising Kids (Winks and Semans), 173, 176
Shakespeare, William, 13, 95, 201
shame, 396
Shaw, George Bernard, 183
She Comes First: The Thinking Man's Guide to Pleasing Women (Kerner), 55
Shelley, Percy Bysshe, 34
Shigella, 326
shortness of breath, 116
Show Me! (Fleischhauer-Hardt and McBride), 79
sickle cell anemia, 116
sights, 33
sildenafil. *See* Viagra
Silva, Jack, 362
Silva, Marie, 362
Silverberg, Cory, 200
simmering, 394
Simon Fraser University, 372
Skene, Alexander, 284
Skene's glands, 284
sleep, 8, 14–15, 211, 391
  apnea, 15, 256–257
  deprivation, 15
  insomnia, 14
  problems, 13
  problems and medication, 14
Slippery Stuff, 325
SM 101 (Wiseman), 342–343
SmartBitchesTrashyBooks.com, 369
smell, 34
Smell and Taste Treatment and Research Foundation, 34
Smith, Bessie, 351
smoking. *See* Tobacco
snoring, 15, 198
  alcohol, 198
  allergies, 198
  earplugs, 198

raising head, 198
sedatives, 198
sleep separately, 198
surgery, 198
tennis ball, 198
tobacco, 198
weight loss, 198
The Social Organization of Sexuality: Sexual Practices in the United States (Laumann), 18
Society for Sex Therapy and Research, xv
Society for the Scientific Study of Sexuality, xv
Something's Gotta Give, 193
The Song of Solomon, 366
The Song of Songs, 366
Sonoma State University, 222
sores
  painful, 131
  painless, 132
sound, 34
soy foods, 211–212, 214
sperm, 20, 48, 58, 82, 84, 95, 109, 111–115, 117–118, 122, 218, 303, 363. *See also* Semen
  motility, 208
  quality, 392
Spiegelhalter, D., 348
Spitzer, Eliot, 185
Spock, Benjamin, 78
spotting, 116–117, 120, 128
Sprinkle, Annie, 58
squirting. *See* Ejaculation, female
St. Louis University, 202
St. Martin's Press, 79
stalking
  statistics, 163
  support for partner victim, 162–163
Stanford, 202
staphylococcus bacteria, 114
statistics, 345
Staxyn, 263. *See* Levitra
Stead, W. T., 96
Stendra. *See* Levitra
Stengel, Casey, 14
Stephens-Davidowitz, Seth, 55, 231, 275
sterilization, 122–123
Stewart, Potter, 357
stomach upset, 263, 265, 295
Stonewall Inn, 349
strangers as partners, 150
Streep, Meryl, 227
stress, 248, 255, 263, 291
  management, 8, 13, 257
  and pregnancy, 174
  relievers, 13
  work, 292
stroke, 119–120, 122, 205, 214, 264–265, 294
substance abuse, 388
sugar pills, 296
suicide, 6
SUNY Albany, 358
SUNY Binghamton, 146, 148
SUNY Stony Brook, 60, 184–185, 372
"Surf City" (Beach Boys), 221